Platelet-Rich Plasma in Tissue Repair and Regeneration

Biao Cheng • Xiaobing Fu
Editors

Platelet-Rich Plasma in Tissue Repair and Regeneration

Technology and transformation application

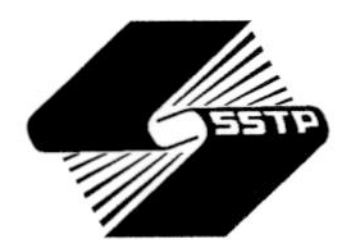

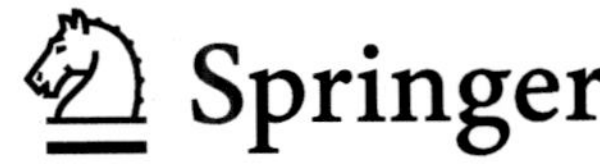

Editors
Biao Cheng
Department of Burn & Plastic Surgery
General Hospital of Southern Theater Command
Guangzhou, China

Xiaobing Fu
Life Science Academy
PLA General Hospital
Beijing, China

ISBN 978-981-99-3195-8 ISBN 978-981-99-3193-4 (eBook)
https://doi.org/10.1007/978-981-99-3193-4

Jointly published with Shanghai Scientific and Technical Publishers
The print edition is not for sale in China (Mainland). Customers from China (Mainland) please order the print book from: Shanghai Scientific and Technical Publishers.

This Springer imprint is published by the registered company Springer Nature Singapore Pte Ltd.
The registered company address is: 152 Beach Road, #21-01/04 Gateway East, Singapore 189721, Singapore

Foreword

Since the concept of PRP was first put forward in the 1950s, in just a few decades of development, concentrated platelets treatment has been widely applied in the fields of many clinical disciplines, such as traditional orthopedics and sports medicine, oral and maxillofacial medicine, and plastic and aesthetics. In recent years, the application of concentrated platelets treatment in ophthalmology, otorhinolaryngology, dermatology, urology, obstetrics and gynecology, reproduction, and other disciplines has attracted more and more attention. The treatment of concentrated platelets has evolved from simply promoting wound healing to initiating the regeneration of various tissues. At the same time, with the wide application of concentrated platelets in the clinical practice, a variety of concentrated platelet products of different traits have gradually been prepared; thus a large number of different nomenclatures of concentrated platelet and application of related derivatives have appeared: from the early platelet gel (PG), platelet-rich plasma (PRP), platelet concentrate (PC), concentrated growth factor plasma rich in growth factors (PRGF), to the later platelet-rich fibrin (PRF), concentrate growth factor (CGF), and platelet lysate (PL). Especially, in recent years, with people's attention to extracellular vesicles, the application of platelet-derived extracellular vesicles has also become a trend. There are also activated PRP and non-activated PRP according to whether PRP is activated. According to the shape, it is divided into PRP gel and liquid PRP; or PRP can be divided into high concentration of white blood cell PRP and low concentration of white blood cell PRP on the basis of the level of white blood cell concentration in PRP. There are also three categories of PRP according to platelet concentration: high, medium, and low; and it is also classified based on whether it contains platelet membrane components.

Although there are many names and types of concentrated platelets, all of these classifications cannot be separated from one key word: platelets. All treatments involved must be based on platelets to work. From the earliest understanding of its hemostasis and coagulation function, to the later discovery of its ability to repair vascular endothelial cells, and release α-granules, dense granules, and other active substances (including growth factor (GF), cytokines, chemokines, extracellular vesicles, miRNA, circRNA, etc.) after activation, the role of concentrated platelets has become more and more complex and extensive. The important role of platelets, especially concentrated platelets, in tissue damage repair and regeneration determines that platelets are the protagonists of the entire biological process.

Another key point is the concentration. Cell therapy must have sufficient active products, and a certain level of platelet extracts determines the reliability of its function. In recent years, we have been exploring basic research and clinical applications of PRP and have gained some understanding. The book will show you the results of some clinical cases and experimental data.

But how to determine the concentration of platelets in concentrated platelet products? Do auxiliary white blood cells need to be added? Is PRP activated or not? Are other components retained and how much is retained? These require a guiding principle to match the needs of clinical use.

Current studies confirm that platelet concentrate products may have a bidirectional regulatory effect. The results of clinical treatments also show this effect. For example, it can be used as a treatment for depigmentation diseases (such as vitiligo) and also has a therapeutic effect on hyperpigmentation disorders (such as chloasma); it can promote collagen production to treat atrophic scars (such as stretch marks) and can also play a role in improving hypertrophic scars (keloids, hypertrophic scars). This subtle regulatory effect may be regulated by the body's internal microenvironment, which plays an important role in the oxidation-reduction balance process to achieve the purpose of treatment.

I followed my teacher, Professor Fu Xiaobing, at the beginning of this century, being engaged in the research of growth factor on tissue repair and regeneration, and gradually began to pay attention to platelets that could release growth factors. More than a decade of research has given me some insights into the functional role of concentrated platelets. This book is a report on the basic research and clinical application of our team in the field of skin soft tissues over the years, involving skin barrier, wound healing, rejuvenation, hair growth, fat grafting, and other aspects. At the same time, I invite several like-minded experts with certain insights into platelets in the fields of bone, joint, rehabilitation, and oral cavity to present their research results and clinical applications to you, hoping the readers to have a more comprehensive understanding of platelets and that readers who are interested in platelets could gain something.

Our research on platelets continues, and we are very excited about some of the new findings (including the effect of platelet-derived extracellular vesicles and platelet-derived mitochondria on tissue repair). The new research results will be published in succession, and I hope you will continue to pay attention to it. Let's work together to consolidate the basic research in the field of platelet regeneration medicine and put it into better application in the clinic.

Xiaobing Fu, M.D., Ph.D.
Life Science Academy
PLA General Hospital
Beijing, China

Biao Cheng, M.D., Ph.D.
Department of Burn & Plastic Surgery
General Hospital of Southern Theater Command
Guangzhou, China

Contents

Contributors

Biao Cheng, M.D., Ph.D. Department of Burn & Plastic Surgery, General Hospital of Southern Theater Command, Guangzhou, China

Liuhanghang Cheng, Ph.D. Department of Burn and Plastic Surgery, PLA General Hospital, Beijing, China

Xiao Cui, Ph.D. Department of Physiotherapy, Guangdong Provincial Hospital of Chinese Medicine, Guangzhou, Guangdong, China

Yunqing Dong Department of Burn and Plastic Surgery, General Hospital of Southern Theater Command, PLA, Guangzhou, China

Xiaobing Fu, M.D, Ph.D. Academician of the Chinese Academy of Engineering (CAE, Division of Medicine and Health), International Academicians of National Academy of Engineering (NAE) of USA and Franch Academy of Medicine, PLA General Hospital and PLA Medical College, Beijing, China

Yuan Gao, M.D. Department of Burn and Plastic Surgery, General Hospital of Southern Theater Command, PLA, Guangzhou, Guangdong, China

Hongchen He, Ph.D. Department of Rehabilitation Medicine, West China Hospital, Sichuan University, Chengdu, Sichuan, China

Liwen Huang, Ph.D. Department of Burn and Plastic Surgery, General Hospital of Southern Theater Command of PLA, Guangzhou, Guangdong, China

Panshi Jin Department of Burn and Plastic Surgery, General Hospital of Southern Theater Command, PLA, Guangzhou, Guangdong, China

Xiaoxuan Lei, Ph.D. Department of Burn and Plastic Surgery, General Hospital of Southern Theater Command, PLA, Guangzhou, Guangdong, China

Linlin Li Department of Plastic Surgery, Dermatology Hospital of Fuzhou, Fuzhou, Fujian, China

Mengru Pang, Ph.D. Department of Burn and Plastic Surgery, The Affiliated Hospital of Guizhou Medical University, Guiyang, Guizhou, China

Qiao Pan, M.D. Department of Burn and Plastic Surgery, General Hospital of Southern Theater Command, PLA, Guangzhou, Guangdong, China

Yan Peng, Ph.D. Department of Burn and Plastic Surgery, General Hospital of Southern Theater of PLA, Guangzhou, Guangdong, China

Guiqiu Shan, Ph.D. Department of Transfusion Medicine, General Hospital of Southern Theater of PLA, Guangzhou, Guangdong, China

Linying Shi, Ph.D. Department of Transfusion Medicine, General Hospital of Southern Theater of PLA, Guangzhou, Guangdong, China

Zhongmin Shi, Ph.D. Department of Orthopaedics, Shanghai Jiao Tong University Affiliated Sixth People's Hospital, Shanghai, China

Ju Tian, M.D. Department of Plastic Surgery, People's Hospital of Zhongshan City, Zhongshan, Guangdong, China

Yali Wang, Ph.D. Department of Blood Transfusion, China-Japan Union Hospital, Jilin University, Changchun, Jilin, China

Zhifa Wang, Ph.D. Department of Stomatology, General Hospital of Southern Theater of PLA, Guangzhou, Guangdong, China

Shikun Wei, Ph.D. Department of Burn and Plastic Surgery, General Hospital of Southern Theater Command, PLA, Guangzhou, Guangdong, China

Xuetao Xie, Ph.D. Department of Orthopaedics, Shanghai Jiao Tong University Affiliated Sixth People's Hospital, Shanghai, China

Pengcheng Xu, Ph.D. Department of Breast Neoplasms Surgery, The 1st Affiliated Hospital of Henan University of Science and Technology, Luoyang, Henan, China

Zhuo Xu, Ph.D. Department of Rehabilitation Medicine, China-Japan Union Hospital, Jilin University, Changchun, Jilin, China

Yu Yang, M.D. Department of Plastic Surgery, The Third Affiliated Hospital of Guangzhou Medical University, Guangzhou, Guangdong, China

Sha Yuan, M.D. Dermatological Department, Hangzhou Meilai Medical Hospital, Hangzhou, Zhejiang, China

Ting Yuan, Ph.D. Department of Orthopaedics, Shanghai Jiao Tong University Affiliated Sixth People's Hospital, Shanghai, China

Xi Yu, Ph.D. Department of Rehabilitation Medicine, West China Hospital, Sichuan University, Chengdu, Sichuan, China

Lei Zhang, Ph.D. Department of Plastic Surgery, Hangzhou Meilai Medical Hospital, Hangzhou, Guangdong, China

Zhaoyuan Zhang, Ph.D. Department of Orthopaedics, Shanghai Jiao Tong University Affiliated Sixth People's Hospital, Shanghai, China

Yiqing Zhou, M.D. Department of Orthopedics, Shanghai Changzheng Hospital, Naval Medical University, Shanghai, China

Meishu Zhu, M.D. Department of Burn and Plastic Surgery, Shenzhen Institute of Translational Medicine, Shenzhen Second People's Hospital, The First Affiliated Hospital of Shenzhen University Health Science Center, Shenzhen, Guangdong, China

Department of Wound Repair, Shenzhen Institute of Translational Medicine, Shenzhen Second People's Hospital, The First Affiliated Hospital of Shenzhen University Health Science Center, Shenzhen, Guangdong, China

Weidong Zhu, Ph.D. Department of Burn and Plastic Surgery, General Hospital of Southern Theater Command, PLA, Guangzhou, Guangdong, China

Yunmin Zhu, M.D. Department of Burn and Plastic Surgery, General Hospital of Southern Theater Command, PLA, Guangzhou, Guangdong, China

Jian Zou, Ph.D. Department of Orthopaedics, Shanghai Jiao Tong University Affiliated Sixth People's Hospital, Shanghai, China

Introduction

1

Biao Cheng and Xiaobing Fu

With the development of regenerative medicine, the medical technology to promote self-repair and regeneration of the body or to reconstruct new tissues and organs to repair, regenerate, and replace damaged tissues and organs involves three main factors, namely, cells (seed cells), active factors, and biological scaffolds. PRP (platelet-rich plasma) is gradually showing its advantages in tissue engineering and regenerative medicine [1]. At the same time, its unique role and some new mechanisms, such as tissue regeneration and immunoregulation, have been gradually revealed and have broad prospects, attracting more and more attention. In particular, the multiple roles of PRP in anti-aging, genetic engineering, tissue engineering, and other aspects (both active factor and secretory cells, as well as scaffold material) deserve our further searching. More than 10 years, its explosive basic and clinical research has confirmed that platelet-rich plasma is indeed the super star of medicine.

1.1 Naming and Classification

In recent 10-year development, people have had a deep understanding of platelet concentrate; however, it has numerous naming and classification; in addition, even if it has the same name, the way of preparation is different in thousand ways, as well as on the activation or not. The application of lead to concentrated platelet treatment is developing rapidly; on the other hand, it is also controversial.

B. Cheng
Department of Burn & Plastic Surgery, General Hospital of Southern Theater Command, Guangzhou, China

X. Fu (✉)
Academician of the Chinese Academy of Engineering (CAE, Division of Medicine and Health), International Academicians of National Academy of Engineering (NAE) of USA and Franch Academy of Medicine, PLA General Hospital and PLA Medical College, Beijing, China

1.1.1 Nomenclature of Platelet Concentrate

Among platelet concentrate products, the term most commonly used is platelet-rich plasma (PRP). Additionally, platelet-rich fibrin (PRF), concentrate growth factors (CGF), platelet lysate (PL), and other forms can never be simply divided into first, second, and third generations [2, 3]; these views are obviously biased; we have been explained in our previous articles [4] and will not be repeated in this article. In this process, platelet concentration is obtained through density gradient centrifugation of the whole blood, followed by repeated freezing and thawing, and the resulting liquid components are known as platelet lysate (PL). It is a method of removing platelet membranes and other cell debris, reducing immunogenicity and preserving a variety of growth factors/cytokines. Due to the simple preparation process, PL does not need to add platelet activator, has strong adaptability to temperature, and has a better preservation time than PRP. Its application is gaining ground, especially in cell culture for stem cell therapy, avoiding the ethical limitations of heterologous serum.

So far, PL has been used in more than 100 clinical studies on stem cell culture. However, due to the different freezing and thawing times, platelet extraction, preparation methods, and other reasons, there are great differences between the results of various studies, and the prepared PL also lacks unified quality standards. In recent years, studies on extracellular vesicles have drawn attention to platelet membrane proteins, which may have their unique roles in many treatments. For example, platelet membrane glycoproteins, as immune receptors and immunogens unique to platelets, should not be ignored in immune regulation and new vascular formation. In this respect, PL shows some defects due to the removal of membrane components. With the development of human understanding, extracellular vesicles and exosomes, which are secreted by cells, have attracted more and more attention, and platelet-derived extracellular vesicles have shown great potential. Therefore, in recent years, this kind of treatment is more commonly referred to as

B. Cheng, X. Fu (eds.), *Platelet-Rich Plasma in Tissue Repair and Regeneration*, https://doi.org/10.1007/978-981-99-3193-4_1

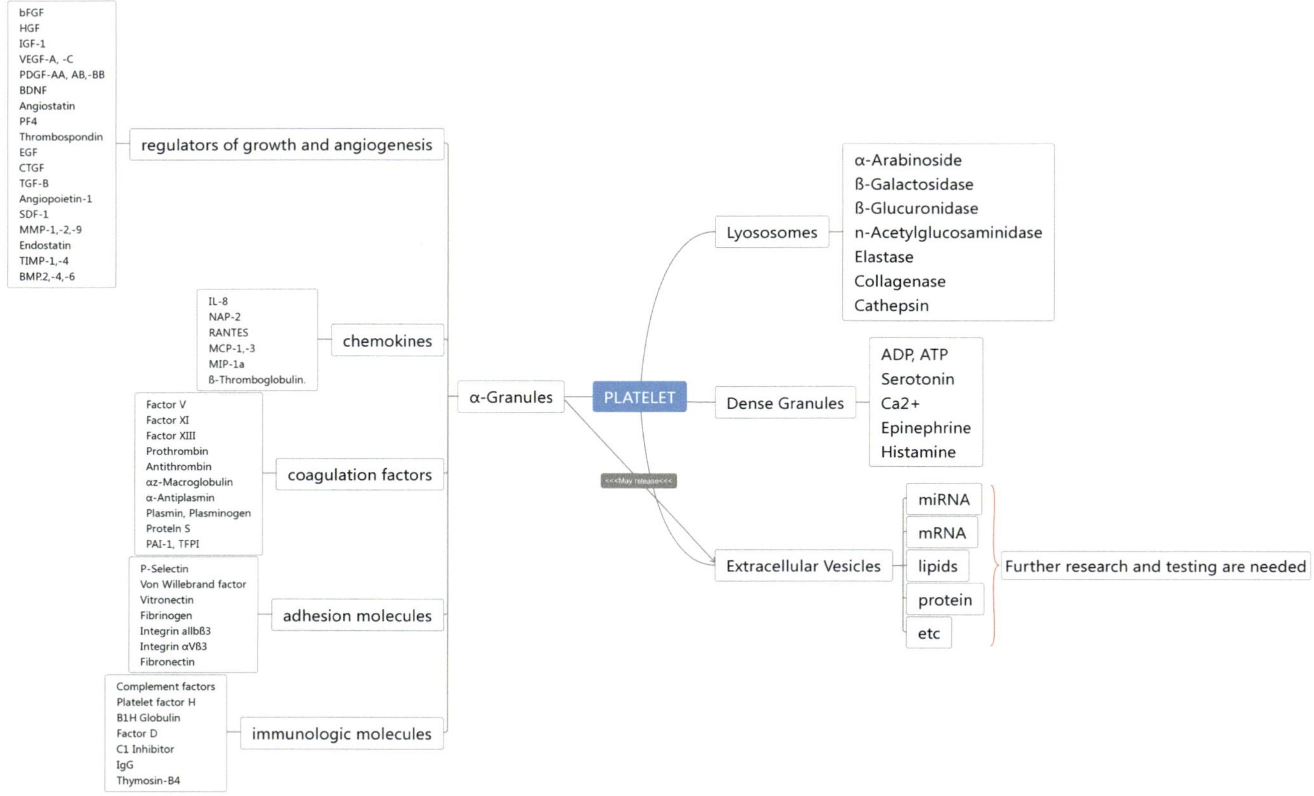

Fig. 1.1 Active component of platelet

platelet-derived biological products (Fig. 1.1). Due to the importance of this type of product in terms of quality control, clinical use of concentrated platelet should be referred to as enriched platelet treatment (EPT) or therapy [4]. The reason for using an enriched version is to emphasize the process and manner in which it was made. We think that all therapy contents have two points:

1. Platelet: Platelets are activated to release a variety of active products, including growth factors, extracellular vesicles, antimicrobial peptides, proteins, RNA, etc. It is these active products that make PRP of great value in clinical application, cell culture, and basic research.
2. Concentrate: Only the Concentration of the active product released by PC (platelet concentrate) can achieve the optimal concentration required by the biological effect, so as to ensure the best clinical effect of the treatment target.

1.1.2 Classification of Platelet Concentrate

In 2009, Dohan proposed a platelet concentrate classification method, which firstly separated traditional PRP and PRF and then further divided them into L-PRP and L-PRF of high concentration leukocytes and P-PRP and P-PRF of low concentration leukocytes according to the concentration of leukocytes. According to this classification method, most clinical PRP can be classified [5].

In 2012, Delong put forward PAW classification system after integrating all existing studies on PRP PAW system which is divided into three parts: the absolute number of platelets, the mode of platelet activation, and whether there are white blood cells (WBC) in PRP. Through PAW system, we can accurately compare the composition of PRP [6].

In 2015, Mautner believed that although the "PAW" classification system took WBC content in PRP as an important observation index, it was not detailed. Simply dividing WBC content into "above baseline" and "below baseline" cannot completely reflect the impact of WBC content in PRP on platelet activity and efficacy. They believed that the classification of PRP should include platelet concentration (absolute number of platelets per milliliter), leukocyte concentration (including neutrophil concentration), erythrocyte concentration, and the concentration of exogenous drugs acting as activators. They suggested using a PLRA (platelet, leukocyte, red blood cells, and activation) classification system with platelet count, white blood cell concentration, red blood cell concentration, and the concentration of exogenous drugs acting as activators [7].

In 2006, Magalon proposed the DEPA (dose of injected platelets, efficiency of production, purity of PRP, and activation of PRP) classification system of PRP: (1) platelet dose,

(2) product efficacy (platelet recovery rate), (3) PRP purity (ratio of platelets, leukocytes, and erythrocytes), and (4) activation process. These parameters can be calculated only after complete counting of cells in whole blood and injected PRP [8].

In 2017, Lana summarized the previous clinical research results of their research team. Lana believed that the differentiation-promoting effect of PRP containing monocytes and PRP without monocytes was related to leukocytes, and the PRP research should focus on monocytes. In addition, attention should also be paid to other parameters during preparation and application/automated manner (machine: M) or handmade (H), spin number (Sp1 or Sp2), red blood cells (RBCs: rich, RBC-R, and poor, RBC-P), platelet concentration (which folds baseline), leukocyte-rich (Lc-R) or poor (Lc-P) and the range, activated (A+) or not (A−), and light activated (L+) or not (L−) [9].

In 2018, the International Society on Thrombosis and Haemostasis (ISTH) and Scientific Standardization Committee (SSC) put forward the consistent recommendations on the application of platelets in regenerative medicine. This classification includes if activated the activation method shall be provided, the total volume used, the frequency of dosing and subcategories of activation, and the platelet concentration and preparation techniques and would include the overall average counts and range (low-high) of platelets and red blood cells and differential leukocyte counts (neutrophils, lymphocytes, and monocytes). The preparation methods are classified into three categories: gravitational centrifugation techniques, standard cell separators, and autologous selective filtration technology (plateletpheresis) [10].

On the basis of this research, in order to compare the results between different groups, Acebes Huerta put forward the factors to be considered when describing PRP products and the tentative naming system in 2019. They believe that quality assessment and precautions are very important. Before PRP is activated or broken, the product should be counted for platelets, white blood cells (WBCs), and red blood cells (RBCs). Good PRP products should not contain red blood cells and white blood cells, or the white blood cell concentration should be lower than a certain value (i.e., <106 wbc/unit) (24). Additionally, we give a lot of emphases on whether the PRP product is applied fresh, activated, or frozen/thawed, based on the relevance that it poses to the appearance of adverse effects [11].

In 2020, Elizaveta believed that PRP classification included platelet count and the role of leukocytes (still controversial). Other variables to be considered include the volume of blood collected (related to the volume of PRP injected), preparation method (centrifugation times, revolutions per minute, centrifugation time, etc.), freshly prepared or freeze-thawed products, activation method (calcium, thrombin, polyacrylamide beads, etc.), activation time (related to the physical state of PRP and the kinetics of growth factor release), and injection frequency. These parameters are closely related to the therapeutic effect of PRP [12].

On account of the continuous updating and discovery of platelets and their released effective components (exosome and miRNA, etc.), various properties (regeneration, immune, etc.) are constantly recognized, which makes the application of enriched platelet therapy (EPT) in various fields constantly bring surprises but also constantly bring worries and doubts about variables. Too fine classification will bring inconvenience in the process of clinical application, and the grade of clinical evidence will decline without careful analysis. How to combine the accuracy of scientific research with the convenience of clinical use is an important issue that needs serious consideration in the future.

1.2 Major Fields of Enriched Platelet Therapy in Clinical Application

Differences in nomenclature and classification make the use and reporting of platelet concentrate and, on the one hand, crazy outbreak and, on the other hand, lack of systematic studies that can be balanced and controlled. Even in terms of safety, it is difficult to obtain mean products due to differences in activator use and traits. In order to avoid blood-borne diseases, autologous concentrated platelet products are mostly used. Patients with platelet dysfunction and contraindications to self-donation will not be able to enjoy the benefits of concentrated platelet therapy. With the expansion of the application range of PRP, successful attempts have been made in clinical application in dermatology; ophthalmology; ear, nose, and throat; obstetrics and gynecology; and sexual medicine in recent years. On the other hand, in the laboratory, the release products and targeted therapy have also made breakthroughs (Fig. 1.2).

At the same time, platelet concentrate can also be combined with a variety of photoelectric equipment (such as plasma radiofrequency, dot array laser, etc.), as well as (stem) cells, hyaluronic acid, fat transplantation, microneedles, surgery, and other methods to reduce the treatment of various types of scar. In general, platelet concentrate can be used as a direct or adjunctive treatment for the scars. He also needs further long-term follow-up to find the most appropriate approach for different scar types [13, 14].

Vascularization of tissue transplantation has always been important and focuses partly on clinical practice. A variety of studies have shown that platelet concentrate can provide nutrients such as plasma for adipose tissue transplantation, secrete growth factors, promote the secretion and paracrine of stem cells, and contribute to the formation of new blood vessels, thus improving the survival rate of tissue transplantation. In the future, the concentration, proportion, and

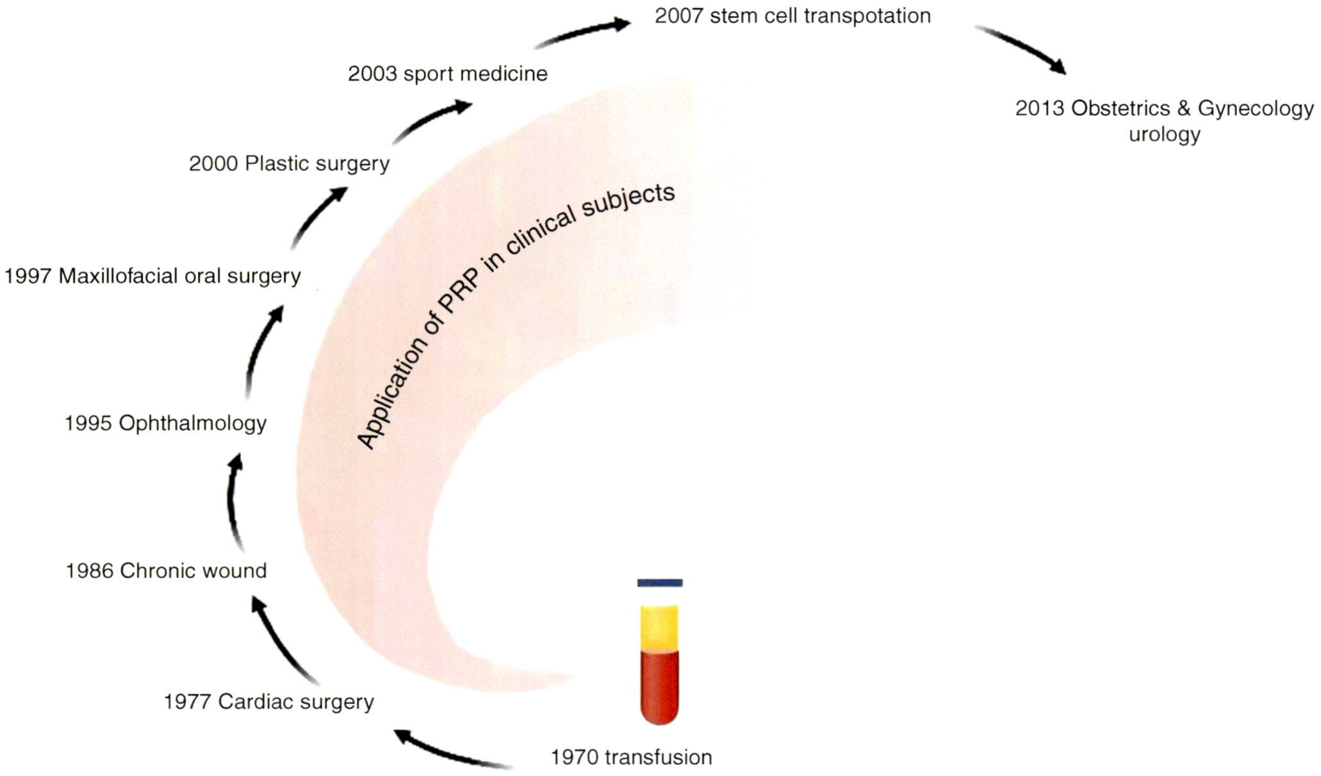

Fig. 1.2 Application of PRP in clinical subjects

activation mode of platelet concentrate transplantation should be further clarified.

Aging involves many aspects of the body, including tissues and organs such as the skin, fat, fascia, bone, and cartilage. In the application of anti-aging, it will mainly develop in the more refined direction of drug administration, optimal concentration, and cost performance, whether nucleated cells are removed or not.

In vitro cell amplification usually requires access to advanced therapeutic drugs for clinical use. It must conform to good manufacturing practices. The use of proven and standardized xeno-free compounds of animal and independent origin (XENo-free) in cell manufacturing is critical for the clinical safety of biological products. Fetal bovine serum (FBS) is a common source of growth factors in experiments. It is usually added to the culture medium to promote cell expansion. However, heterogeneous carbohydrates and proteins in fetal bovine serum may cause clinical side effects. Substitution of FBS for cell products has long been strongly recommended in Europe and the USA.Human platelet concentrate may become an alternative source of growth factors, and it is safe, abundant, suitable and inexpensive. In previous studies, human growth factor extracted through repeated freeze-thaw cycles has been successfully used to amplify cells in vitro. Mixing preparations from multiple single donors minimize product variability [15, 16]. It is more ethical for platelet concentrate to provide a culture medium with an indistinguishable origin for stem cell therapy.

The application of platelet-rich plasma in tissue engineering materials has been a research hotspot in recent years, and it will be an important direction of future research as a cell scaffold. At present, some scholars have studied platelet-rich plasma combined with other drugs or biomaterials to construct degradable tissue engineering to complete the repair and regeneration of soft tissue [17]. The variety of forms of platelet concentrate (gel or liquid, such as platelet lysate and platelet which secrete exosome) also makes its application in tissue engineering become extremely flexible and can be loaded with different biodegradable biomaterials (hydrogel, acellular matrix, etc.) according to the needs of tissue regeneration. However, the active time of platelet concentrate is short; storage and sustained release have always been the focus of research. In addition, for standardized use, we recommend that researchers and clinicians fully describe the type of platelet concentrate they use, the preparation method (centrifugal force, centrifugal time) [18], and the concentration, dose, and mode of activation (activated or not? Activator? Ultrasonic? Photoelectric?). Also of great concern is the time window of the application.

1.3 Rational Thinking of Enriched Platelet Therapy in Clinical Application

In recent years, the clinical application of enriched platelet therapy has been very widespread, extending to infertility, sclerosis, and other difficult diseases and even developing to the treatment of tumors. However, scholars believe that the treatment of cancer should be cautious [19]. With the effects of platelet concentrate on immune regulation, especially the regulation of innate and adaptive immune functions, local oxygen regulation, and *redox* rebalancing, platelets may become therapeutic targets for many diseases. But all should follow medical ethics and evidence-based medicine.

Although the application of enriched platelet therapy in clinical medicine has achieved exciting results, we should be aware of this explosive growth. In some cases, the use of autologous platelet concentrate is not completely safe. Although deriving from autologous tissue itself is safe, its safety will be reduced in the process of extraction and preparation. Pain, swelling, and bruising are temporary and reversible compared to common side effects. Indeed, there have been reports of skin reaction to calcium preparations and even anaphylactic shock [20]. Moreover, a case report of a healthy woman with severe complications of permanent blindness in one eye after receiving PRP injection [21] and pigmentation caused by platelet concentration [22] was also reported. Although it is still uncertain whether these are caused by platelet concentrate itself, activators, or other factors, how to avoid and reduce the occurrence of such things in the process of clinical treatment is still a problem that we need to continue to pay attention to. Only in this way can we make the application of platelet concentrate scientific, reasonable, and long-term.

References

1. Kawase T. Platelet-rich plasma and its derivatives as promising bioactive materials for regenerative medicine: basic principles and concepts underlying recent advances. Odontology. 2015;103:126–35.
2. Sunitha Raja V, Munirathnam Naidu E. Platelet-rich fibrin: evolution of a second-generation platelet concentrate. Indian J Dent Res. 2008;19(1):42–6.
3. Pascoal MC, dos Santos NM, Completo AG, et al. Tensile strength assay comparing the resistance between two different autologous platelet concentrates (leucocyte-platelet rich fibrin versus advanced-platelet rich fibrin): a pilot study. Int J Implant Dent. 2021;7:1.
4. Cheng B. Problems and reflections of concentrated platelet products in traumatic surgery. J Trauma Surg. 2018;20(11):7–11.
5. Dohan Ehrenfest DM, Bielecki T, Del Corso M, et al. Shedding light in the controversial terminology for platelet-rich products: platelet-rich plasma (PRP), platelet-rich fibrin (PRF), platelet-leukocyte gel (PLG), preparation rich in growth factors (PRGF), classification and commercialism. J Biomed Mater Res A. 2010;95(4):1280–2.
6. DeLong JM, Russell RP, Mazzocca AD. Platelet-rich plasma: the PAW classification system. Arthroscopy. 2012;28(7):998–1009.
7. Mautner K, Malanga GA, Smith J, et al. A call for a standard classification system for future biologic research: the rationale for new PRP nomenclature. PM R. 2015;7(4 Suppl):S53–S9.
8. Magalon J, Chateau AL, Bertrand B, et al. DEPA classification: a proposal for standardising PRP use and a retrospective application of available devices. BMJ Open Sport Exerc Med. 2016;2(1):e000060.
9. Lana J, Purita J, Paulus C, et al. Contributions for classification of platelet rich plasma - proposal of a new classification: MARSPILL. Regen Med. 2017;12(5):565–74.
10. Paul H. The use of platelets in regenerative medicine and proposal for a new classification system: guidance from the SSC of the ISTH. J Thromb Haemost. 2018;16(9):1895–900.
11. Acebes-Huerta A, Arias-Fernandez T, Bernardo A, et al. Platelet-derived bio-products: classification update, applications, concerns and new perspectives. Transfus Apher Sci. 2019;59:102716. https://doi.org/10.1016/j.transci.2019.102716.
12. Kon E, Di Matteo B, Delgado D, Cole BJ, Dorotei A, Dragoo JL, Filardo G, Fortier LA, Giuffrida A, Jo CH, Magalon J, Malanga GA, Mishra A, Nakamura N, Rodeo SA, Sampson S, Sánchez M. Platelet-rich plasma for the treatment of knee osteoarthritis: an expert opinion and proposal for a novel classification and coding system. Expert Opin Biol Ther. 2020;20(12):1447–60.
13. Makki M, Younes AEKH, Fathy A, et al. Efficacy of platelet-rich plasma plus fractional carbon dioxide laser in treating posttraumatic scars. Dermatol Ther. 2019;32(5):e13031.
14. Abellan Lopez M, Bertrand B, Kober F, et al. The use of higher proportions of platelet-rich plasma to enrich microfat has negative effects a preclinical study. Plast Reconstr Surg. 2020;145(1):130–40.
15. Mohammadi S, Nikbakht M, Malek Mohammadi A, et al. Human platelet lysate as a Xeno free alternative of fetal bovine serum for the in vitro expansion of human mesenchymal stromal cells. Int J Hematol Oncol Stem Cell Res. 2016;10(3):161–71.
16. Yamahara K, Sudo T, Hamada A, et al. Adult bovine platelet lysate-derived serum "NeoSERA" is safe, less ethical and powerful alternative to fetal bovine serum for the culture of mesenchymal stem cells. Cytotherapy. 2019;21(5):S80–1.
17. Naderi N, Griffin MF, Mosahebi A, et al. Adipose derived stem cells and platelet rich plasma improve the tissue integration and angiogenesis of biodegradable scaffolds for soft tissue regeneration. Mol Biol Rep. 2020;47(3):2005–13.
18. Croisé B, Paré A, Joly A, et al. Optimized centrifugation preparation of the platelet rich plasma: literature review. J Stomatol Oral Maxillofac Surg. 2020;121(2):150–4.
19. Luzo ACM, Fávaro WJ, Seabra AB, et al. What is the potential use of platelet-rich-plasma (PRP) in cancer treatment? A mini review. Heliyon. 2020;6(3):e03660.
20. Latalski M, Walczyk A, Fatyga M, et al. Allergic reaction to platelet-rich plasma (PRP): case report. Medicine (Baltimore). 2019;98(10):e14702.
21. Kalyam K, Kavoussi SC, Ehrlich M, et al. Irreversible blindness following periocular autologous platelet rich plasma skin rejuvenation treatment. Ophthal Plast Reconstr Surg. 2017;33(3S Suppl 1):S12–6.
22. Uysal CA, Ertas NM. Platelet-rich plasma increases pigmentation. J Craniofac Surg. 2017;28(8):e793.

Overview of Platelet-Rich Plasma

2

Biao Cheng and Ju Tian

Platelet-rich plasma (PRP) is a blood product concentrate obtained by centrifugation of whole blood that is characterized by a high concentration of platelets (4–6 times their normal values) [1]. PRP contains a small amount of plasma (plasma is not necessary) which contains a variety of proteins. The core of PRP is platelets. After platelets are activated, they release super-physiological concentrations of growth factors, cytokines, a variety of proteins, exosomes, platelet microparticles, and other biologically active substances, which promote tissue regeneration and repairing.

In the past two decades, PRP has been widely used in many clinical departments such as orthopedics, orthopedics, sports medicine, oral and maxillofacial surgery, heart surgery, gynecology, ophthalmology, burns and plastic surgery, dermatology, otolaryngology, etc. and other applications. It has achieved good results in promoting tissue regeneration and repairing and is called a panacea. PRP has been widely used in the fields of plastic and cosmetic surgery to promote wound healing; prevent scar hyperplasia, facial rejuvenation, and hair regeneration; improve the survival rate of transplanted fat; treat acne scars; and promote bone and cartilage tissue nerve regeneration [2].

2.1 History, Development, and Current Status of Platelet-Rich Plasma

Since the 1970s, the study of platelet-rich plasma in wound repair has been carried out. The concept is developed from fibrin glue [3]. In 1977, Harke [4] prepared PRP for the first time and successfully combined it. It is used in cardiac surgery. In 1993, Hood added thrombin and calcium ions to PRP, proposed the concepts of platelet gel (PG) and platelet-rich plasma (PRP), and found that PRP is rich in platelets, whose number is higher than that of whole blood. The number is more than three times higher [5]. It is worth noting that the current concept of fibrin glue generally refers to a gel prepared from platelet-poor plasma (PPP) [6]. In 1998, Marx and others applied autologous PRP in the reconstruction of mandibular bone grafts [7]. Subsequently, Choukroun of France developed another platelet concentrate, which is called platelet-rich fibrin (PRF) [8]. At present, there are many conceptual descriptions of platelet concentrate products in the literature, and the classification is also inconsistent. The preparation methods are often different, which can easily cause confusion and bring inconvenience to reading literature and conducting related research. The more common concepts related to platelet concentrate products include PRP (platelet-rich plasma), PRGF (plasma-rich growth factors), PRF (plasma-rich fibrin), CGF (concentrated growth factors), (PRP gel), platelet gel, PRP clot, etc. According to the application form of platelet concentrate products, they are divided into inactive PRP and activated PRP. According to the number of white blood cells, they are divided into leukocyte-poor PRP (also called pure PRP or P-PRP) and leukocyte-rich PRP (L -PRP), leukocyte-poor PRF (P-PRF), leukocyte-rich PRF (L-PRF).

In short, platelet concentrate products are plasma rich in platelets, the platelet content of which is several times higher than that of normal whole blood. The core role of these platelet concentrate products is platelets, whose platelet content is several times higher than that of normal whole blood. Plasma contains a variety of proteins, and after platelet activation, it releases super-physiological concentrations of growth factors, cytokines, multiple proteins, exosomes, platelet microparticles, and other biologically active substances to promote tissue regeneration and repair, so it may be more accurate to call it enriched platelet products(EPP). With the deepening of the understanding of the factors affecting the number of platelets in platelet concentrate products, the

B. Cheng (✉)
Department of Burn & Plastic Surgery, General Hospital of Southern Theater Command, Guangzhou, China

J. Tian
Department of Plastic Surgery, People's Hospital of Zhongshan City, Zhongshan, Guangdong, China

B. Cheng, X. Fu (eds.), *Platelet-Rich Plasma in Tissue Repair and Regeneration*, https://doi.org/10.1007/978-981-99-3193-4_2

difference in composition after activation, spatial conception, and different functions, as well as the continuous expansion and change of its application range and mode, there should be a comprehensive and innovative thinking on platelet concentrate treatment technology.

In the past, many names of PRP have their own characteristics, but they are inseparable from the basis of "concentration" and "enrichment," targeting different tissues (bone, cartilage, muscle, fat, skin, etc.) and different purposes (proliferation, migration, and differentiation promotion). Filling/stenting, vascularization, phagocytosis, and oxidation-reduction stress may require different forms of platelet concentrates. Therefore, it is more reasonable to call it enriched platelet therapy (EPT). As this treatment technology, PRP, PRF, CGT, etc. are all its connotations and in accordance with the signal pathways and key proteins that need to be initiated for repair after tissue damage, choosing the appropriate form of platelet concentrate product (whether it contains neutrophils or lymph? Is it exogenous or activated in the body? etc.?) is of great significance to further enrich the treatment methods and improve the clinical treatment effect.

Among the many application forms of EPT, the concept of PRP is currently widely used in the literature. It is liquid before activation and gelatinous after activation, which is called PRP gel. PRP can reduce the incidence of infection, reduce hospitalization time and postoperative drainage, promote wound healing, and reduce the occurrence of complications. At present, the well-documented application of PRP in plastic and cosmetic surgery began in 2001. Powell et al. reported in 2001 that pure platelet-rich plasma was sprayed under the skin flap before the wound was closed after deep facial lift. The patient used PRP on one side of the face and found that PRP has anti-inflammatory properties to reduce edema and ecchymosis [9]. In 2001, Man et al. used PRP (platelet gel) combined with PPP (fibrin glue) to apply to the face and neck to lift the abdomen. Other operations have been found to shorten the operation time, reduce drainage and compression dressing, reduce postoperative pain and swelling, improve wound healing, and shorten postoperative recovery time [10]. Bhanot used PRP in 20 cases of cosmetic surgery (face lift, breast plastic surgery, or neck lift) in 2002, showing that PRP gel can effectively prevent capillary bleeding in surgical operations and shorten the recovery time [11]. Subsequently, PRP has been widely used in plastic surgery fields such as promoting wound healing, preventing scar hyperplasia, promoting skin regeneration, improving wrinkle rejuvenation, promoting hair growth, increasing the survival rate of transplanted fat, treating acne and acne scars, and promoting bone and cartilage tissue nerve regeneration. In 2012, Sanchez DJ proposed the application of PRP to regenerative medicine [12]. Regenerative medicine promotes the body's self-repair and regeneration by studying the body's normal tissue characteristics and functions, wound repair and regeneration mechanisms, and stem cell differentiation mechanisms and methods or by constructing new tissues and organs to maintain, repair, regenerate, or improve damaged tissues and tissues. PRP can play an important role in promoting organ function.

The concept of PRP is widely used, but it lacks an accurate definition. Most of the literature defines PRP as the high-concentration platelet-rich plasma obtained after centrifugation of whole blood. It can be prepared with autologous blood (Fig. 2.1) (most of which are prepared with autologous blood) or allogeneic blood. For the concentration of white blood cells and red blood cells contained, there are no specific requirements for concentrations such as fibrinogen. This definition obviously cannot meet the needs of experiments and clinical trials. First of all, in addition to the density gradient centrifugation method, the preparation method for obtaining PRP can also be obtained using a fully automatic plasma separation and exchange device. This method is mainly used for the collection of blood bank platelets and clinical component blood transfusion. Secondly, the existing concept does not have a unified standard for the concentration of platelets in PRP but only emphasizes concentrated or super-physiological concentration. Most scholars refer to platelets that are 3–5 times the average platelet concentration in the blood as PRP [13]. Some scholar think it is better to increase the concentration factor to 8–10 times [14]. However, due to the large difference in platelets in individual human whole blood (150,000–350,000/μl), if PRP is defined according to the platelet concentration factor, the platelets in each individual PRP prepared will be very different, which is not conducive to comparison with each other for standardized treatment. The currently recognized minimum platelet concentration in qualified PRP is $1 \times 10^6/\mu l$ ($1000 \times 10^9/l$) [13]. Finally, PRP also contains a variety of functional components such as plasma, white blood cells, red blood cells, and fibrin, which will affect the function of PRP. According to related studies, there are more than 1000 proteins in PRP [15], which does not include the number of active ingredi-

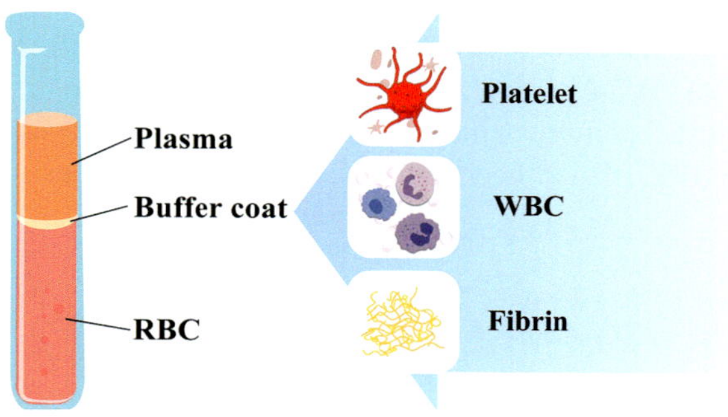

Fig. 2.1 PRP was extracted from whole blood. (Drawn by Keyao Jia)

ents such as exosomes, platelet microparticles, and microRNA. The complexity of PRP components makes its concept and classification extremely difficult.

At present, there are many descriptions of the concept of platelet concentrate products in the literature, and the classification is also inconsistent [16]. The preparation methods are often different, which can easily cause confusion and cause inconvenience to reading the literature and engaging in related research. The concept of PRP is widely used. It includes many contents. According to whether it is activated or not, it is divided into inactive PRP and activated PRP. Inactive PRP is liquid. After PRP is added with an activator, it forms a PRP gel, which can be placed at 37 °C. In the water bath, with the passage of time, the gel gradually shrinks and releases biologically active substances. PRP can also be divided into pure PRP and leukocyte-rich PRP according to its components. Pure PRP contains fewer white blood cells, and leukocyte-rich PRP contains more white blood cells that cause the closed specific gravity, but the specific number of white blood cells is still unclear.

Based on the results of existing studies, there is no doubt about the efficacy of PRP. The key is to choose the appropriate preparation method and use pattern and its indications. However, for diseases with clear curative effects of PRP, there are often problems of uncertainty in curative effect. Most of the reasons are due to the diversity of PRP preparation methods and different evaluation methods, resulting in non-comparable PRP and uneven quality. Future research needs to solve the main problem not whether PRP is effective but how to obtain a high repeatability rate, and the most effective clinical treatment and achieve PRP preparation and treatment standardization.

2.2 Composition and Role of PRP

Platelet-rich plasma includes platelets, white blood cells and plasma, and other components, and its core substance is platelets. Platelets are small, biologically active cytoplasm shed from mature megakaryocytes in the bone marrow. They are small in size and have no nucleus but intact plasma membrane and organelles, with a diameter of 2–4 μl.

Platelets are secretory cells, usually dormant, and have no regular shape. There are two forms: one is inactive and has a biconvex disc shape, and the other is activated. After being activated, the shape changes and occurs. Aggregate and extend the pseudopodia, release the particles, the shape is more irregular, and release the contents of the particles through exocytosis. There are dozens of protein molecules with important biological activities.

Platelet cells contain alpha granules, dense granules, lysosomes, mitochondria, glycogen granules, endoplasmic reticulum, microtubules, microfilaments, and Golgi apparatus. α-Granules constitute the major granule population in terms of size and number. They contain adhesion and growth factors, such as transforming growth factor-β (TGF-β), platelet-derived growth factor (PDGF), vascular endothelial growth factor (VEGF), basic fibroblast growth factor (bFGF), epidermal growth factor (EGF), and insulin-like growth factor (IGF). Dense particles have a small diameter and a small number, and they exhibit strongly electron-dense cores surrounded by clear spaces enclosed by single membranes and store pro-aggregating factors. Lysosomes are only present in part of the platelets, and the number is small. In addition, platelets also contain a variety of genetic materials, including DNA, RNA, mRNA, miRNA, LnRNA, cirRNA, etc. When platelets are activated, shorter RNA will also be released with the release of vesicles(Fig. 2.2) and transferred

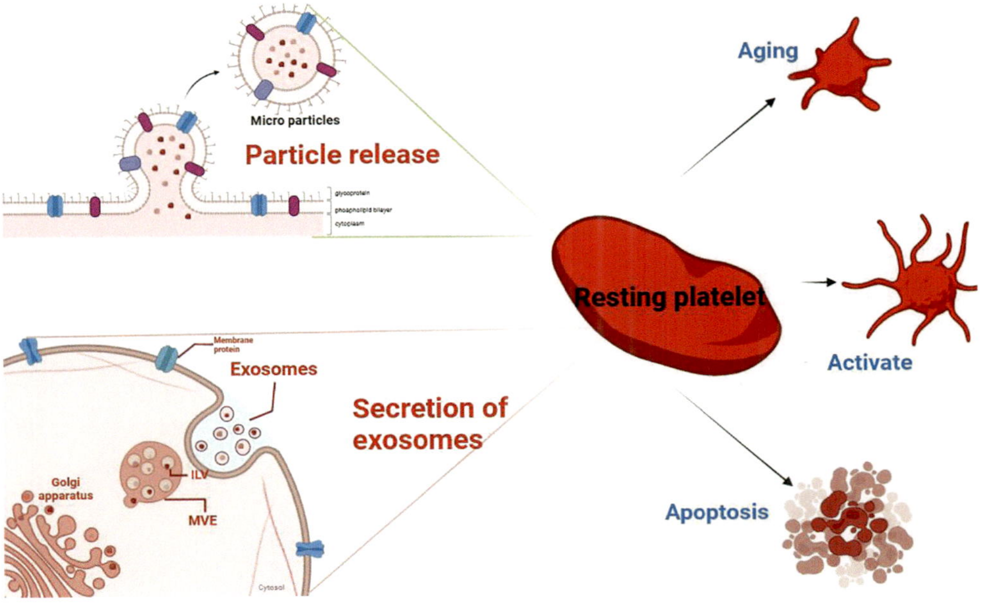

Fig. 2.2 Platelets release extracellular vesicles in various states. (*MVE* multivesicular endosomes, *ILV* intraluminal vesicles)

to target cells for functional regulation. The relevant sorting and acting mechanism need to be further studied.

2.3 Current Preparation Methods and Principles

Different preparation methods are used to obtain different products. Platelet-rich plasma can be divided into unactivated PRP and activated PRP according to its application form. Activated PRP can be divided into PRP gel and PRP release (liquid); PRP coagulation glue means that when platelets are activated to release growth factors, the released fibrinogen is polymerized into fibrin and connected into a network to form a gel-like substance with a certain erectile property and strength visible to the naked eye. PRP releases usually refer to the supernatant containing growth factors and active proteins released into plasma or serum after activation of platelets.

The preparation of PRP is divided into automatic plasma exchange method and density gradient centrifugation method. At present, density gradient centrifugation is used for preparation, and there are a variety of commercial preparation systems available for selection. We found that the factors that affect PRP preparation include centrifugal force, centrifugation time, number of centrifugation, temperature, age, gender, the type of anticoagulant, platelet count of the donor, etc. [17–20]. When using the density gradient centrifugation method, some scholars [21] believe that single centrifugation can achieve the effect, but more scholars agreed two density gradient centrifugation methods. There is no uniform standard for the two centrifugal force and times. Increase the centrifugal forces and time. Centrifugation time can increase the degree of enrichment, but it will cause self-activation, which will cause platelet destruction. Most scholars believe that after the first low-speed centrifugation, high-speed centrifugation is performed again, and the platelet recovery rate in the obtained PRP is higher. Arora et al. compared three kinds of centrifugal force and centrifugation time to prepare PRP and evaluated the effect of preparation using seven indexes such as platelet enrichment rate and growth factor release and pointed out that the centrifugal force should be specified when preparing platelets instead of using revolutions per minute [22]. Because in the case of the same number of revolutions and time, as the centrifugal radius changes, the centrifugal force will change accordingly.

Although the descriptions in the literature are very different, the process is absolutely unfavorable. First, a test tube containing an anticoagulant is used to acquire the patient's blood, and the first centrifugation is performed at a constant acceleration to separate the red blood cells from other blood components. After the first centrifugation step, whole blood is divided into three layers: the upper layer mainly contains plasma and platelets; the middle thin layer is called the albuginea layer, which is rich in white blood cells and platelets; and the bottom layer is mainly composed of red blood cells. When it is necessary to prepare pure PRP (leukocyte-poor and platelet-rich plasma), transfer the upper layer and the superficial layer to another sterile centrifuge tube. When it is necessary to prepare PRP rich in white blood cells, it is necessary to transfer the entire buffy coat layer and a small amount of red blood cells to another centrifuge tube. During the second centrifugation, the centrifugal force should be sufficient to facilitate the formation of platelet pellets at the bottom of the centrifuge tube. After the second centrifugation, the upper part of the platelet-poor plasma is taken out, and the platelet precipitation is mixed with the remaining plasma to obtain PRP. Of course, when the blood volume is small, only a small amount of buffy coat can be produced. How to accurately control the white blood cell content is a technical problem.

Various factors affect the PRP platelet concentration gradient, such as platelet size and biological differences between individuals and hematocrit variability. But the most critical factor affecting the concentration of platelets is the operation after the second centrifugation, because some red blood cells inevitably get mixed into the platelet precipitate, and the surface of these remaining red blood cells can adsorb platelets and white blood cells. A short time of manual mixing is not enough to completely resuspend the platelets. About 20% of the platelets are still adsorbed in the RBC particles, so it is important to resuspend the platelets sufficiently [18, 23].

And now existing activation methods include (Fig. 2.3) the following:

1. The most commonly used method: Adding thrombin and/or calcium ions—PRP.
2. Whole blood was collected in a tube without anticoagulant and centrifuged for activation—PRF.
3. Multiple freeze-thaw cycles were used to lysate platelets—PL.
4. Sonication is used to lysate platelets—PRP.
5. Using pulsed electric field to activate platelets—PRP.
6. Using centrifugation: Removal of white blood cells, preparation of precursor, F2 activation, and mixing steps to produce new agents that can be used for soft tissue filling—PRGF.
7. Using light to activate platelet—PRP.

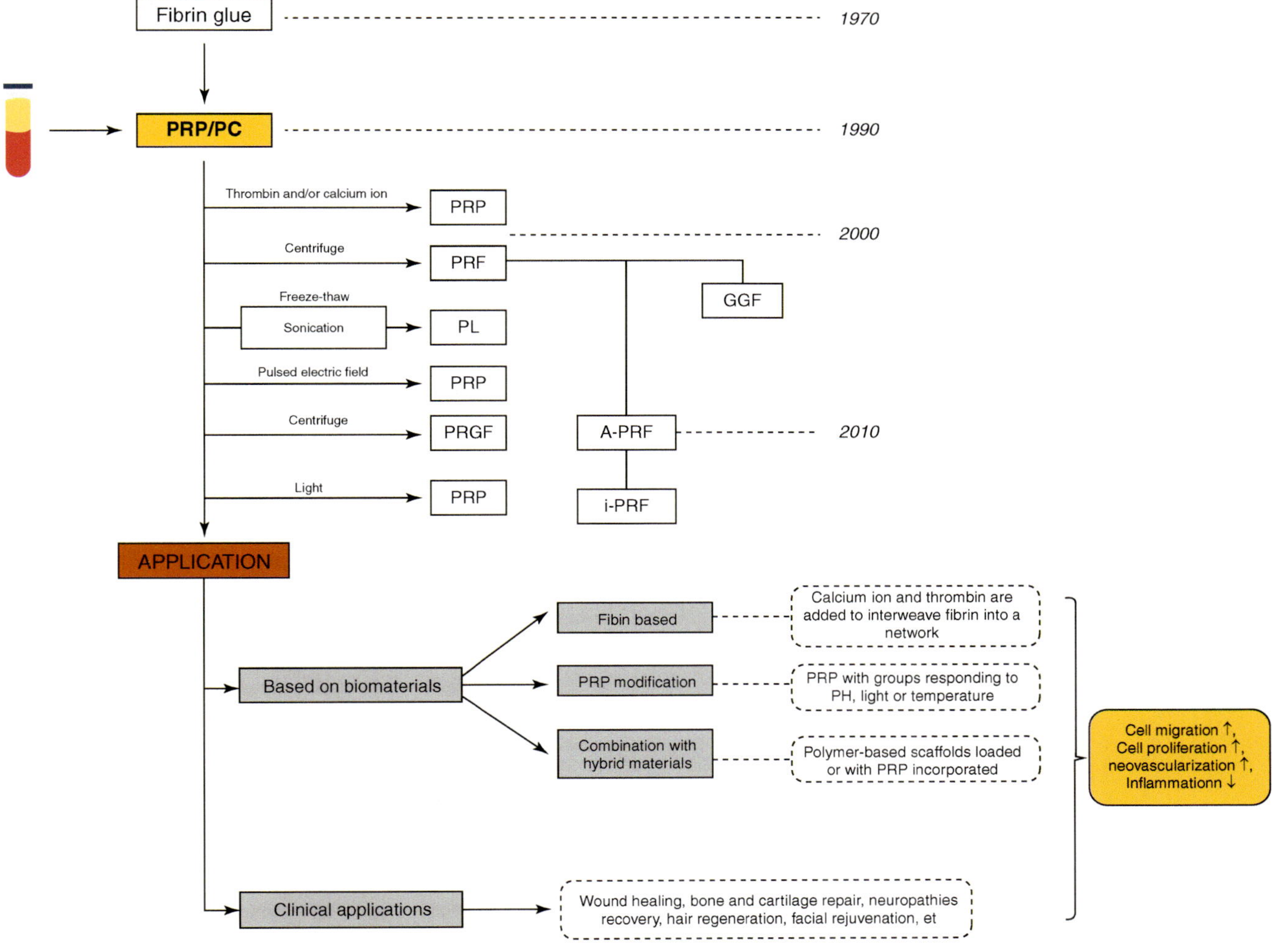

Fig. 2.3 Activation mode and application of PRP

References

1. Carrillomora P, Gonzálezvillalva A, Macíashernández SI, et al. [Platelets-rich plasma: a versatile tool for regenerative medicine?]. Cirugía Y Cirujanos. 2013;81(1):74.
2. Hausauer AK, Humphrey S. The physician's guide to platelet-rich plasma in dermatologic surgery part II: clinical evidence. Dermatol Surg. 2020;46(4):447–56.
3. Naik B, Karunakar P, Jayadev M, Marshal VR. Role of platelet rich fibrin in wound healing: a critical review. J Conserv Dent. 2013;16:284–93.
4. Harke H, Tanger D, Furst-Denzer S, et al. [Effect of a preoperative separation of platelets on the postoperative blood loss subsequent to extracorporeal circulation in open heart surgery (author's transl)]. Anaesthesist. 1977;26(2):64–71.
5. Hood AG, Hill AG, Reeder GD, et al. Perioperative autologous sequestration: a new physiologic glue with wound healing properties. Am Acad Cardiovasc Perfusion. 1993;14:126–9.
6. Burnouf T, Goubran HA, Chen TM, et al. Blood-derived biomaterials and platelet growth factors in regenerative medicine. Blood Rev. 2013;27:77–89.
7. Marck RE, Middelkoop E, Breederveld RS, et al. Considerations on the use of platelet-rich plasma, specifically for burn treatment. J Burn Care Res. 2014;35(3):219–27.
8. Dohan DM, Choukroun J, Diss A, et al. Platelet-rich fibrin (PRF): a second-generation platelet concentrate. Part I: technological concepts and evolution. Oral Surg Oral Med Oral Pathol Oral Radiol Endod. 2006;101(3):e37–44.
9. Powell DM, Chang E, Farrior EH. Recovery from deep-plane rhytidectomy following unilateral wound treatment with autologous platelet gel: a pilot study. Arch Facial Plast Surg. 2001;3:245–50.
10. Man D, Plosker H, Winland-Brown JE. The use of autologous platelet-rich plasma (platelet gel) and autologous platelet-poor plasma (fibrin glue) in cosmetic surgery. Plast Reconstr Surg. 2001;107(1):239.
11. Bhanot S, Alex JC. Current applications of platelet gels in facial plastic surgery. Facial Plast Surg. 2002;18:27–33.
12. Sánchez-González DJ, Méndez-Bolaina E, Trejo-Bahena NI. Platelet-rich plasma peptides: key for regeneration. Int J Pept. 2012;2012(3):532519.
13. Marx RE. Platelet-rich plasma (PRP) what is PRP and what is not PRP? Implant Dent. 2001;10(4):225–8.

14. Peerbooms JC, van Laar W, Faber F, et al. Use of platelet rich plasma to treat plantar fasciitis: design of a multi centre randomized controlled trial. BMC Musculoskelet Disord. 2010;11(1):69–70.
15. Senzel L, Gnatenko DV, Bahou WF. The platelet proteome. Curr Opin Hematol. 2009;16(5):329.
16. Alves R, Grimalt R. A review of platelet-rich plasma: history, biology, mechanism of action, and classifications. Skin Appendage Disord. 2018;4(1):18–24.
17. Jo CH, Roh YH, Kim JE, et al. Optimizing plateletrich plasma gel formation by varying time and gravitational forces during centrifugation. J Oral Implantol. 2013;39:525–53.
18. Amable PR, Carias RBV, Teixeira MVT, et al. Platelet-rich plasma preparation for regenerative medicine: optimization and quantification of cytokines and growth factors. Stem Cell Res Ther. 2013;4:67.
19. Sonker A, Dubey A. Determining the effect of preparation and storage: an effort to streamline platelet components as a source of growth factors for clinical application. Transfus Med Hemother. 2015;42:174–80.
20. Mazzocca AD, MB MC, Chowaniec DM, et al. Platelet-rich plasma differs according to preparation method and human variability. J Bone Joint Surg Am. 2012;94(4):308–16.
21. Bausset O, Giraudo L, Veran J, et al. Formulation and storage of platelet-rich plasma homemade product. Bioresour Open Access. 2012;1(3):115–23.
22. Arora S, Doda V, Kotwal U, et al. Quantification of platelets and platelet derived growth factors from platelet-rich-plasma (PRP) prepared at different centrifugal force (g) and time. Transfus Apher Sci. 2016;54(1):103–10.
23. Dhurat R, Sukesh M. Principles and methods of preparation of platelet-rich plasma: a review and author's perspective. J Cutan Aesthet Surg. 2014;7(4):189.

PRP and Skin Barrier

3

Xiao Cui, Guiqiu Shan, Sha Yuan, and Biao Cheng

Skin is the largest organ of the human body as well as the first defensive barrier of our body being in contact with the environment (Fig. 3.1). The appearance and function of the human skin change profoundly with the increase of age (intrinsic aging) and the accumulation of external factors (extrinsic aging). Photoaging is the primary cause of extrinsic aging, and some environmental factors could make the skin vulnerable. It is well documented that radiation from solar ultraviolet (UV), infrared, and visible light could produce oxidative stress, photoaging, and photocarcinogenesis [1]. In recent years, research also focused on the assessment of injury that environmental contaminants may cause to the skin. Signs of skin aging include dryness, pigmentation disorders, wrinkles, and sagging skin. Histologically, the characteristics of aging skin are excessive damage of the epidermis, atypical hyperplasia and inflammatory cells of keratinocytes, flattening of the dermis-epidermis junction, atrophy of the dermis, disorder of collagen fiber arrangement, elastic degeneration, a small number of fibroblasts, irregular hyperplasia of accessory glands [2], and so on. In a word, with aging, the skin barrier function is diminished, and cellular replacement in the skin and mechanical protection continually decreases. Therefore, skin health and maintaining or restoring a young appearance is the priority choice in people's life.

X. Cui
Department of Physiotherapy, Guangdong Provincial Hospital of Chinese Medicine, Guangzhou, Guangdong, China

G. Shan
Department of Transfusion Medicine, General Hospital of Southern Theater of PLA, Guangzhou, Guangdong, China

S. Yuan
Dermatological Department, Hangzhou Meilai Medical Hospital, Hangzhou, Zhejiang, China

B. Cheng (✉)
Department of Burn & Plastic Surgery, General Hospital of Southern Theater Command, Guangzhou, China

When the skin barrier is damaged, the ability of resistance to external pathogenic microorganisms is weakened, which can induce and aggravate many skin diseases. After the skin barrier is broken, necrotic keratinocytes release damage-related molecules that will activate the natural immune system and trigger skin inflammation. In addition, epidermal Langerhans cells can induce immune tolerances, while dermal dendritic cells have immune activation function. Therefore, when the skin barrier function completes Langerhans cell recognition, skin symbiotic bacteria do not cause immune response, but when after the skin barrier function is impaired, bacteria, fungi, and viruses that are usually on the surface of the skin enter into the dermis, where they are identified by dendritic cells which present antigen, activate the immune system, and induce inflammation. If the skin barrier function is damaged, many immune-related skin diseases such as eczema, atopic dermatitis, and psoriasis can be aggravated. Therefore it is very important to protect the skin barrier.

At present, there are many methods of skin rejuvenation, such as dermal filler, Botox injection, laser treatment and chemical peeling, etc., with different effects and side effects. In order to further improve the clinical efficacy, people began to seek methods in the field of regenerative medicine to prevent, reduce, or reverse the clinical symptoms of skin aging. Platelet-rich plasma (PRP) stands out in this respect and has achieved positive results in clinic. It can stimulate the syn-

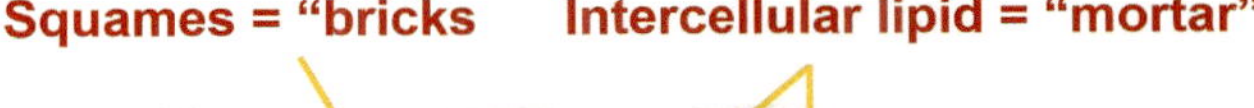

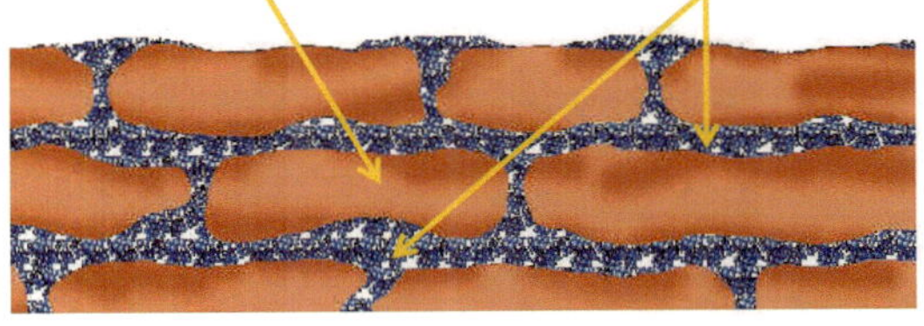

Fig. 3.1 The skin barrier

B. Cheng, X. Fu (eds.), *Platelet-Rich Plasma in Tissue Repair and Regeneration*, https://doi.org/10.1007/978-981-99-3193-4_3

Table 3.1 Possible mechanism of PRP on skin barrier

Skin barrier	Possible mechanism of PRP
Physical barrier	1. Promote the proliferation of skin fibroblasts and collagen synthesis
	2. Remodel the ECM
	3. Promote the synthesis of hyaluronic acid
	4. Increase G1 cell cycle regulatory factors to regulate cell metabolism and accelerate tissue renewal
	5. Enhance the densification of epidermal structure
Chemical barrier	1. Improve the skin gland secretion function
	2. Anti-bacterial and anti-inflammatory activity
	(a) Mediate the internalization of phagocytes to various pathogens
	(b) Release chemokines to promote the aggregation of inflammatory cells
	(c) Release antibacterial peptides involved in the bacteriostatic process directly
	(d) Leukocytes in PRP regulate inflammatory response
Pigment barrier	1. Pigmentation is regulated by melanocytes, keratinocytes and fibroblasts
	2. Regulate tyrosine kinase receptor activity through bFGF and HGF signaling pathway
	3. Supplement antioxidant enzymes to remove free radicals and abnormal pigment deposition
Immune barrier	1. Secrete chemokines and recruit a variety of immune cells to participate in the immune response
	2. Enhance the antigen presentation of dendritic cells
	3. Coordinate the directed differentiation of T cells and activate B cells to produce a variety of key antibody subtypes
Nerve barrier	1. Regulate neurotrophic factors release and cell migration to promotes axon regeneration
	2. Regulate the inflammatory microenvironment around injured nerves, provide suitable ECM and promote nerve regeneration
	3. Promote angiogenesis, guide axons growth and Schwann cells migration
	4. Reduce the side effects of denervation of Schwann cells and activate it to promote axonal regeneration

PRP platelet rich plasma, *ECM* extracellular matrix, *bFGF* b fibroblast growth factor, *HGF* hepatocyte growth factor

thesis of collagen, make the epidermis thickened, improve skin color, reduce or lighten wrinkles, and repair other signs of aging on the face, which has attracted wide attention of clinical and scientific researchers. PRP protects the body and maintains the homeostasis of the skin from the aspects of skin barrier (including physical barrier, chemical barrier, pigment barrier, immune microbial-barrier, and nerve barrier) (Table 3.1) and many aspects related to skin function.

3.1 PRP and Skin Physical Barrier

The cuticle cells of the skin and the mixed lipids filled between cells constitute the skin physical barrier. This barrier function is called brick-wall structure: the cuticle cells are bricks, and the filled lipids are called mortar to form a defense wall, which can not only protect the body from external damage but also prevent the loss of water, electrolyte, and other substances in the body. If the skin physical barrier is damaged, PRP can play a more comprehensive repair role.

3.1.1 PRP Promotes the Proliferation of Skin Fibroblasts and Collagen Synthesis

Activation of dermal fibroblasts is essential for the regeneration of the aging skin [3]. In vitro experiments, the proliferation of keratinocytes and fibroblasts was observed to be enhanced when cultured at the appropriate PRP concentration, while exosomes of PRP could increase the proliferation and mobility of fibroblasts to a greater extent (compared with PRP) [4]. At the same time, the hepatocyte growth factor (HGF), vascular endothelial growth factor (VEGF), monocyte chemotactic protein 1, neutrophil-activated protein 78, and granulocyte macrophage colony-stimulating factor secretion increased; the type I collagen peptide and the expression of type I collagen increase. In photoaging, the animal models and human facial skin aging treatment before and after contrast are found, the skin collagen fiber was close, the total area of the elastic fiber increased, the mature collagen fibers increased obviously, and the type I and III collagen synthesis increased obviously [3, 5]. Studies have confirmed the mRNA expression of platelet-derived growth factor (PDGF) in fibroblasts and keratinocytes at the affected site. PDGF can increase the transformation of fibroblasts to muscle fibroblasts in the damaged sites, promote the synthesis of collagen and epithelial formation in the damaged tissues, and promote the growth and repair of tissues [6, 7]. PDGF in PRP is a powerful mitogen, which activates the mitosis of senescent damaged local cells by binding to the receptors on fibroblasts, endothelial cells, and macrophages, so as to increase the number of regenerated cells [8]. It can also promote the proliferation and migration of endothelial cells, so as to play the role of angiogenesis [9] and the production of transforming growth factor-β (TGF-β). TGF-β can promote the proliferation of undifferentiated mesenchymal cells, which can not only directly affect the protein synthesis of fibroblasts to extracellular matrix but also stimulate fibroblasts to synthesize a large number of collagen matrix and regulate collagen synthesis, especially the synthesis of type I and type III collagen to start and secrete collagenase [10]. At the same time, TGF matrix can effectively inhibit the decomposition of collagen by MMP-1, MMP-3, and MMP-9 of matrix metalloproteinases (MMPs). In addition, the epidermis performs the barrier functions of the skin, and the cuticle is primarily responsible for these barrier functions. PDGF also stimulates the production of insulin growth factor-1 (IGF-1) [11]. IGF-1 can increase the activity of keratinocytes and promote keratinization. Therefore, PRP has the ability to increase skin elasticity through keratinocytes, fibroblast proliferation, and collagen production.

3.1.2 PRP Remodels the ECM

Remodeling extracellular matrix (ECM) is a necessary condition for skin rejuvenation, and PRP leads to remodeling of ECM, which requires activation of dermal fibroblasts, which are essential for aging skin. PRP contains a variety of high concentrations of growth factors and cell adhesion molecules; when it is injected into damaged skin tissue, aging can induce MMP-1, MMP-2, and MMP-3 expression in human skin fibroblasts [3], promote photoaging ECM component (including aging harmful fragments and skin collagen and connective tissue) removal, and, through a variety of molecular mechanisms, induce synthesis of new collagen by dermal fibroblasts and enhance the skin elasticity.

3.1.3 PRP Promotes the Synthesis of Hyaluronic Acid

The ability of PRP to stimulate hyaluronic acid (HA) synthesis is another possible reason for improving skin aging. HA affects the skin's ability to retain moisture by binding to and retaining water molecules. And the water molecules cause the skin to swell and fill up. As a result, increased levels of HA improve the appearance of the skin [12].

3.1.4 PRP Increases G1 Cell Cycle Regulatory Factors to Regulate Cell Metabolism and Accelerate Tissue Renewal

The fibroblast growth factor (FGF) in PRP can promote mitosis of mesoderm cells, promote cell movement, and make cells transform and proliferate from G0 phase to G1 phase. At the same time, a large number of collagen and fibroblasts are produced, which constitute the extracellular matrix, promote reepithelialization and angiogenesis [13], and accelerate tissue renewal.

3.1.5 PRP Enhances the Densification of Epidermal Structure

The tight junctions between the keratinocytes are anchored in their cytoskeleton, contributing to the physical barrier. Studies have shown that during the skin development of the newborn suckling mouse, PRP intervention therapy significantly escalated the expression levels of early loricrin and involucrin of the epidermal tissues [14]. In addition, PRP contains a large amount of cell adhesion proteins, such as cellulose, fibronectin, and vitronectin, which aggregates the growth factors released by platelets to play a role locally, and can also serve as a scaffold for new cells and tissues to promote the repair of the aging skin and at the same time increase the expression of cyclin A protein to tighten the skin [14].

3.2 PRP and Skin Chemical Barrier

The chemical barrier consists of lipids, degradation products of filaggrin (FLG), and antimicrobial peptides. Skin aging results in a decrease in the number of nerves and blood vessels in the epidermis and dermis, and skin metabolism slows down. The number of skin glands (including lipid glands and sweat glands) is reduced, and their secretion ability is degraded, resulting in rough, dry, sensitive skin. These signs are related to impaired enzymatic processes, partly due to the decrease in the water content of stratum corneum (SC) [15]. The intercellular lipid determines the permeability of the stratum corneum. However, chronological aging leads to the decrease of intercellular lipid secretion, which increases the permeability of SC and water loss. With high protease activity, the production of natural moisturizing factor (NMF) formed from the proteolysis of FLG is decreased. This part of functional repair can be achieved by enhancing epidermal structure density and secreting growth factor and active protein to activate gland function by PRP, which is aforementioned.

Also, the skin is colonized by an abundant and diverse community of microbes, which plays an essential role in the cell cycle of the keratinocytes and in the immune networks of the skin that have systemic implications. When the balance of the cutaneous microbiome is broken and the barrier function is diminished, it may cause acne, dermatitis, eczema, and other skin inflammatory and immune diseases. For the aged epidermis, susceptibility to irritant contact dermatitis and, often, severe xerosis and impaired permeability to the drug are increased [16]. As the emergence of drug-resistant bacteria makes it increasingly difficult for antibiotics to treat bacterial infections, people begin to find new opportunities for antimicrobial pathways from the host itself. Studies have reported that PRP has procured preferable effects in the treatment of certain skin diseases. The mechanism of its anti-bacterial and anti-inflammatory activity could (1) mediate the internalization of phagocytes to various pathogens [17], (2) release chemokines to promote the aggregation of inflammatory cells, and (3) release platelet-derived antibacterial peptides

(PDAPs) involved in the bacteriostatic process directly. It has been reported that PDAPs contain at least four families of antimicrobial proteins, Kinocidins, defensins, antimicrobial peptide derivatives, and proteolytic derivatives [17], such as thrombin-induced platelet microbicidal protein-1 (tPMP-1), platelet factor-4 (platelet factor 4, PF4), and regulated activation protein (regulated upon activation of normal T cell expressed and secreted (RANTES); connective tissue-activating peptide-3 (CTAP-3), thymosin-β4 (T-β4), fibrin peptide-A (fibrinopeptide-A, FP-A), FP-B, etc. have strong killing effects on *Staphylococcus aureus*, *Escherichia coli*, *Candida albicans*, *Bacillus subtilis*, *Lactococcus*, *Cryptococcus neoformans* [18, 19], etc. Trier et al. [20] also found that platelets repeatedly recognize *Staphylococcus aureus* and react to it repeatedly: when platelets interact with *Staphylococcus aureus*, δ particles release ADP and ATP. α-Particles release PMPs and Kinocidins. ADP repeatedly stimulates the ADP receptors P2X1 and P2Y12 on the platelet surface and continuously activates surrounding resting platelets to promote the release of PMPs and Kinocidins. This self-amplifying cascade effect plays an important role in activating platelet host defense, which is not achieved by other antibacterial drugs. (4) Leukocytes in PRP are involved in the regulation of inflammatory response. At present, there is still a lot of controversies about whether to retain leukocytes in PRP preparation. Because leukocytes may aggravate inflammatory reactions, there is potential damage to healthy tissues. For example, neutrophils in leukocytes may produce excessive MMPs and IL during the inflammatory phase of injury repair, thus causing muscle damage. But its advantages cannot be ignored. For example, neutrophils are the main defense system against pathogenic microorganisms and local inflammatory response, which release a large number of protease and active oxygen to fight against microorganisms [21]; mononuclear and multinuclear granulocytes can anchor local inflammatory response to promote tissue repair process; neutrophils of appropriate concentration can also control infection [22]. In the cell experiment, it was found that PRP containing leukocytes significantly promoted the growth of rabbit bone marrow mesenchymal stem cells and cartilage formation. Histological examination showed that the cartilage repair effect of the combination of PRP containing leukocytes and rabbit bone marrow mesenchymal stem cells in vivo was better than that of PRP group without leukocytes. Therefore, when considering the function of leukocytes in PRP, it may be necessary to focus on the repair of different diseases or tissues in order to make them play the best role. PRP with a certain concentration of leukocytes is often used to prevent infection in joint replacement and other surgical operations [23].

3.3 PRP and Skin Pigment Barrier

In order to prevent solar radiation from causing photoaging, the skin utilizes a special and complex pigmentation mechanism to resist damage. Exposure to solar radiation increases the production of reactive oxygen species (ROS) and causes damage to DNA, proteins, and lipids [24]. The antioxidant levels in the skin reduced. Skin pigmentation protects cells from the harmful effects of ultraviolet radiation (UVR) in the environment and repairs DNA damage. Melanin can reduce the skin's absorption of UV and remove the ROS produced during UV exposure. Skin pigmentation is a fragile function, and many physiological and external events can modify skin pigmentation, leading to hyperpigmentation or hypopigmentation, such as altered hormone levels, aging, skin diseases, and environmental stimuli and stresses. In recent years, PRP began to participate in the treatment of orbital pigmentation [25] and chloasma and combined with vitamin D in the treatment of vitiligo pigmentary disorders [26] and achieved good clinical results, but the specific mechanism is not clear; it may be that PRP is involved in the regulation of skin pigment metabolism.

From several key cells involved in skin pigmentation, PRP could regulate pigmentation by affecting key cellular players: melanocytes and keratinocytes in the epidermis and fibroblasts in the dermis, which are closely related to melanogenesis. Skin pigmentation is mainly due to the accumulation of melanin particles in keratinocytes. The synthesis of melanin (melanogenesis) begins with the formation of melanosomes in melanocytes. After four steps of maturation, melanosomes are transferred into keratinocytes and transported and reorganized in the supranuclear area to form melanin caps called microparasols, which protect the keratinocyte nuclei from UVR damage [27]. The paracrine signal regulating melanogenesis is transmitted by keratinocytes and dermal fibroblasts adjacent to melanocytes. The close relationship between these cell types is very important in the regulation of skin pigmentation. There is highly interaction among them, and they communicate with each other through secretion factors (such as amsh, SCF, KGF, and bFGF) and their receptors to regulate skin pigmentation [28, 29]. PRP may be involved in the regulation of melanogenesis by these three kinds of cells, which makes the abnormal pigmentation process tend to recover. Our research team focused on the effects of PRP on HaCaT keratinocytes [30] and melanocytes [31]. PRP treatment can protect UVB (ultraviolet B)-damaged HaCaT cells and PIG1 cells. This effect is achieved by enhancing the oxidative defense ability of cells (increasing the activities of antioxidant enzymes glutathione peroxidase (GSH-Px), superoxide dismutase (SOD), and catalase (CAT)). It can significantly reduce the content of malondialdehyde (MDA) and reactive oxygen species (ROS) in cells, inhibit apoptosis (which downregulate the expression of Bcl-2 and Bax and upregulate the expression of cyclin B, PI3K, AKT, and ERK), and promote DNA damage repair (which significantly decrease the expression level of intracellular γ-H2AX). Notably, PRP pre-treatment also significantly reduced the expression of pro-inflammatory cytokines IL-1β, TNF-α, and IL-6 in HaCaT cells [30]. It is important to note that PRP treatment inhibited UVB-induced melanogenesis via the PI3K/Akt/GSK3β signal pathway [31].

In terms of signal pathways, melanogenesis in the human skin is a tightly regulated process. Although the signaling pathway of melanin generation is mostly converged to the microphthalmia-associated transcription factor (MITF) [32, 33], it involves the regulatory link of tyrosine kinase active receptor in the process of melanin generation, and PRP may play a role in regulating bFGF and HGF signaling pathways as the following:

1. bFGF signaling pathway:FGF-2 can act on melanocyte proliferation [34] and also on melanin synthesis [35]. Melanocytes do not express bFGF. After UV induction, keratinocytes secrete bFGF, which binds to its receptor (FGFR) on melanocytes, resulting in activation of MAPK pathway, allowing phosphorylation of signal transducer and activator of transcription 3 (STAT3) to phosphorylate, thus enhancing the expression of Paired Box 3 (PAX3), a transcription factor that regulates the expression of MITF [36].
2. HGF signaling pathway: HGF is produced and released by human keratinocytes [37]. HGF binds to its receptor c-Met on melanocytes and subsequently activates the MAPK signaling pathway and enhances melanocyte proliferation [29]. When these two signaling pathways are abnormal, PRP may interfere with melanin formation by secreting related growth factors. In vitro studies have also observed the important effects of TGF-β and EGF on melanin formation, which may also be the role of PRP.

Previous studies have confirmed the presence of SOD, CAT, and GSH-Px [38] in PRP, which are endogenous antioxidant enzymes in the human body and can remove free radicals and melanin deposition in the human body. Our results suggested that PRP was capable of scavenging oxidation products by improving the activity levels of enzyme antioxidants [30, 31]. This may also be the reason why PRP improves the appearance of pigmentation. Although there have been clinical reports that PRP has no obvious effect on improving abnormal facial pigmentation, its potential to repair the skin pigmentation barrier is worth looking forward to. Furthermore, recent studies have shown that aging human melanocytes drive skin aging through paracrine telomere dysfunction [39]. This suggests that the study of abnormal pigment metabolism goes far beyond cosmetic needs and may require more attention to its relevance to aging.

3.4 PRP and Skin Immune Barrier

The skin is often considered to be the body's largest immune/endocrine organ (about 15% of body weight, with an average surface area of about 2 m^2). In reaction to changing external and also internal environment, the skin can generate signals to produce rapid (neural) or slow (humoral or immune) responses at the local and systemic levels and restore or maintain local and global homeostasis in relation to hostile environment. In the case of UVR, the main effects of UVR on skin are DNA damage, oxidative stress, harmful effects on ECM, inflammation, and immunosuppression. It activates the neuroendocrine system by nerve transmission or by cutaneous originating chemical mediators, and the photoaging process of the skin can be thought of as a chronic injury that exceeds the ability of the skin to repair itself [40]. UVR also induces immunosuppression and immune tolerance through the action of immunomodulatory molecules such as TNF-α, prostaglandin PG E2, and IL-10 [41].

It is known that platelets can promote the self-regulation of the body's immune system, and PRP may participate in the immune regulation of the skin barrier through activated platelets: Platelets can secrete a large number of chemokines after activation in the body, recruiting a variety of immune cells to participate in the immune response. When vascular injury causes bacterial infection, human platelets express multiple Toll-like receptors (TLRs), which can induce enhanced expression of p-selectin (CD62P) and platelet glycoprotein GPIib-Gpiiia complex on platelet surface [42]. CD62P binds to p-selectin glycoprotein lig 1 (PSGL-1) and promotes the rapid formation of platelet-neutrophil complexes, which activate host cells and recruit neutrophils to the site of injury and infection, which formed neutrophil extracellular traps (NETs) [43].

Platelets can enhance the antigen presentation of dendritic cells (DCs). Platelets rapidly bind to C3 proteins of *Listeria monocytogenes* via GPIb, enhancing DCs' ability to capture pathogens [44]. In addition, cytotoxic CD8+T cells were enhanced when platelet bacterial complex was effectively presented to T and B cells by DCs [45]. Therefore, platelets regulate the types of microbial antigen-presenting cells (APC) and antigen-presenting responses to promote the coordination of innate and adaptive immune responses, which is crucial for antimicrobial host defense. Platelets coordinate the directed differentiation of T cells (such as Th17 cells [46], which play an important role in recruiting and promoting neutrophils to the site of infection) and activate B cells to produce a variety of key antibody subtypes. At the same time, normal platelets (CD154+) can stimulate

CD4 + T cells to significantly induce the formation of B cell germinal centers and produce large amounts of immunoglobulin [47].

3.5 PRP and Skin Nerve Barrier

The nerve barrier of the skin is closely related to other barrier functions. For example, the effects of UV on the skin can activate the neuroendocrine system through neurotransmitters or skin-derived chemical mediators, and the skin and central neuroendocrine responses can also be activated in response to environmental stress. Skin tissues that may participate in skin neuroendocrine response include epidermal keratinocytes, Langerhans cells, melanocytes, and dermal cells such as fibroblasts, macrophages, mast cells, and lymphocytes. Exogenous factors can not only change the skin immune response but also affect the interaction between the skin immune system and neuroendocrine response [48]. Chronological aging leads to a series of skin changes: firstly, the epidermal and dermal layers become thinner; secondly, the atrophy of glands affected sweat secretion and sebum production; and thirdly, the proliferation and desquamation of keratinocytes decreased [49]. Likewise, the skin will also lose sensitivity due to the reduction of sex hormone secretion and the number of nerve endings.

It is well known that there are four important processes involved in nerve regeneration and repair: dedifferentiation of Schwann cells, secretion of neurotrophic factors, formation of blood vessels around injured nerves, and reconnection between regenerated axons and target organs. PDGF in PRP is the mitogen of Schwann cells and a nutrient factor required for the survival of neurons. It promotes axon regeneration by regulating the release of neurotrophic factors and cell migration [50, 51]. The inflammatory response of the host to the transplanted nerve has a great influence on the nerve regeneration process. The inflammatory response leads to nerve cell apoptosis, which in turn reduces the ability of the nerve to regenerate. GFs in PRP can overcome the inflammatory microenvironment around injured nerves, provide appropriate extracellular matrix for injured nerves, play the role of anti-apoptosis and neuroprotection, and promote nerve regeneration [52, 53]. It has been confirmed that blood vessels can act as a basis or signal to guide the growth of axons and migration of Schwann cells, because macrophages can sense the hypoxic environment at the nerve junction and can produce a strong paracrine effect on endothelial cells through VEGF, promoting and supporting the angiogenesis process [54, 55]. PRP-Exos may also promote PRP-induced angiogenesis by activating Erk and Akt signaling pathways [56]. When antibodies of VEGF and PRP were combined to the damaged nerve, the effect of PRP on nerve regeneration was weakened, indicating that VEGF is one of the factors secreted by PRP to promote nerve regeneration [57, 58]. Meanwhile, TGF-β, an important growth factor in PRP, can reduce the side effects of denervation of Schwann cells and activate Schwann cells to promote axonal regeneration [59, 60].

In addition to providing nutrition for supplementing skin growth factors and promoting angiogenesis, PRP can also release a variety of antiaging ingredients to repair skin nerve barrier. Some studies suggest that platelets can secrete a variety of proteins and immunomodulators. After GDF11 protein in rodent plasma was shown to reverse muscle and brain aging [61–63], GDF11 in human plasma was also shown to have an antiaging effect and was highly concentrated in platelets [64]. The existence of tissue inhibitors of metalloproteinases (TIMPs) in PRP can reduce the degradation of extracellular matrix, thereby reducing the degradation of collagen, increasing collagen synthesis, and reducing the symptoms of delaying skin aging [65]. A US study has shown that the blood-derived factor TIMP2 in young mice is resistant to aging changes in older mice and suggests that human umbilical cord blood has a similar effect to that of activating old tissues [66]. Our research team has demonstrated that PRP contains antiaging components GDF11 and TIMP2 [38]. This suggests that the antiaging effect of PRP depends not only on growth factors but also on antiaging proteins. PRP contains multiple RNA-binding proteins that are involved in cell growth and control the expression of aging-related proteins and regulate oxidative stress response. PRP has been shown to release RNA-binding proteins [67], such as heat shock proteins (HSPs), when activated by thrombin. Existing literature has confirmed the occurrence of HSP 27, HSP 60, HSP 70, and HSP 90 in PRP [68]. Heat shock proteins can act as molecular chaperones, coordinate immunity, and participate in cell apoptosis, which can improve the stress capacity of cells and thus achieve antiaging effect. PRP also contains other cell types that have the potential to promote tissue healing. For example, CD34+ cells derived from circulating blood mononuclear cells create an optimal microenvironment for tissue healing. Therefore, using PRP to directly implant a variety of active substances into aging skin, PRP continuously activates the functional expression of aging cells; promotes skin tissue regeneration, cell proliferation, differentiation, and rearrangement; and is a new method to explore antiaging skin.

3.6 PRP and Skin Microbial Barrier

The epidermal surface of the skin is colonized with a stable natural microbiome, including bacteria, fungi, viruses, and other microorganisms. Among them, are Actinobacteria with an abundance of Gram-positive bacteria, such as *Staphylococcus*, *Propionibacterium*, and *Corynebacterium* species. The composition of microbial communities depends on the skin site, but the relative abundance of bacterial taxa is also affected by the skin microenvironment. Sebaceous sites are dominated by lipophilic *Propionibacterium*, while the area with abundant sweat glands could provide a moist environment, thus allowing *Staphylococcus* and *Corynebacterium* to multiply in large numbers. Bacterial commensal colonization of the human skin is vital for the defense training and maintenance of the skin's innate and adaptive immune functions. Such *Staphylococcus* epidermidis, the natural cutaneous microbiome, mediated innate immune alertness by inhibiting the colonization of pathogenic *Staphylococcus aureus* and inducing the expression of AMPs. Meanwhile, it may increase expression of TJ proteins occludin and ZO-1, which could enhance epidermal barrier function. It should also be noted that epidermis pH and the skin immune system strictly regulated the composition of the microbiome. Therefore, the epidermal barrier efficacy is based on the cooperative interaction between the chemical barrier, the skin immune system, and the skin microbiota. The skin microbiome participates in transmission of xenobiotic environmental signals to the functional immune network of the skin [69].

Intravia and his colleagues' study investigates the antibacterial properties of two different platelet concentration preparations (PRPLP and PRPHP) through a time-kill assay. PRPLP, PRPHP, PBS, whole blood, and cefazolin were added to experimental reaction tubes, each containing a single bacterial inoculum of *Staphylococcus aureus* (*S. aureus*), *Staphylococcus epidermidis* (*S. epidermis*), methicillin-resistant *Staphylococcus aureus* (MRSA), or *Propionibacterium acnes* (*P. acnes*), and assessed at five time points (0, 1, 4, 8, and 24 h). Compared to whole blood, both PRP products showed a significant decrease ($p < 0.05$) in bacterial growth (*S. aureus*, *S. epidermis*, MRSA, and *P. acnes* at 8 h and *S. epidermis*, MRSA, and *P. acnes* after 24 h). Differences in platelet and white blood cell concentrations did not cause distinction in antibacterial activity [70]. Prysakde studies a direct correlation between *C. acnes* recoveries and granulocyte counts were observed. The greatest antimicrobial activity with the leukocyte-rich, high platelet PRP preparation is combined with an antibiotic in the injectate [71].

Our studies to explore the antimicrobial activity of platelet-rich plasma (PRP) against *Propionibacterium (P) acnes* in vitro. The bacteriostatic experiment in vitro of PRP was performed by paper disk diffusion method (also known as Kirby-Bauer method). The erythromycin solution was used as positive control, and the negative control was platelet-poor plasma (PPP). PRP was sensitive to *Propionibacterium acnes*, and the inhibitory zone diameter in the disk diffusion test was 15.37 ± 0.747 mm, which had statistical significance when compared to PPP ($p < 0.05$) (Fig. 3.2 and 3.3). According to the standards of grade division in antibiotic susceptibility test, the inhibitory effect of PRP on *Propionibacterium acnes* was highly sensitive. PRP has a good antibacterial effect on *Propionibacterium acnes*, which constitutes the principal pathogenic cause for acne development.

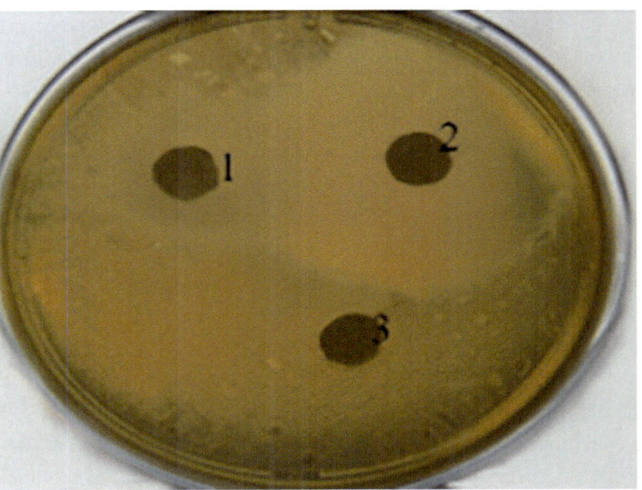

Fig. 3.2 Antibacterial effect of *Propionibacterium acnes* (disk diffusion method): (1) PRP, (2) erythromycin, and (3) PPP

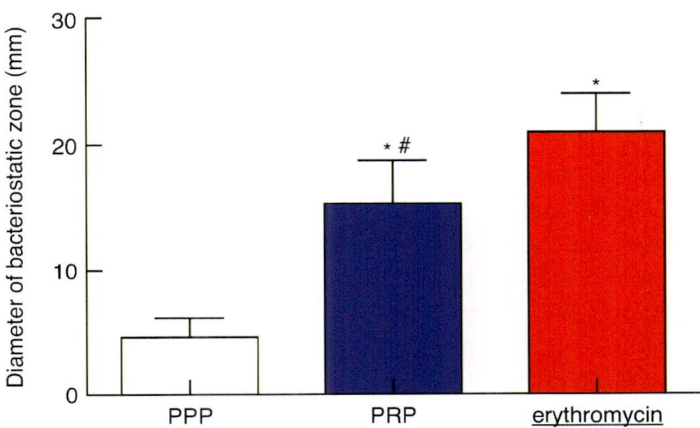

Fig. 3.3 The compared bacteriostatic effect of PRP and erythromycin with PPP ($p < 0.05$)

Platelets, as an important component of the host against infection, play an important role in the antibacterial mechanism in its own way: (1) produce antibacterial oxygen metabolites, (2) promote the complement binding of bacteria, (3) internalize and eliminate pathogens from the blood, (4) exert antibody-dependent cytotoxicity, (5) strengthen the bactericidal mechanism of leukocytes, and (6) degranulate and release various cationic antimicrobial peptides, most of which are classical chemokines with direct antibacterial properties.

This experiment has still some deficiencies: first of all, it is used in the experiment the acne propionic acid bacillus strains (ATCC6919) standard, it has to do with clinical isolates which may be a degree of differences, and further research should use clinical isolates of acne propionic acid bacillus, to explore the relationship between the PRP and antibiotics against infection, including the synergy between them. In the experiment, the size of antibacterial zone obtained by disk diffusion method is not only affected by the antibacterial activity of the drug itself but also by the stability of the drug in the process of disk production and the rate of drug diffusion in AGAR. Under these influences, the results may be far from the actual situation. Therefore, more experiments and clinical observations are needed to prove that disk diffusion method is used to explore the antibacterial activity of PRP against *Propionibacterium acnes*.

3.7 PRP Influencing the Skin Structure, Barrier Cornified Envelope Development of Newborn Suckling Mouse

Speaking of the barrier function of the skin, stratum corneum (SC) is the major barrier that prevents the exogenous stimulations and antigens from entering the organism and the internal water-electrolyte form being lost. The cornified envelope (CE) formed inside the stratum corneum is the foundation of skin barrier. Stratum corneum is the basis for the other barriers (physical barrier, chemical barrier, pigment barrier, immune microbial barrier, and nerve barrier).

The infants could reach the same skin structure with adults completely at the age of about 3 years old; in the meantime, the lower skin barrier function is easy to arouse the endogenous immune reaction and skin injury in case of exogenous stimulation to evoke a series of diseases related to the barrier function disorders of the skin. According to the clinical report, the pathogenesis of various skin diseases is related to the functional declines and disorders. Research on skin barrier is increasingly noted, and therapeutic tools of enhancing the barrier function of the skin have become the key points to prevent and cure various skin diseases.

Due to the rich growth factors and active protein, etc., PRP can not only improve the water content of the skin but also strengthen the immune protection capability of the skin against the external world, reduce the stimulation to the skin from the external objects, and restore the skin to the optimum state.

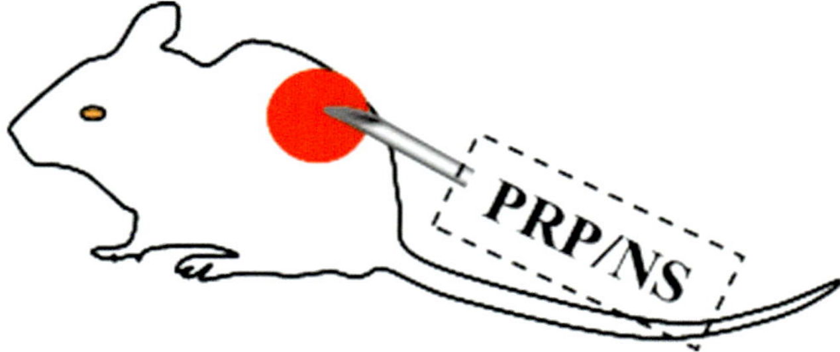

Fig. 3.4 C57BL/6 suckling mice were injected intradermal with a 1 ml syringe at a concentration of 109 PRP or normal saline, about 0.05 mL per mouse, 2 days per time

Therefore, the newborn C57BL/6 suckling mouse model is adopted in this research to observe the PRP's intervention in the development process of skin structure and cornified envelope.

Forty newborn C57BL/6 suckling mice were randomly divided into an experimental group with PRP and a control group with normal saline, with 20 mice for each group. In the central area of the back, each mouse in the experimental group received intradermal injection of 0.05 ml PRP whose platelet concentration is 10/ml on a single point, while the control group received an equivalent amount of normal saline (Fig. 3.4).

Take five animal samples, respectively, from each group at day 3, day 5, day 6, and day 10 for the paraffin-embedded routine HE of full-thickness skin tissue and Masson staining to inspect the interest protein of immunohistochemistry technique, make histological observation and shooting on the tissue slice, and adopt the Image J software to measure the gray level of the skin and IOD value expressed by interest protein, the IPP (Integrated Performance Primitives) software to measure the thickness of dermal layer and cuticular layer, and the SPSS (Statistical Package for the Social Sciences) statistical software to make analysis and calculation on the data.

PRP has significantly improved the development process of cuticular layer and dermal layer in the skin tissue structure of newborn suckling mice. Also, the PRP intervention therapy has promoted the early cutin to form the cellular multiplication and differentiation; in the meantime, the PRP intervention therapy has escalated the expression levels of early Ioricrin and Involucrin of the skin tissue for the newborn suckling mouse to a marked degree.

PRP plays a significant role in promoting the growth of early cuticular and dermal structures of the suckling mouse as well as improving the barrier function of the skin to be mature and complete (Tables 3.2 and 3.3).

PRP significantly promoted the increase and development of epidermis and dermis thickness in the early stage of neonatal rat skin tissue. In the PRP experimental group, the secretion of new collagen in the dermis tissue of neonatal rats was significantly increased, and the collagen arrangement was more inclined to the mature skin tissue (Fig. 3.5). At the same time, the detection results of keratin K1 (Fig. 3.6), Ioricrin, and Involucrin in the epidermal tissues of newborn mice during skin development showed that PRP intervention significantly promoted the proliferation and differentiation of early keratinocytes. Moreover, PRP intervention significantly upregulated the expression levels of Ioricrin and Involucrin in the skin tissues of newborn rats at days 3, 5, and 7 and reached a plateau at day 10 (Fig. 3.7 and 3.8).

Therefore, according to the research and observation on the development of PRP in newborn mice, PRP can significantly promote the development of epidermis and dermis structure in early suckling mice and the process of skin barrier function toward maturity and integrity. To enhance the skin barrier function, cure and protect the occurrence and

Table 3.2 The variation of thickness of the epidermis in infant mice (unit:um)

	The thickness of the epidermis (μm)	
Day	NS	PRP
Day 3	422.77 ± 12.47	435.07 ± 10.53[a]
Day 5	440.79 ± 11.33	459.98 ± 9.05[a]
Day 7	471.25 ± 9.86	497.25 ± 8.12[a]
Day 10	498.24 ± 12.85	516.74 ± 14.36[a]

[a]Showed statistical difference compared with control group, $p < 0.05$ ($n = 20$, M ± SD)

Table 3.3 The variation of thickness of the corium in infant mice (unit:um)

	The thickness of the dermis (μm)	
Day	NS	PRP
Day 3	717.94 ± 9.85	743.71 ± 11.42[a]
Day 5	1098.87 ± 15.23	1168.19 ± 16.03[a]
Day 7	1676.55 ± 13.46	1820.33 ± 10.77[a]
Day 10	1703.19 ± 7.25	1716.74 ± 12.13[a]

[a]Showed statistical difference compared with control group, $p < 0.05$ ($n = 20$, M ± SD)

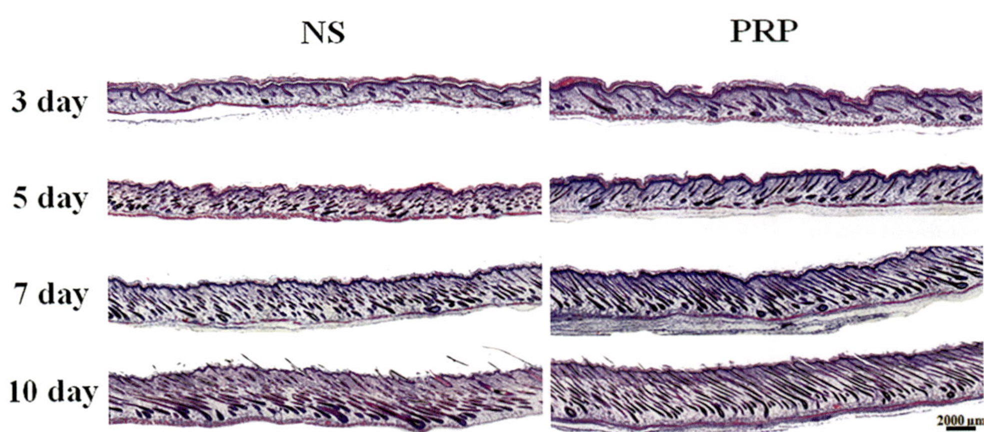

Fig. 3.5 The result of Masson staining of skin tissue of C57BL/6 suckling mice after birth, bar: 2000 μm

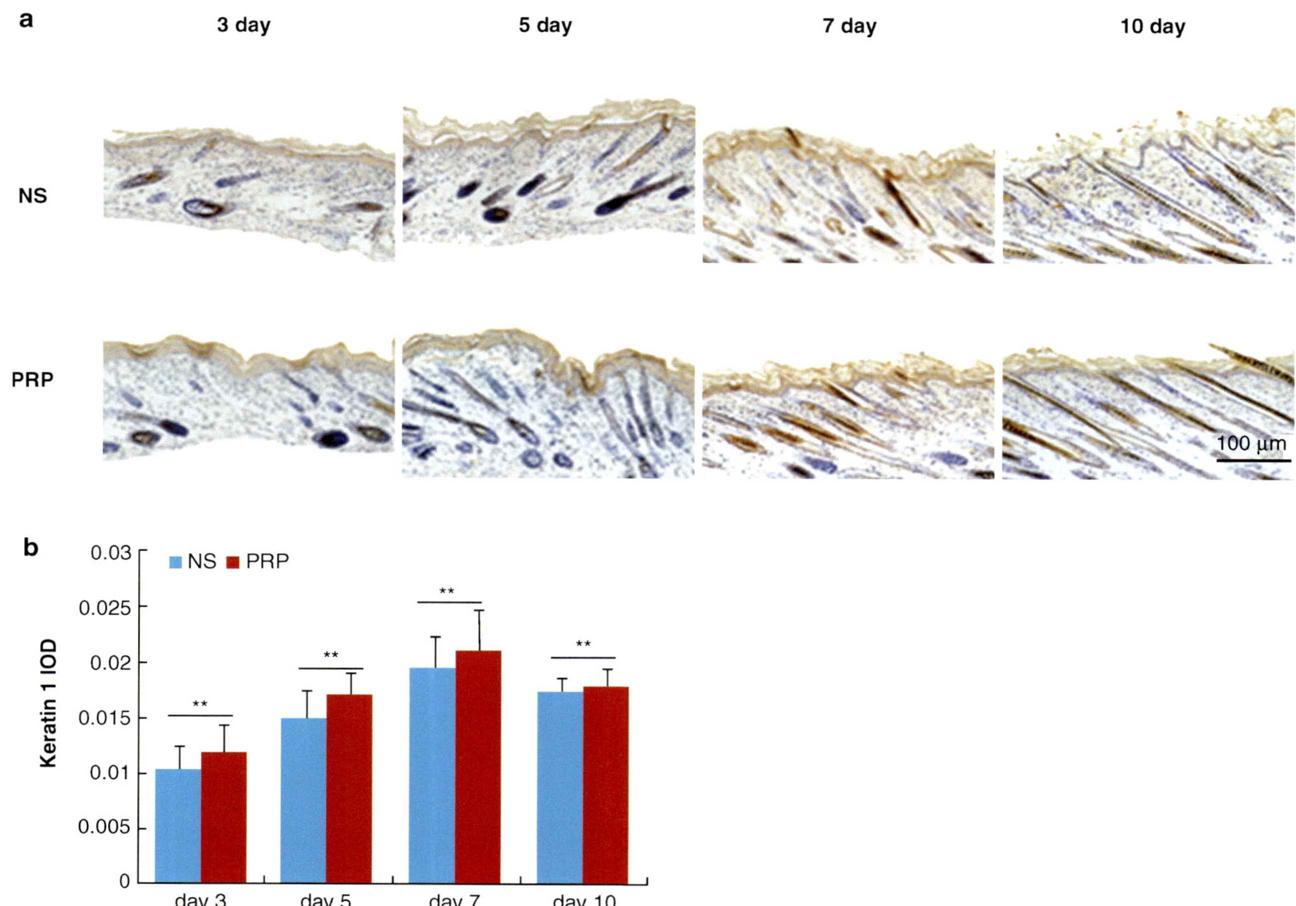

Fig. 3.6 (**a**) Immunohistochemical detection of K1 expression in the skin tissues of neonatal rats at day 3, day 5, day 7, and day 10 in the control group and PRP group; (**b**) statistical results of IOD values of K1 expression in skin tissues of neonatal rats in NS control group and PRP experimental group on different days. Bar: 100 μm, $^{**}p < 0.01$

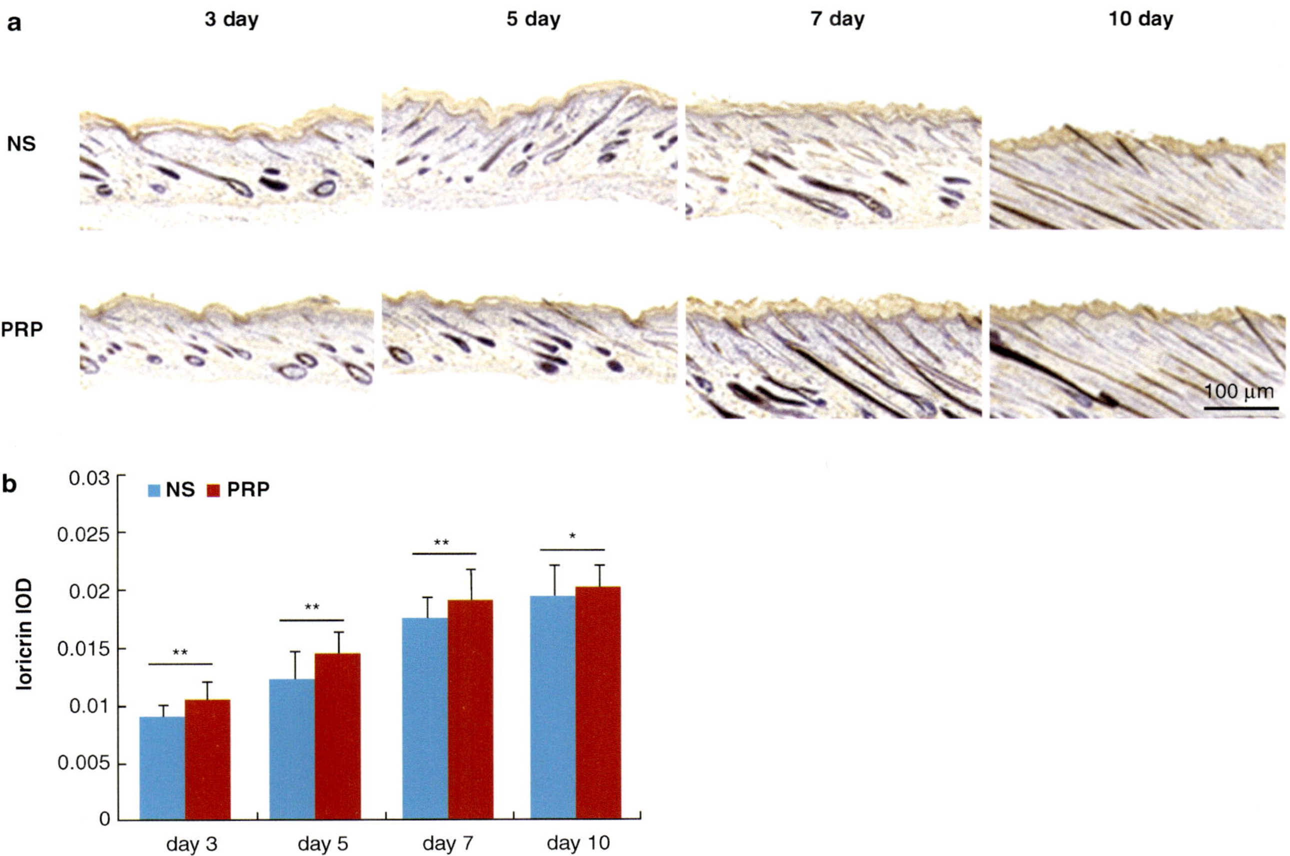

Fig. 3.7 (**a**) Ioricrin expression was detected by immunohistochemistry in the skin tissues of neonatal rats at day 3, day 5, day 7, and day 10 in the control group and PRP group; (**b**) statistical results of IOD values of Ioricrin expression in skin tissues of neonatal rats in NS control group and PRP experimental group on different days. Bar: 100 μm, $^{**}p < 0.01$

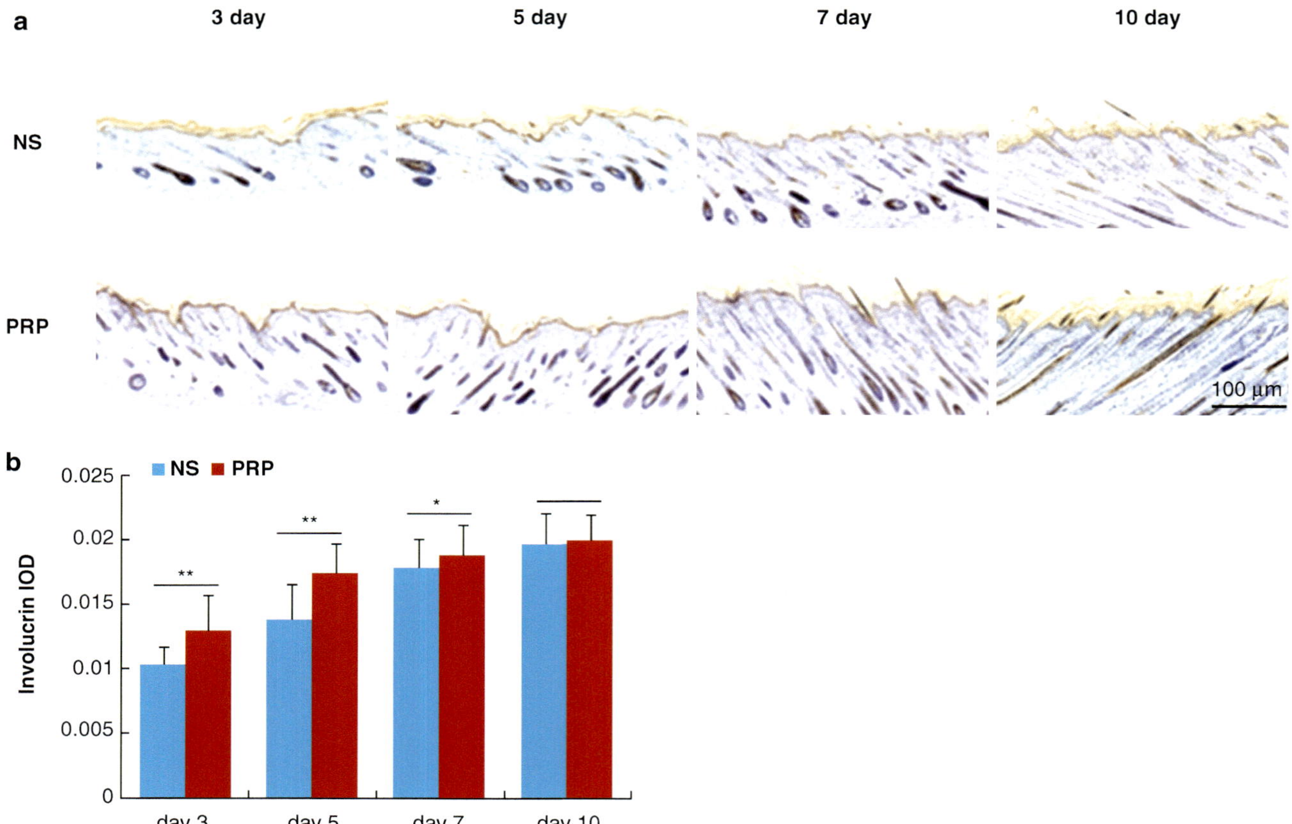

Fig. 3.8 (**a**) The expression of Involucrin in the skin tissues of neonatal rats was detected by immunohistochemistry on day 3, day 5, day 7, and day 10 in the control group and PRP group; (**b**) statistical results of IOD values of Involucrin expression in skin tissues of neonatal rats in NS control group and PRP experimental group on different days. Bar: 100 μm, $^{**}p < 0.01$

development of a variety of skin-related diseases to provide new treatment direction.

3.8 PRP and Its Clinical Application in Skin Barrier

Acne is defined as the pilosebaceous unit of chronic inflammatory disease, which is typically classified as noninflammatory (open and closed blackhead acne) and inflammatory (papules and pustules). Acne may be controlled and treated by local treatment or systemic oral medication to prevent permanent scar formation, limit the duration of the disorder, and minimize morbidity. Topical products have the advantage of being applied to the affected area directly, thus decreasing systemic absorption and increasing the exposure of the pilosebaceous units to the treatment. However, the side effects of skin irritation cannot be ignored. PRP has shown good efficacy in the treatment of acne. Patients with moderate to severe facial acne received local injection of autogenous PRP (the platelet concentration in the PRP ranged from 700,000,000 to 1,000,000,000 platelets per ml). Prior to treatment, calcium gluconate was added at a ratio of 1:9 (calcium gluconate/plasma) to activate platelets. All participants completed the study and were followed up for 1–3 months. The serial photographs were evaluated prior to and following treatment. The observed treatment showed excellent or marked improvement after the first- or third-time treatment (Figs. 3.9, 3.10, and 3.11). No patient was reported to show no improvement.

In conclusion, the current research on the therapeutic mechanism of PRP in beauty is no longer just focused on the role of growth factors in PRP, but we are increasingly aware of the role played by other bioactive ingredients. PRP is not only a repository of biological scaffolds and growth factors but also a trigger for tissue regeneration and repair. PRP may repair the skin barrier function by participating in the regulation of skin immunity and neuroendocrine, change the activity of cells and tissues through the influence on the cell cycle, regulate the pigment metabolism, improve the skin quality, lighten the complexion, restore the skin elasticity, and balance the sebum secretion,

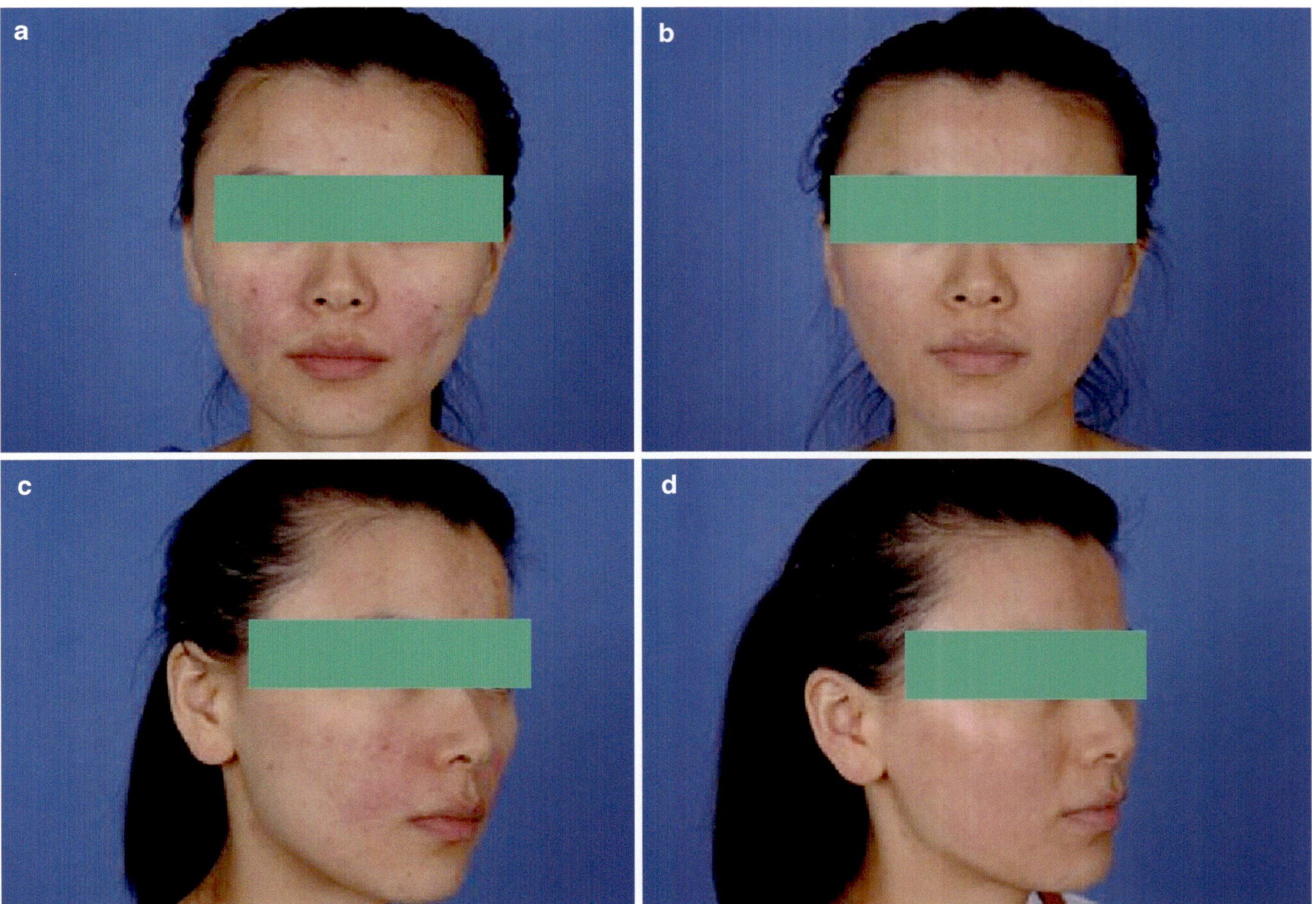

Fig. 3.9 ablative erbium fractional laser with PRP treatment of acne vulgaris. (**a**, **c**)Acne vulgaris; (**b**, **d**)1 month after ablative erbium fractional laser with PRP treatment acne vulgaris

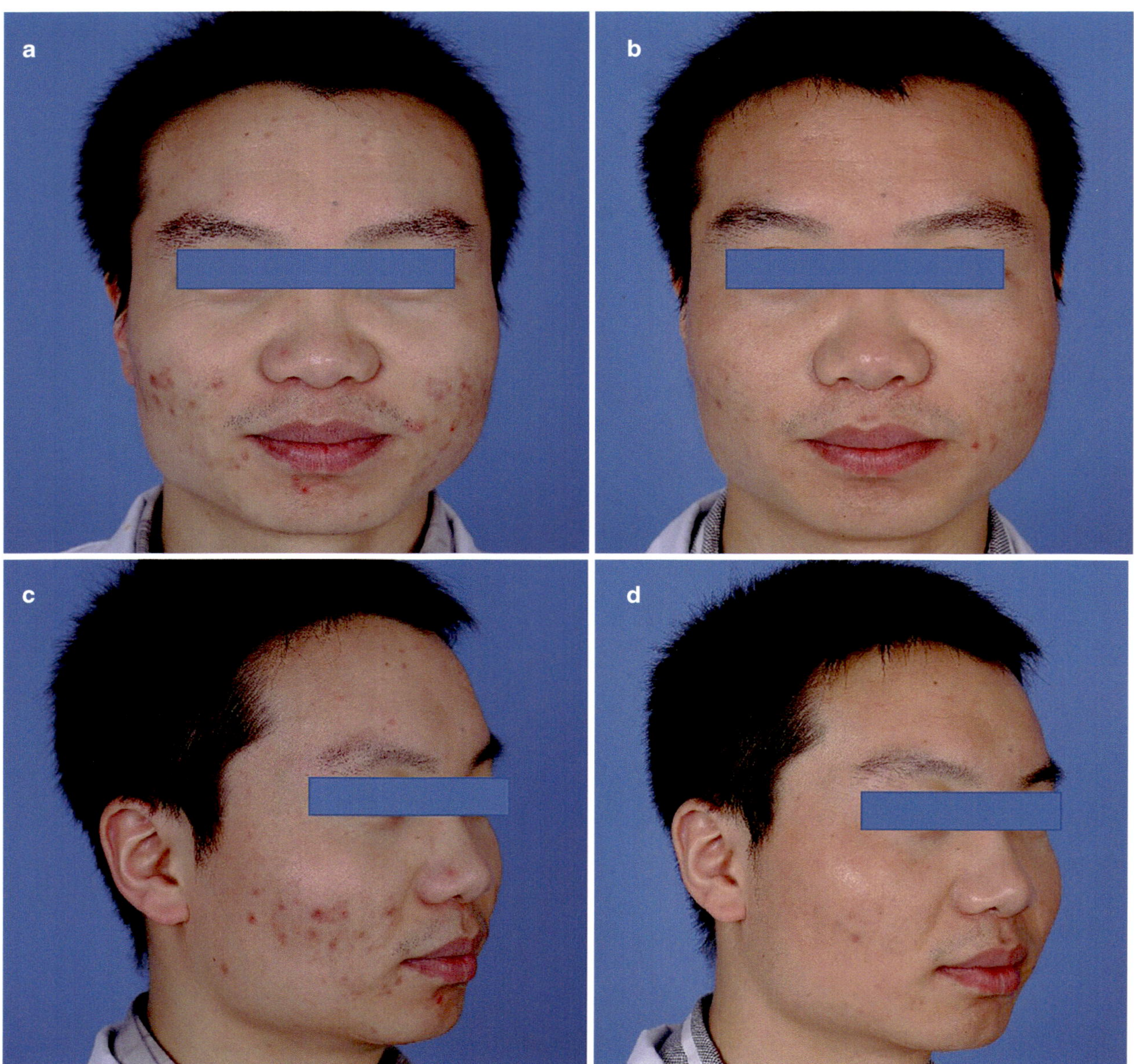

Fig. 3.10 Ablative erbium fractional laser with PRP treatment of acne vulgaris. (**a**, **c**) Acne vulgaris; (**b**, **d**) 3 months after ablative erbium fractional laser with PRP treatment of acne vulgaris

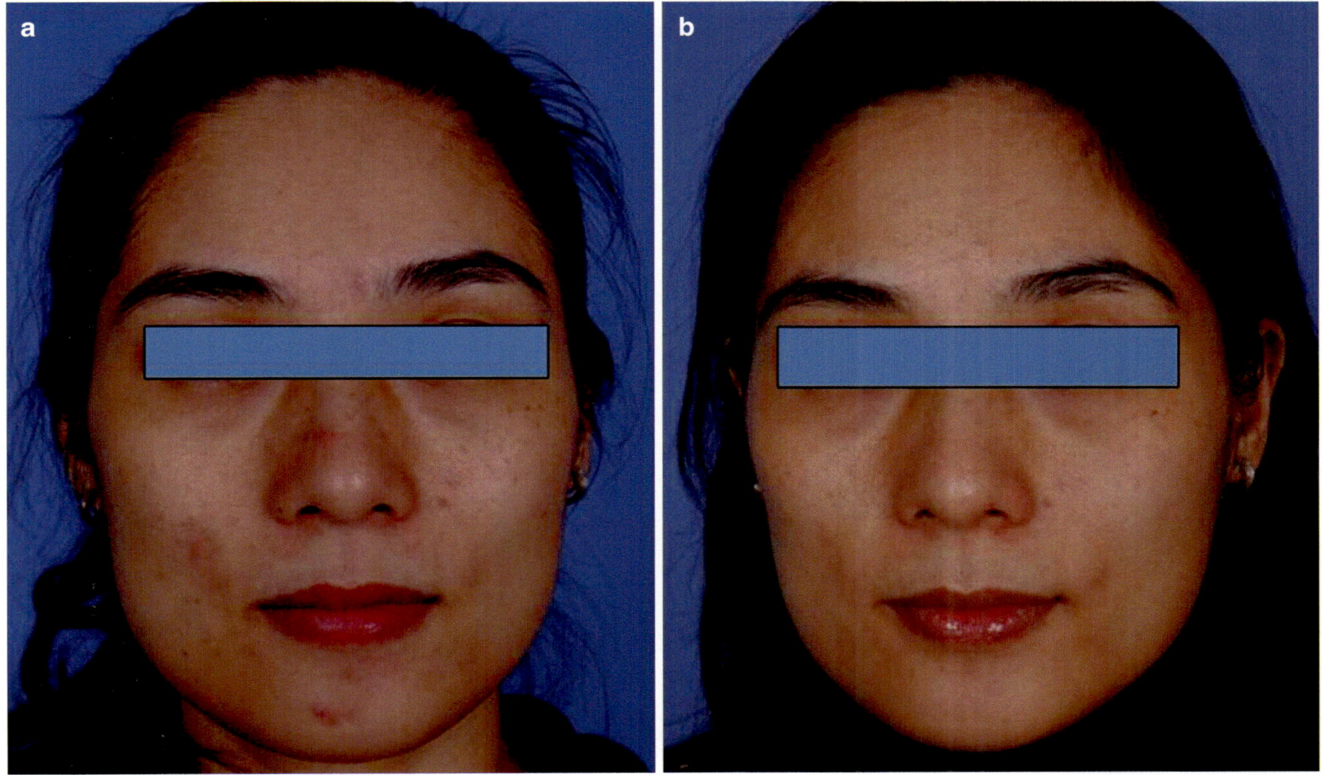

Fig. 3.11 Ablative erbium fractional laser with PRP treatment of acne vulgaris. (**a**) Acne vulgaris; (**b**) 1 month after ablative erbium fractional laser with PRP treatment of acne vulgaris

so as to achieve the skin rejuvenation. However, we are far from satisfied with this, PRP still has great potential to be exploited, and the mechanism of PRP still needs to be further explored.

References

1. Birch-Machin MA, Bowman A. Oxidative stress and ageing. Br J Dermatol. 2016;175(Suppl 2):26–9.
2. Krutmann J, Bouloc A, Sore G, et al. The skin aging exposome. J Dermatol Sci. 2017;85:152–61. https://doi.org/10.1016/j.jdermsci.2016.09.015.
3. Abuaf O, Yildiz H, Baloglu H, et al. Histologic evidence of new collagen formulation using platelet rich plasma in skin rejuvenation: a prospective controlled clinical study. Ann Dermatol. 2016;28:718–24.
4. Guo SC, Tao SC, Yin WJ, et al. Exosomes derived from platelet-rich plasma promote the re-epithelialization of chronic cutaneous wounds via activation of YAP in a diabetic rat model. Theranostics. 2017;7(1):81–96.
5. Sclafani AP, Mccormick SA. Induction of dermal collagenesis, angiogenesis, and adipogenesis in human skin by injection of platelet-rich fibrin matrix. Arch Facial Plast Surg. 2012;14(2):132–6.
6. Corrral C, Siddiqui A, Wu L, et al. Vascular endothelial growth factor is more important than basic fibroblastic growth factor during chemic wound healing. Arch Surg. 1999;134:200–5.
7. Cho JM, Lee YH, Baek RM, et al. Effect of platelet-rich plasma on ultraviolet b-induced skin wrinkles in nude mice. J Plast Reconstr Aesthet Surg. 2011;64(2):e31–9.
8. Eppley BL, Woodell JE, Higgin J. Platelet quantification and growth factor analysis from platelet-rich plasma: implications for wound healing. Plast Reconstr Surg. 2004;114:1502–4.
9. Heldin CH, Westermark B. Mechanism of action and in vivo role of platelet-derived growth factor. Physiol Rev. 1999;79:1283–316.
10. Appleton L. Wound healing: future directions. Drugs. 2003;6(11):10–67.
11. Lynch SE, Nixon JC, Colvin RB, et al. Role of platelet-derived growth factor in wound healing: synergistic effects with other growth factors. Proc Natl Acad Sci U S A. 1987;84:7696–700.
12. Yuksel E, Sahin G, Aydin F, et al. Evaluation of effects of platelet-rich plasma on human facial skin. J Cosmet Laser Ther. 2014;16:206–8.
13. Xie J, Bian H, Qi S, et al. Effects of basic fibroblast growth factor on the expression of extracellular matrix and matrix metalloproteinase-1 in wound healing. Clin Exp Dermatol. 2008;33:176–82.
14. Yuan S (2018) Research on platelet - rich plasma (PRP) promoting the skin structure, barrier function and hair follicle development of newborn suckling mouse. Guangzhou Medical University, p. 3.
15. Tončić RJ, Kezić S, Hadžavdić SL, et al. Skin barrier and dry skin in the mature patient. Clin Dermatol. 2017;36:109–15. https://doi.org/10.1016/j.clindermatol.2017.10.002.
16. Dąbrowska AK, Spano F, Derler S, et al. The relationship between skin function, barrier properties, and body-dependent factors. Skin Res Technol. 2018;24:165–74. https://doi.org/10.1111/srt.12424.
17. Kuehnert MJ, Roth VR, Haley NR, et al. Transfusion-transmitted bacterial infection in the United States, 1998 through 2000. Transfusion. 2001;41(12):1493–9.

18. Krijgsveld J, Zaat SA, Meeldijk J, et al. Thrombocidins, microbicidal proteins from human blood platelets, are C-terminal deletion products of CXC chemokines. J Biol Chem. 2000;275(27):20374–81.
19. Xiong YQ, Bayer AS, Yeaman MR. Inhibition of intracellular macromolecular synthesis in Staphylococcus aureus by thrombin-induced platelet microbicidal proteins. J Infect Dis. 2002;185(3):348–56.
20. Trier DA, Gank KD, Kupferwasser D, et al. Platelet antistaphylococcal responses occur through P2X1 and P2Y12 receptor-induced activation and kinocidin release. Infect Immun. 2008;76(12):5706–13.
21. Lopez-Vidriero E, Goulding KA, Simon DA, et al. The use of platelet rich plasma in arthroscopy and sports medicine: optimizing the healing environment. Arthroscopy. 2010;26(2):269–78.
22. Li H, Li B. PRP as a new approach to prevent infection: preparation and in vitro antimicrobial properties of PRP. J Vis Exp. 2013;(73):50351.
23. Moojen DJ, Everts PA, Schure RM, et al. Antimicrobial activity of platelet-leukocyte gel against Staphylococcus aureus. J Orthop Res. 2008;26(3):404–10.
24. Kammeyer A, Luiten RM. Oxidation events and skin aging. Ageing Res Rev. 2015;21:16–29. https://doi.org/10.1016/j.arr.2015.01.001.
25. Mehryan P, Zartab H, Rajabi A, et al. Assessment of efficacy of platelet-rich plasma (PRP) on infraorbital dark circles and crow's feet wrinkles. J Cosmet Dermatol. 2014;13:72–8.
26. Raheem T, Mohammed B, El-Sayed N. Vitamin D and platelet rich plasma (PRP) in the treatment of vitiligo. Fayoum Univ Med J. 2019;3:60–70.
27. Lebleu A, Court E, Menon G, et al. Role of p150Glued subunit of dynactin in the structure and maintenance of keratinocyte microparasol. Journal Of Investigative Dermatology. In: 75 varick st, 9th flr, new york, ny 10013–1917, vol. 133. USA: Nature Publishing Group; 2013. p. S113–3.
28. Yamaguchi Y, Hearing VJ. Physiological factors that regulate skin pigmentation. Biofactors. 2009;35:193–9.
29. Costin GE, Hearing VJ. Human skin pigmentation: melanocytes modulate skin color in response to stress. FASEB J. 2007;21:976–94.
30. Cui X, Ma Y, Wang H, et al. The anti-photoaging effects of pre- and post-treatment of platelet-rich plasma on UVB-damaged HaCaT keratinocytes. Photochem Photobiol. 2020;97:589. https://doi.org/10.1111/php.13354.
31. Ma Y, Xuan M, Dong Y, et al. Platelet-rich plasma protects human melanocytes from oxidative stress and ameliorates melanogenesis induced by UVB irradiation. Biosci Biotechnol Biochem. 2020;85(7):1686–96. https://doi.org/10.1093/bbb/zbab085.
32. Vachtenheim J, Borovansky J. "Transcription physiology" of pigment formation in melanocytes: central role of MITF. Exp Dermatol. 2010;19:617–27.
33. Cheli Y, Ohanna M, Ballotti R, et al. Fifteen-year quest for microphthalmia-associated transcription factor target genes. Pigment Cell Melanoma Res. 2010;23:27–40.
34. Halaban R, Langdon R, Birchall N, et al. Basic fibroblast growth factor from human keratinocytes is a natural mitogen for melanocytes. J Cell Biol. 1988;107:1611–9.
35. Puri N, van der Weel MB, de Wit FS, et al. Basic fibroblast growth factor promotes melanin synthesis by melanocytes. Arch Dermatol Res. 1996;288:633–5.
36. Dong L, Li Y, Cao J, et al. FGF2 regulates melanocytes viability through the STAT3-transactivated PAX3 transcription. Cell Death Differ. 2012;19:616–22.
37. Hirobe T. Role of keratinocyte-derived factors involved in regulating the proliferation and differentiation of mammalian epidermal melanocytes. Pigment Cell Res. 2005;18:2–12.
38. Tian J, Cheng LHH, Cui X, et al. Application of standardized platelet-rich plasma in elderly patients with complex wounds. Wound Repair Regen. 2019;16(6):1457–65.
39. Victorelli S, Lagnado A, Halim J, et al. Senescent human melanocytes drive skin ageing via paracrine telomere dysfunction. EMBO J, 2019, 38:e101982.
40. Zamarrón A, Lorrio S, González S, et al. Fernblock prevents dermal cell damage induced by visible and infrared a radiation. Int J Mol Sci. 2018;19:1–15. https://doi.org/10.3390/ijms19082250.
41. Christensen L, Suggs A, Baron E. Ultraviolet photobiology in dermatology. Adv Exp Med Biol. 2017;996:89–104. https://doi.org/10.1007/978-3-319-56017-5_8.
42. Carestia A, Kaufman T, Rivadeneyra L, et al. Mediators and molecular pathways involved in the regulation of neutrophil extracellular trap formation mediated by activated platelets. J Leukoc Biol. 2016;99(1):153–62.
43. Li FX, Zhang ZH, Li XM, et al. Advances in research on the neutrophil extracellular traps in inflammatory diseases. Military Med J Southeast China. 2021;23(4):378–82.
44. Broadley SP, Plaumann A, Coletti R, et al. Dual-track clearance of circulating bacteria balances rapid restoration of blood sterility with induction of adaptive immunity. Cell Host Microbe. 2016;20(1):36–48.
45. Mudd JC, Panigrahi S, Kyi B, et al. Inflammatory function of CX3CR1+ CD8 T cells in treated HIV infection is modulated by platelet interactions. J Infect Dis. 2016;214(12):1808–16.
46. Gerdes N, Zhu L, Ersoy M, et al. Platelets regulate CD4(+) T-cell differentiation via multiple chemokines in humans. Thromb Haemost. 2011;106(2):353–62.
47. Elzey BD, Grant JF, Sinn HW, et al. Cooperation between platelet-derived CD154 and CD4+ T cells for enhanced germinal center formation. J Leukoc Biol. 2005;78(1):80–4.
48. Slominski AT, Zmijewski MA, Plonka PM, et al. How UV light touches the brain and endocrine system through skin, and why. Endocrinology. 2018;159(5):1992–2007. https://doi.org/10.1210/en.2017-03230.
49. Rinnerthaler M, Bischof J, Streubel MK, et al. Oxidative stress in aging human skin. Biomol Ther. 2015;5:545–89. https://doi.org/10.3390/biom5020545.
50. Takeshi OYA, Ying-Luan ZHAO, Takagawa K, et al. Platelet-derived growth factor-B expression induced after rat peripheral nerve injuries. Glia. 2002;38:303.
51. Oudega M, Xu XM, Guenard V, et al. A combination of insulin-like growth factor-I and platelet-derived growth factor enhances myelination but diminishes axonal regeneration into Schwann cell grafts in the adult rat spinal cord. Glia. 1997;19:247.
52. Moussaa M, Lajeunesseb D, Hilalc G, et al. Platelet rich plasma (PRP) induces chondroprotection via increasing autophagy anti-inflammatory markers, and decreasing apoptosis in human osteoarthritic cartilage. Exp Cell Res. 2017;352:146.
53. Rao SN, Pearse DD. Regulating axonal responses to injury: the intersection between signaling pathways involved in axon myelination and the inhibition of axon regeneration. Front Mol Neurosci. 2016;9(33):1.
54. Werner S, Grose R. Regulation of wound healing by growth factors and cytokines. Physiol Rev. 2003;83:835–70.
55. Hsu C, Chang J. Clinical implications of growth factors in flexor tendon wound healing. J Hand Surg. 2004:29:551–63.
56. Zhang W, Dong X, Wang T, et al. Exosomes derived from platelet-rich plasma mediate hyperglycemia-induced retinal endothelial injury via targeting the TLR4 signaling pathway. Exp Eye Res2019 12;189:107813.
57. Sánchez M, Garate A, Delgado D, et al. Platelet-rich plasma, an adjuvant biological therapy to assist peripheral nerve repair. Neural Regen Res. 2017;12(1):47.
58. Sánchez M, Anitua E, Delgado D, et al. Platelet-rich plasma, a source of autologous growth factors and biomimetic scaffold for peripheral nerve regeneration. Expert Opin Bio Ther. 2017;17(2):197.

59. Zheng C, Zhu Q, Liu X, et al. Effect of platelet-rich plasma (PRP) concentration on proliferation, neurotrophic function and migration of Schwann cells in vitro. J Tissue Eng Regen Med. 2016;10:428.
60. Teymur H, Tiftikcioglu YO, Cavusoglu T, et al. Effect of platelet-rich plasma on reconstruction with nerve autografts. Kaohsiung J Med Sci. 2017;33:69.
61. Rodgers BD, Eldridge JA. Reduced circulating GDF11 is unlikely responsible for age-dependent changes in mouse heart, muscle, and brain. Endocrinology. 2015;156(11):3885.
62. Sinha M, Jang YC, Oh J, et al. Restoring systemic GDF11 levels reverses age-related dysfunction in mouse skeletal muscle. Science. 2014;344:649–52.
63. Loffredo FS, Steinhauser ML, Jay SM, et al. Growth differentiation factor 11 is a circulating factor that reverses age-related cardiac hypertrophy. Cell. 2013;15:828–39.
64. Bueno JL, Ynigo M, De MC, et al. Growth differentiation factor 11 (GDF11)-a promising anti-ageing factor - is highly concentrated in platelets. Vox Sang. 2016;111(4):434–6.
65. Senzel L, Gnatenko DV, Bahou WF. The platelet proteome. Curr Opin Hematol. 2009;16(5):329.
66. Castellano JM, Mosher KI, Abbey RJ, et al. Human umbilical cord plasma proteins revitalize hippocampal function in aged mice. Nature. 2017;544(7651):488.
67. Coppinger JA, Cagney G, Toomey S, et al. Characterization of the proteins released from activated platelets leads to localization of novel platelet proteins in human atherosclerotic lesions. Blood. 2004;103(6):2096–104.
68. Jayachandran M, Miller VM. Human platelets contain estrogen receptor α, caveolin-1 and estrogen receptor associated proteins. Platelets. 2003;14(2):75–81.
69. Lefèvre-Utile A, Braun C, Haftek M, Aubin F. Five functional aspects of the epidermal barrier. Int J Mol Sci. 2021;22:11676.
70. Intravia J, Allen DA, Durant TJ, et al. In vitro evaluation of the anti-bacterial effect of two preparations of platelet rich plasma compared with cefazolin and whole blood. Muscles Ligaments Tendons J. 2014;4(1):79–84.
71. Prysak MH, Lutz CG, Zukofsky TA, Katz JM, Everts PA, Lutz GE. Optimizing the safety of intradiscal platelet-rich plasma: an in vitro study with Cutibacterium acnes. Regen Med. 2019;14(10):955–67.

Platelet-Rich Plasma and Wound Healing

4

Pengcheng Xu and Yunqing Dong

This chapter focuses on the research progress of platelet-rich plasma in wound healing, from bench to bedside. Combined with the basic science and clinical application, it reveals the application effect and mechanism of platelet-rich plasma on common clinical wounds, including pressure ulcers, electric injuries, Achilles tendon wounds, venous ulcer of the lower extremity, and chronic refractory wounds and radiotherapy wounds.

4.1 The Mechanism of Platelet-Rich Plasma in Promoting Wound Healing

Wound is the damage of normal skin or tissue caused by external factors such as surgery, external force, heat, electric current, chemical substances, low temperature, and internal factors such as local blood supply disturbance. It is often accompanied by the damage of skin integrity and the loss of a certain amount of normal tissue, and the normal function of skin is damaged [1].Wound healing is a complex biological process which is controlled by many kinds of cells, cytokines, and extracellular matrix. It is affected by systemic factors (such as diabetes, hypertension, etc.) and local factors (such as local blood supply, infection, etc.) [2].

The collection of platelet-rich plasma (PRP) refers to the method of concentrating platelets in plasma to a level higher than that in whole blood. PRP is the platelet plasma obtained by centrifugation when the platelet concentration reaches 3–6 times of the patient's own platelet concentration, which contains a variety of bioactive substances such as cytokines to promote tissue repair and regeneration. At present, it has become an important part of regenerative medicine [3]. In recent years, with the emergence of the concept of PRP and the study of its mechanism, PRP has been successfully applied in orthopedics, burn and plastic surgery, dermatology, and other disciplines. With the development of tissue engineering, genetic engineering, and stem cell culture, the application of PRP shows greater advantages. The research and application of PRP in wound repair is one of the important fields of PRP research. The clinical application of PRP in pressure ulcer, electric injury, Achilles tendon injury, venous ulcer of the lower extremity, chronic refractory wound, radiotherapy wound, and so on has achieved satisfactory curative effect [4].

4.1.1 The Process and Mechanism of Wound Healing

Wound repair is a series of repair activities to restore the integrity of the body surface and maintain the stability of the body through its own regeneration ability. This complex process involves inflammation, re-epithelialization, neovascularization, and activation of histiocytes [5], followed by synthesis and degradation of extracellular matrix. The biological activity of cells is determined by extracellular matrix (external factor) and cell receptor (internal factor). All these processes are regulated by cytokines and growth factors. The repair process can be divided into blood clot stage, inflammation stage, proliferation stage, and remodeling stage [6]. Each stage interweaves with each other to complete the wound healing. In the process of wound healing, platelets are not only involved in the coagulation process but also an important source of growth factors and various cytokines, which can increase the speed of wound healing and improve the quality of wound healing.

After trauma, the tissue first enters the coagulation process: local vasoconstriction reduces blood flow; the exposure of collagen fibers and the activation of vasoactive factors

P. Xu (✉)
Department of Breast Neoplasms Surgery, The 1st Affiliated Hospital of Henan University of Science and Technology, Luoyang, Henan, China

Y. Dong
Department of Burn and Plastic Surgery, General Hospital of Southern Theater Command, PLA, Guangzhou, China

B. Cheng, X. Fu (eds.), *Platelet-Rich Plasma in Tissue Repair and Regeneration*, https://doi.org/10.1007/978-981-99-3193-4_4

attract platelet aggregation to form blood clot, which provides the matrix for the adhesion and migration of donor cells [7]. Subsequently, platelets release more vasoactive substances, which make the blood vessels further contract and attract more platelet aggregation. At the same time, these bioactive substances can further induce inflammatory cells and fibroblasts to migrate to the wound surface, and the body then enters the wound healing stage.

Wound repair immediately entered the inflammatory phase [8]. After the immune system is activated, neutrophils infiltrate the wound and phagocytize the invading pathogenic microorganisms at first. Then monocytes infiltrated and transformed into macrophages, which could phagocytize the necrotic tissue cell fragments [9]. The inflammatory cells infiltrating the wound can also release cytokines and various growth factors to promote wound repair and make it enter the proliferative phase [10].

In the proliferative phase, the basal cells proliferate and gradually move inward which can stimulate the growth of granulation tissue. Granulation tissue is composed of vascular endothelial cells, macrophages, and fibroblasts, gradually filling the tissue defects. Then the granulation tissue is gradually in the process of epithelialization so that the wound was finally completely covered by epithelial cells [11]. At the same time, extracellular matrix also promotes cell adhesion, migration, and proliferation. The interaction between them promotes the proliferation and migration of keratinocytes.

The new granulation tissue and epithelial cells go a step further transformation, and the wound enter the remodeling stage after the epithelialization of the wound [12]. At this stage, the collagen matrix replaces the temporary extracellular matrix, and the arrangement of collagen fibers changes which enhances the strength of new connective tissue. The vascular structure formed and tended to be stable, making the wound color gradually close to the normal state. This process lasts for a long time and is susceptible to the influence of the early stage, resulting in negative wound healing, leading to chronic refractory wound or excessive scarring. It involves imbalance of inflammatory stage, abnormal vascular microenvironment, and dysfunction of epithelial effector cells.

4.1.2 Theoretical Basis of PRP Application in Wound Repair

Wound healing is a complex biological process and has its own rules. It finishes by early inflammatory reaction, middle granulation tissue hyperplasia, late re-epithelialization, and tissue shaping. Under normal circumstances, this process can successfully complete the wound repair. However, in adverse conditions, such as severe trauma, burns, infection, insufficient blood supply to the lower extremities, and imbalance of the diabetic microenvironment, the biological process of wound healing can be altered, resulting in difficulty in wound healing, even the formation of chronic refractory ulcers, which need to rely on external control [13]. After more than 20 years of clinical application and basic research, we found that the application of PRP in wound repair is effective [14].

PRP contains high concentration of platelets, leukocytes, and a large number of proteins [15]. Activated platelets can release a variety of active ingredients to participate in tissue repair mechanisms, such as cell chemotaxis, cell proliferation, angiogenesis, matrix deposition, immune regulation and tissue remodeling, etc., which has a wide range of tissue formation abilities and can initiate and regulate the wound healing of tissues [16]. In addition, leukocytes can prevent infection and fibrin can construct the three-dimensional structure needed for tissue repair locally [17, 18].

Studies have shown that platelets are involved in all stages of wound healing [19]. (1) In the blood clotting stage, thrombin and intracellular calcium ions are released to activate coagulation factor and start coagulation chain reaction, which makes a-granule release growth factors and accelerate wound repair of tissue [20]. (2) In the inflammatory stage, a large number of activated platelets are accumulated in the wound surface. The growth factors secreted by them act on neutrophils, monocytes, macrophages, and fibroblasts to guide the wound repair. At the same time, a large number of PDGF (platelet-derived growth factor), TGF (transforming growth factor), and FGF (fibroblast growth factor) stimulate fibroblasts to produce collagen and promote angiogenesis [21]. (3) In the proliferative phase, fibroblasts continuously transplanted to the wound area. Driven by PDGF and TGF, fibroblasts proliferate and synthesize granulation tissue, which secret fibrin to constitute the temporary matrix [22]. (4) During the molding stage, platelet growth factor assisted in the re-epithelialization and final remodeling of the wound. Therefore, platelet plays an important role in all stages of wound healing by providing a large number of synergistic growth factors [23].

From what has been discussed above, PRP has unique advantages in wound repair. (1) As an autologous platelet concentrate, the proportion of growth factors in PRP is similar to the one in normal physiological concentration. It is an important factor that PRP can promote repair of tissue more quickly [24]. (2) PRP contains a lot of fibrins, which provides a good scaffold for repairing cells and can also contract the wound [25]. (3) PRP can be made into a gel by the action of thrombin and applied to the wound surface, which not only provides a moist environment but also is conducive to wound healing. It can also make the growth factor limited to the wound for a long time and avoid the shortcomings of the liquid recombinant growth factor reagent which is widely used in clinical practice and is easy to lose and evaporate in the wound [26]. (4) PRP is self-derived, which fundamentally avoids the concerns of immune rejection, transmission of diseases, and the possibility of changing human genetic structure caused by exogenous growth factors [14].(5) Because of the similar sedimentation coefficient of leukocytes, monocytes, and platelets in blood, PRP produced by centrifugation also contains a large number of leukocytes and monocytes, which can better prevent infection. (6) PRP is easy to make. It only needs to take blood from the patient's vein (mostly from the jugular vein or elbow vein) and has little trauma to the patient. At the same time, the cost is low so that it can reduce the medical expenses. (7) So far, no adverse reactions of PRP have been found.

4.2 Clinical Application of PRP in Wound Repair

Up to now, PRP has been widely used in clinical treatment and its efficacy has been widely recognized. PRP also played a positive role in wound repair, especially in the outcome of refractory wounds.

4.2.1 The Treatment of PRP in Osteonecrosis and Soft Tissue Defect After Tibiofibular Fracture Combined with Diabetes Mellitus

A 59-year-old male patient with diabetes and high blood pressure did not touch the dorsal artery of the left tibia and fibula after operation. He underwent repeated debridement of VSD (ventricular septal defect) external fixator, completely removed the necrotic tissue, and cleared the unhealthy granulation. After infection control and wound bed preparation, PRP was injected to repair the wound. It can be seen that 1 week after injection, the wound granulation tissue in the injection area grows well and is fresh, the wound shrinks, the epithelial tissue grows synchronously with the reduction and healing of the wound, and the wound closure speed is faster. After about 2 months of treatment, the wound was basically completely healed and the patient was discharged, as shown in Fig. 4.1.

4.2.2 The Treatment of PRP in Infected Soft Tissue Defect After Trauma Debridement

A 31-year-old male patient, who was in good health and had undergone debridement of VSD, had no obvious healing trend after routine dressing change, so he was treated with PRP injection. After 1 week of treatment, the wound became smaller and the granulation tissue increased. About 1 month after treatment, the wound healed, as shown in Fig. 4.2.

4.2.3 The Treatment of PRP in Soft Tissue Defect After Trauma Debridement

A 62-year-old female patient with hypertension took hormone drugs for a long time after debridement of left anterior tibial trauma. After dressing change and debridement in many hospitals, no obvious granulation growth was found. After treatment of PRP, the wound gradually became smaller and granulation tissue increased. After three times of treatment of PRP, the wound healed, as shown in Fig. 4.3.

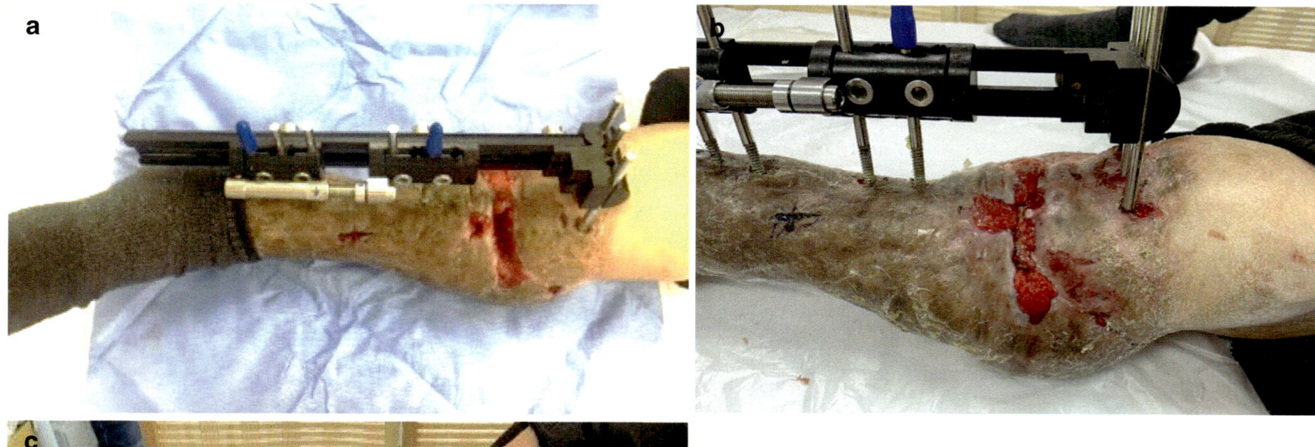

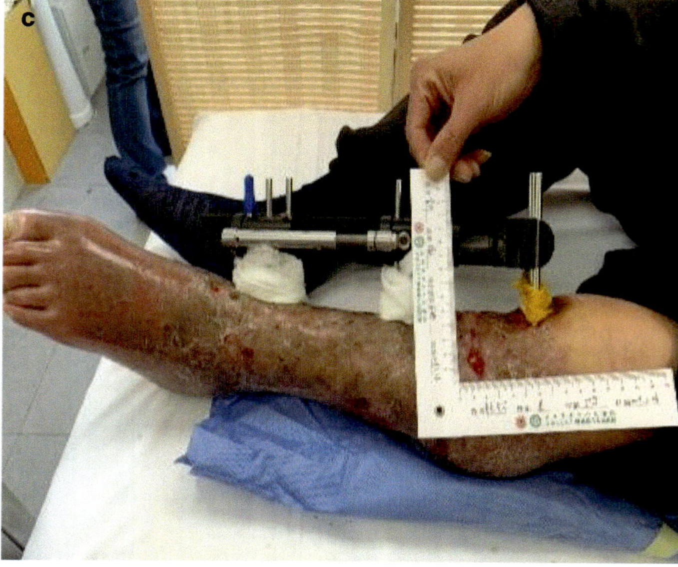

Fig. 4.1 (**a**) After the infection was effectively controlled and the wound bed was ready, the patient was treated with PRP injection. (**b**) One week after the treatment of PRP, granulation grew rapidly. (**c**) One month after the treatment of PRP, the patient was discharged after the wound was basically completely healed

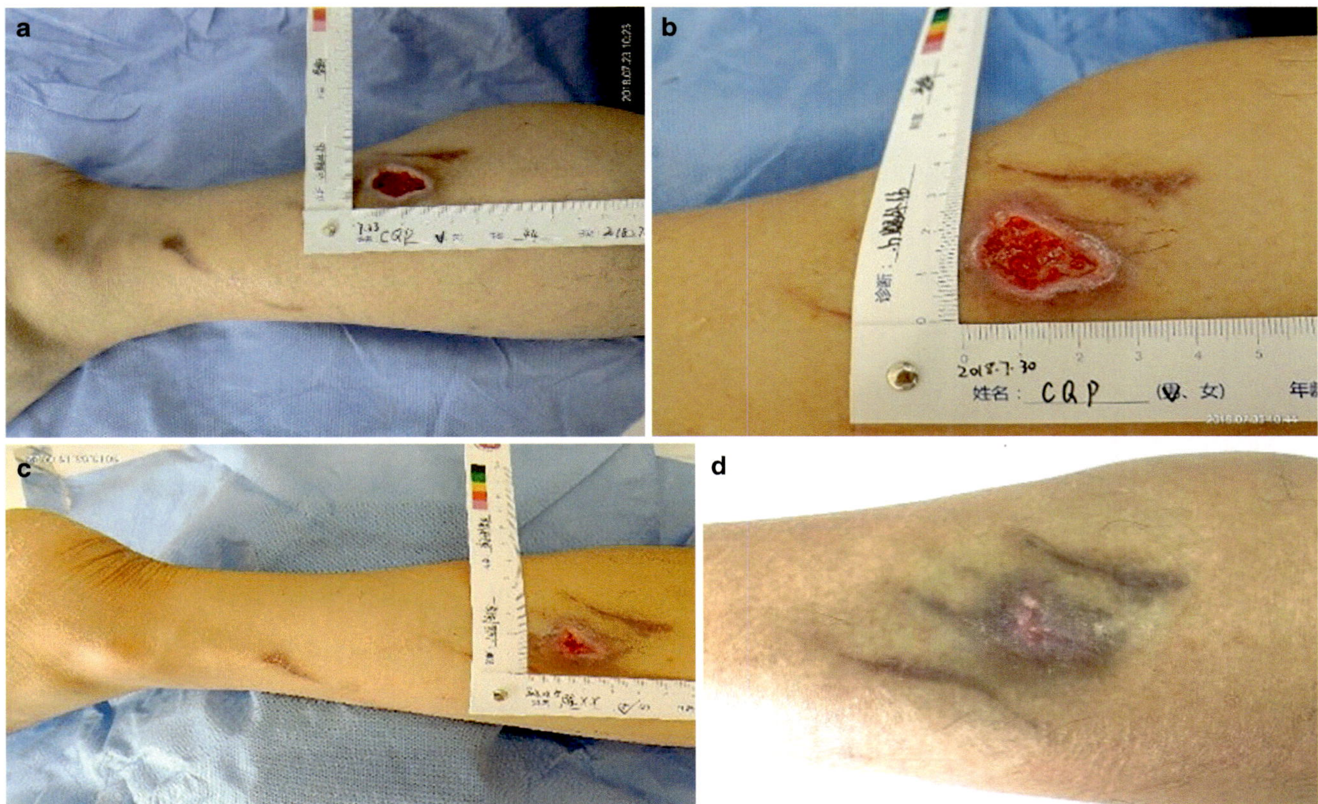

Fig. 4.2 (**a**) After the infection was effectively controlled and the wound bed was ready, the patient was treated with PRP injection. (**b**) One week after the treatment of PRP, granulation grew rapidly. (**c**) Three weeks after the treatment of PRP. (**d**) One month after the treatment of PRP, the wound was basically completely healed

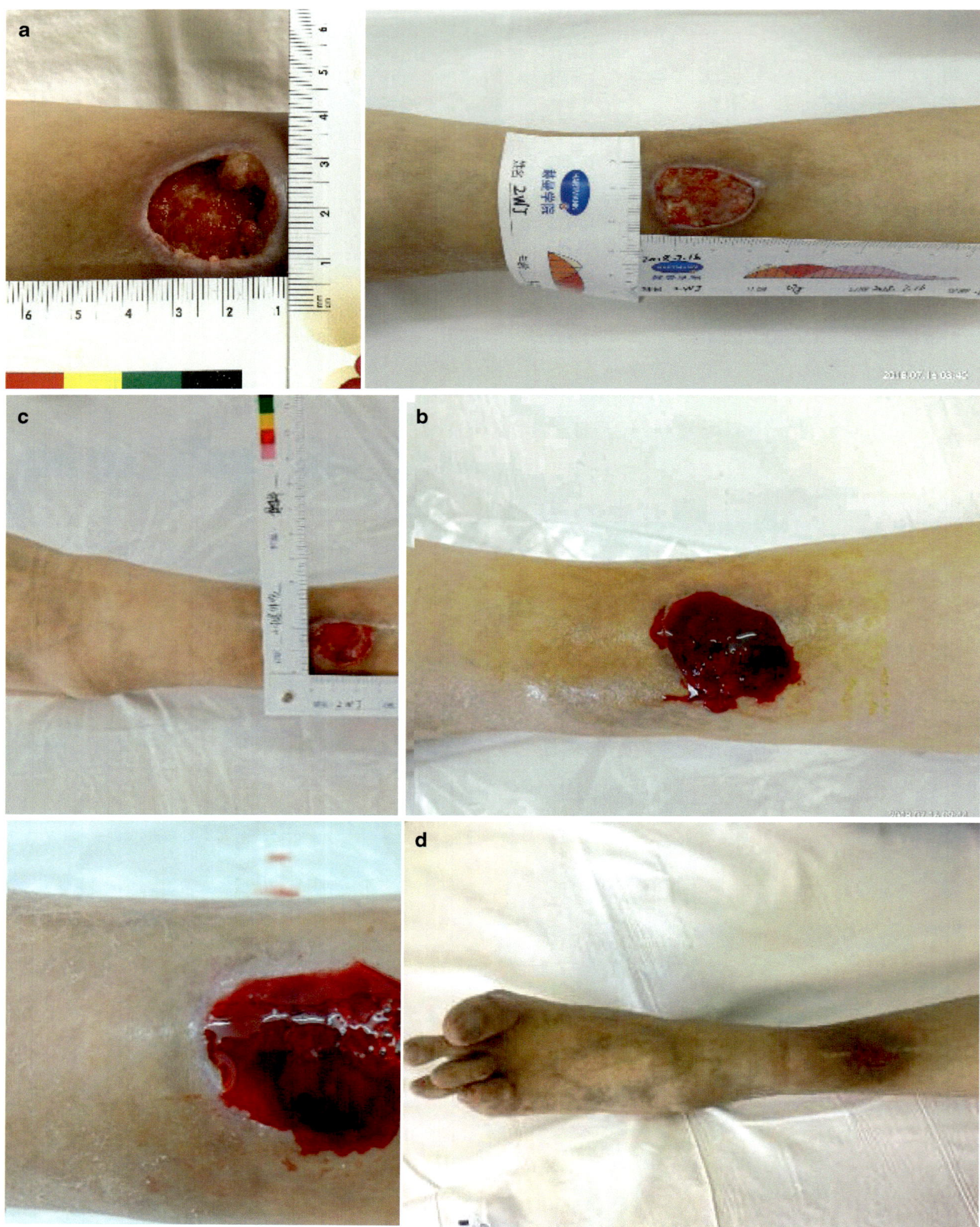

Fig. 4.3 (**a**) The granulation of the wound grew slowly and was treated with PRP for the first time. (**b**) After half a month, the wound was basically filled with granulation tissue and had an obvious shrinking trend and was treated with PRP for the second time given. (**c**) One month later, the wound narrowed further and was treated with PRP for the third time. (**d**) Two months after the treatment of PRP, the wound was basically completely healed

4.3 Basic Study of PRP in Wound Repair

As an autocomponent, PRP is rich in a variety of effector molecules, and its clinical application is undoubtedly safe and effective. A large number of clinical data show that PRP is involved in wound repair and regeneration, but its mechanism of action remains to be further improved. In this chapter, we summarize some of the preliminary basic researches of our team.

4.3.1 PRP Is Involved in all Stages of Wound Healing

Yunqing Dong et al. repaired full-thickness skin defects in C57 mice with PRP or normal saline, respectively. There were 15 C57BL/6 mice, weighing 20–25 g, male. A full-thickness skin defect with an area of 1 cm^2 was made on both sides of the back. One side was randomly selected as the experimental group. The wound was treated with 0.1 ml PRP everyday, and the other side was the control group. The same amount of normal saline was injected, and then the wound was covered with 3M film close to the skin. The wound healing on both sides was compared by gross and histological observation at 3, 5, 7, and 10 days after operation.

4.3.1.1 General Observation of Wound Healing

On post injury days (PID) 3, 5, and 7, the wounds in the two groups were reduced, but the contraction rate in the PRP group was significantly higher than that in the control group. On PID 10, the wounds in the experimental group were all healed, while the wounds in the control group were still not completely covered by the skin, as shown in Fig. 4.4.

Hematoxylin eosin staining was performed on the specimens taken on PID 10. It can be seen that the PRP group has entered the mature stage of wound repair. The wound contains a large number of mature capillaries. The complete epidermal layer is closely connected with the dermis to form the basal layer. The normal saline group also forms an obvious epidermal layer, but the new epithelium in the PRP group is significantly thicker. At the same time, skin accessory organs such as hair follicles and sebaceous glands were found in the wound of PRP group, which was closest to normal skin tissue [27]. Masson staining was performed on the specimens taken on PID 10. In PRP group, collagen was recombined; collagen fiber bundles were significantly thickened and arranged more regularly and orderly, while the content of wound collagen in normal saline group was also increased, but the arrangement was still disordered. Histological analysis shows that PRP group can better help wound re-epithelialization and collagen regeneration, so as to further promote wound healing [28], as shown in Fig. 4.5.

Immunohistochemical analysis was performed on PID 3 and 5. It can be found that the wound healing speed and quality in PRP group are significantly better than those in control group.

This experimental study showed that the expressions of TNF-α and IL-1β in PRP group were lower than those in the control group. They are pro-inflammatory factors. If they are still high at this time, it indicates that the wound is still in a continuous inflammatory reaction, and the inflammatory cells are in an excessive accumulation and activation state, which will lead to the uncontrolled immune regulation mechanism, aggravate the degree of tissue injury, prolong the inflammatory period, and lead to poor wound healing [29].

The expression of TGF-β1 in PRP group was higher than that in the control group. TGF-β1 can make fibroblastic and inflammatory cells aggregate to the wound and induce granulation tissue growth, epithelialization, and collagen deposition. It is a kind of multifunctional growth factor that plays an important role in wound repair [30].

The expression of VEGF in PRP group was higher than that in control group. VEGF can promote the increase of vascular permeability, the migration and proliferation of vascular endothelial cells, and the formation of mature blood vessels [31]. The expression of CD34 in PRP group is higher than that in control group. CD34 plays an important role in

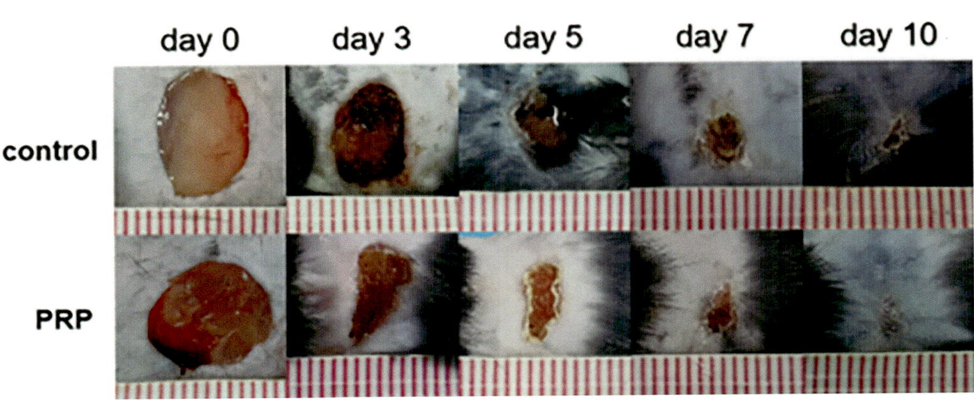

Fig. 4.4 The effect of PRP on wound healing quality was analyzed at histological level

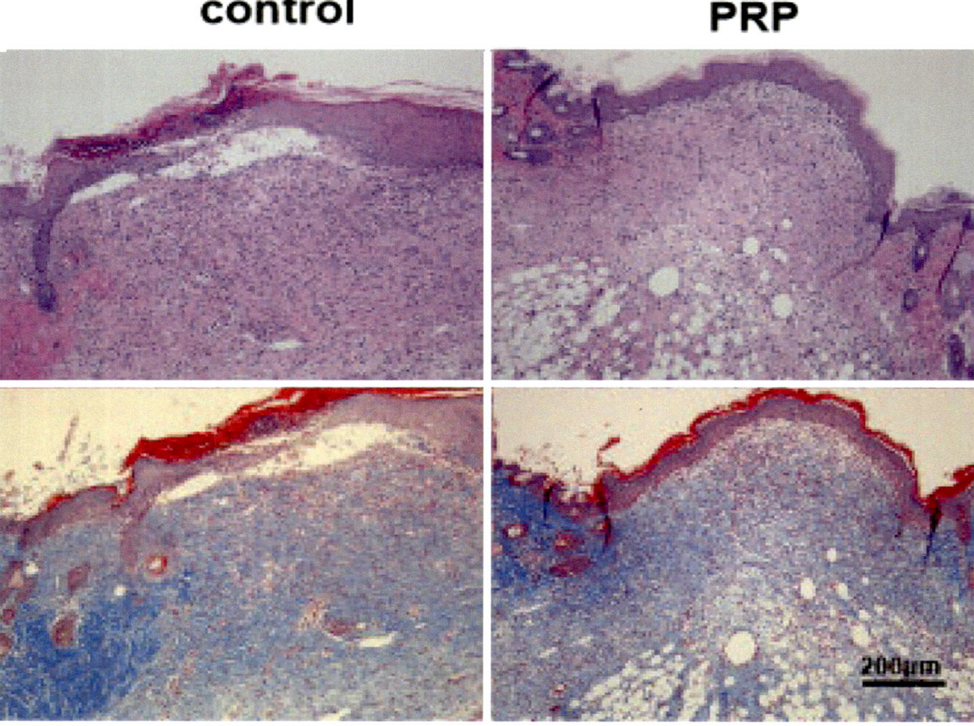

Fig. 4.5 PRP is involved in wound inflammation, angiogenesis, and tissue remodeling

mediating intercellular adhesion. It can participate in the transportation and colonization of hematopoietic stem cells, inflammatory response, and lymphocyte homing [32], as shown in Fig. 4.6.

4.3.2 PRP Participates in Wound Re-epithelialization by Regulating the Function of Epidermal Stem Cells (ESCs)

A study by Pengcheng Xu et al. [33], published in the Burns & Trauma, found that PRP can significantly promote skin wound healing, which is related to the regulation of local inflammation and the promotion of angiogenesis and so on. In particular, in this study, PRP was found to regulate the function of epidermal stem cells to participate in the process of wound re-epithelialization. The application of PRP improved the survival rate of primary cultured ESCs and activated their migration and proliferation. These effects were accompanied by changes in the ratio of keratin 10 to keratin 14, which ultimately promoted the transformation of ESCs into skin effector cells, contributing to the acceleration of wound reepithelialization and wound closure.

Furthermore, the authors investigated the possible mechanism of PRP regulating human epidermal stem cells to promote wound re-epithelialization at transcriptome level. In this study, the authors cultured human ESC from prepuce tissue and divided them into control group and PRP group according to random number table method. Transcriptome sequencing and data analysis were performed on the two groups of samples by RNA sequencing technology. The differentially expressed genes were analyzed by the Gene Ontology (GO) and Kyoto Encyclopedia of Genes and Genomes (KECG). The results showed that there were 449 differentially expressed genes between the two groups, including 354 upregulated genes and 95 downregulated genes. Among them, 18 were significantly increased and 5 were significantly decreased. GO and KECG analysis showed that the differentially expressed genes were mainly enriched in epidermal construction and keratinization process and may be closely associated with keratin 19, keratin 10, and S100A7, which are related to re-epithelialization.

This study preliminatively explored the mechanism network of PRP regulating human ESC function and promoting wound re-epithelialization and found that PRP may be related to the transcriptional regulation of several genes, such as keratin 19, keratin 10, and S100A7. Further exploration of the possible regulatory network will provide more evidence support for its subsequent clinical application.

In addition, it can be seen from the references that wound healing is also related to a variety of other growth factors in PRP. For example, PDGF has a chemotactic effect on mesenchymal stem cells and fibroblasts locally and has a good synergistic effect with TGF-β to stimulate the differentiation of fibroblasts, collagen synthesis, and vascular regeneration.

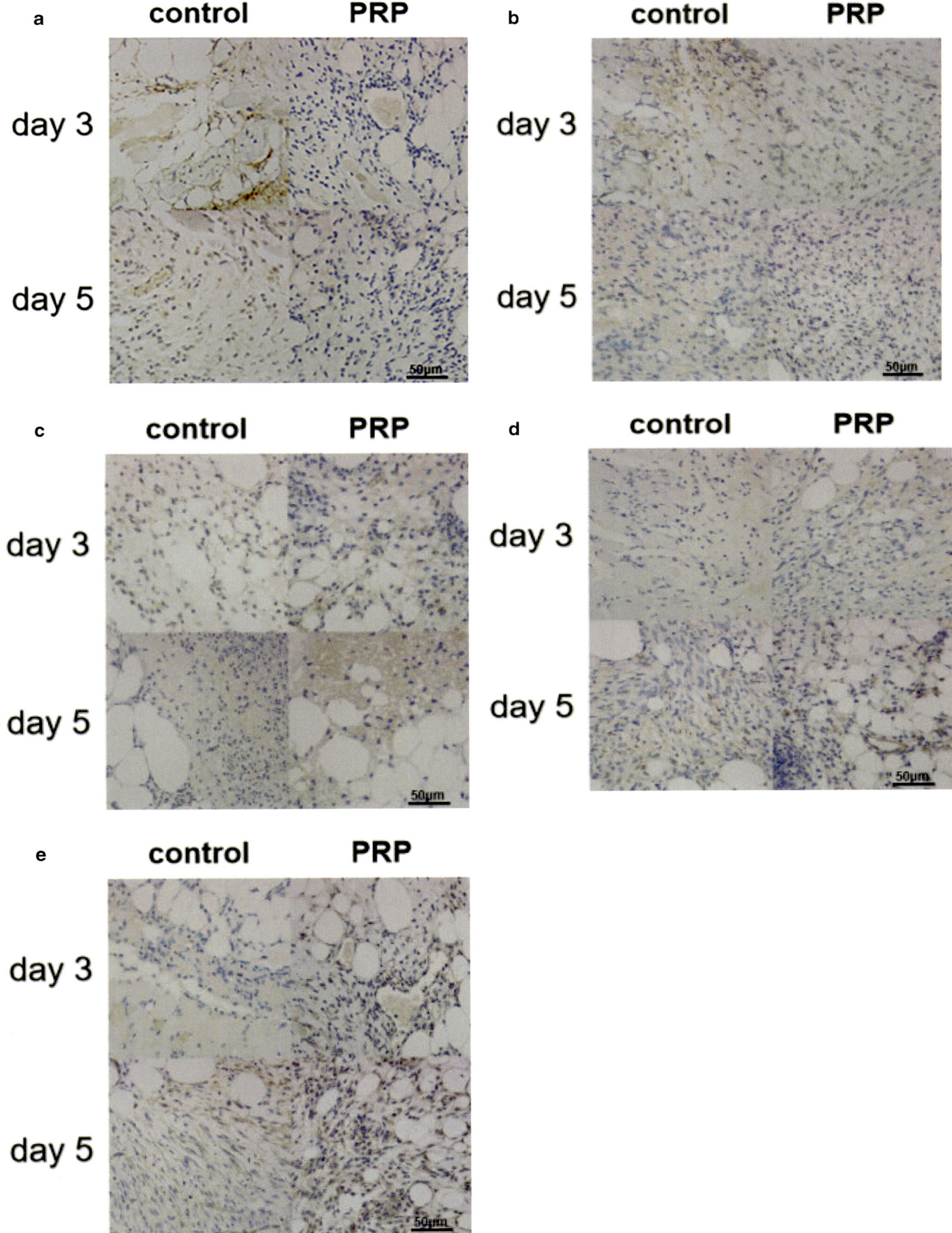

Fig. 4.6 (**a**) Comparison of TNF-α exexpression levels between PRP group and control group. (**b**) Comparison of IL-1β expression levels between PRP group and control group. (**c**) Comparison of TGF-β1 expression levels between PRP group and control group. (**d**) Comparison of VEGF expression levels between PRP group and control group. (**e**) Comparison of CD34 expression levels between PRP group and control group

IGF can enhance collagen synthesis and promote fibroblastization. FGF can stimulate the growth of surface fibroblasts, muscle cells, endothelial cells, and epidermal cells and promote vascular regeneration, collagen synthesis, and wound contraction.

In conclusion, PRP has a good regulatory effect on wound healing, especially chronic wounds. The continuous improvement of its mechanism research will gradually clarify the internal factors of PRP to coordinate the positive outcome of wound repair and promote the wide application of PRP in clinical practice. PRP is characterized by being taken from and applied to patients, and its safety and effectiveness are well known to all. However, due to the personalized preparation system, especially in the application of chronic wounds, the wound microenvironment is extremely complex under the influence of local pathogenic factors and the patient's own condition, which will lead to uncontrollable healing quality and the possibility of recurrence. Therefore, we should continue to explore and optimize the preparation methods and quality control standards, so that the standard procedures are more standardized.

References

1. Landén Ning X, Dongqing L, Mona S. Transition from inflammation to proliferation: a critical step during wound healing. Cell Mol Life Sci. 2016;73:3861–85.
2. Eming Sabine A, Paul M, Marjana T-C. Wound repair and regeneration: mechanisms, signaling, and translation. Sci Transl Med. 2014;6:265sr6.
3. Jie F, Xin W, Wen J, et al. Platelet-rich plasma therapy in the treatment of diseases associated with orthopedic injuries. Tissue Eng Part B Rev. 2020;26:571–85.
4. Krister J, Gao N, Henrik S, et al. The humanistic and economic burden of chronic wounds: a protocol for a systematic review. Syst Rev. 2017;6:15.
5. Shin CJ, Leigh M, Yian CS, et al. Drug therapies and delivery mechanisms to treat perturbed skin wound healing. Adv Drug Deliv Rev. 2019;149–150:2–18.
6. Janis Jeffrey E, Bridget H. Wound healing: part I. Basic science. Plast Reconstr Surg. 2016;138:9S–17S.
7. Joseph A, Mark T, Paul H, et al. Effect of platelet-rich plasma on healing tissues in acute ruptured Achilles tendon: a human immunohistochemistry study. Lancet. 2015;385:S19.
8. Morton Laurel M, Phillips Tania J. Wound healing and treating wounds: differential diagnosis and evaluation of chronic wounds. J Am Acad Dermatol. 2016;74:589–605; quiz 605–6.
9. Gisselle E, Alejandro E, Gabriel A, et al. Pure platelet-rich plasma and supernatant of calcium-activated P-PRP induce different phenotypes of human macrophages. Regen Med. 2018;13:427–41.
10. Foster Timothy E, Puskas Brian L, Mandelbaum Bert R, et al. Platelet-rich plasma: from basic science to clinical applications. Am J Sports Med. 2009;37:2259–72.
11. Jiangong N, Zhe C, Bailu P, et al. Keratinocyte growth factor/fibroblast growth factor-7-regulated cell migration and invasion through activation of NF-kappaB transcription factors. J Biol Chem. 2007;282:6001–11.
12. Jang YC, Arumugam S, Gibran NS, et al. Role of alpha(v) integrins and angiogenesis during wound repair. Wound Repair Regen. 1999;7:375–80.
13. Christina L, Richard S. Wound management for the 21st century: combining effectiveness and efficiency. Int Wound J. 2016;13:5–15.
14. Fernanda ML, Talita S, Cherici CIC, et al. Platelet-rich plasma (PRP): methodological aspects and clinical applications. Platelets. 2015;26:101–13.
15. Maria TA, Rita AA, Gilles D, et al. Platelet-rich plasma to treat experimentally-induced skin wounds in animals: a systematic review and meta-analysis. PLoS One. 2018;13:e0191093.
16. Thomas G, Frelinger Andrew L, Michelson Alan D. Platelet physiology. Semin Thromb Hemost. 2016;42:191–204.
17. Boswell Stacie G, Cole Brian J, Sundman Emily A, et al. Platelet-rich plasma: a milieu of bioactive factors. Arthroscopy. 2012;28:429–39.
18. Dohan Ehrenfest David M, Lars R, Tomas A. Classification of platelet concentrates: from pure platelet-rich plasma (P-PRP) to leucocyte- and platelet-rich fibrin (L-PRF). Trends Biotechnol. 2009;27:158–67.
19. Chun Q. The molecular biology in wound healing & non-healing wound. Chin J Traumatol. 2017;20:189–93.
20. Seeger Mark A, Paller Amy S. The roles of growth factors in keratinocyte migration. Adv Wound Care. 2015;4:213–24.
21. Price B, Robert F. Platelet alpha-granules: basic biology and clinical correlates. Blood Rev. 2009;23:177–89.
22. Rosaria DPM, Linda S, Amelia C, et al. Platelet derivatives in regenerative medicine: an update. Transfus Med Rev. 2015;29:52–61.
23. Mussano F, Genova T, Munaron L, et al. Cytokine, chemokine, and growth factor profile of platelet-rich plasma. Platelets. 2016;27:467–71.
24. Marx Robert E. Platelet-rich plasma: evidence to support its use. J Oral Maxillofac Surg. 2004;62:489–96.
25. Katrin R, Frank R, Goessler Ulrich R, et al. Current status of genetic modulation of growth factors in wound repair. Int J Mol Med. 2006;17:183–93.
26. Yajuan Y, Jian S, Guizhen F, et al. Use of autologous platelet rich fibrin-based bioactive membrane in pressure ulcer healing in rats. J Wound Care. 2019;28:S23–30.
27. Yuanyuan Z, Weihao Y, Huiling L, et al. Injectable supramolecular gelatin hydrogel loading of resveratrol and histatin-1 for burn wound therapy. Biomater Sci. 2020;8:4810–20.
28. van Zuijlen PPM, Ruurda Joris JB, van Veen HA, et al. Collagen morphology in human skin and scar tissue: no adaptations in response to mechanical loading at joints. Burns. 2003;29:423–31.
29. Daijun Z, Tengfei L, Song W, et al. Effects of IL-1β and TNF-α on the expression of P311 in vascular endothelial cells and wound healing in mice. Front Physiol. 2020;11:545008.
30. Gad Shereen B, Hafez Mona H, El-Sayed Yasser S. Platelet-rich plasma and/or sildenafil topical applications accelerate and better repair wound healing in rats through regulation of proinflammatory cytokines and collagen/TGF-β1 pathway. Environ Sci Pollut Res Int. 2020;27:40757–68.
31. Etulain J, Mena HA, Negrotto S, et al. Stimulation of PAR-1 or PAR-4 promotes similar pattern of VEGF and endostatin release and pro-angiogenic responses mediated by human platelets. Platelets. 2015;26:799–804.
32. Fernando GA, Miranda DT, Castiglia GC, et al. Platelet-rich plasma diminishes calvarial bone repair associated with alterations in collagen matrix composition and elevated CD34+ cell prevalence. Bone. 2010;46:1597–603.
33. Pengcheng X, Yaguang W, Lina Z, et al. Platelet-rich plasma accelerates skin wound healing by promoting re-epithelialization. Burns Trauma. 2020;8:tkaa028.

Platelet-Rich Plasma and Scar

5

Mengru Pang and Biao Cheng

The common causes of scars are infection, surgery, injuries, and inflammation. Scars in the forehead, eye, nose, cheek, and other prominent parts will have a serious impact on the patients' mental health and social activities. Scars in some specific parts may even cause dysfunction resulting in a severe reduction in the patient's quality of life. How to effectively improve the appearance and texture of scars has always been the direction of many plastic surgeons.

Accurate classification of scars is critical for determining appropriate treatment strategies. It is generally classified into hypertrophic scars, keloids, or atrophic scars, in addition to some traditional treatment methods, such as surgical resection and intralesional injection of glucocorticoid/5-fluorouracil (5-FU), microdermabrasion, etc. Nowadays, in order to meet the needs of patients for short-time treatment and short-time recovery—no effect on daily life and social interaction—and, meanwhile, the requirements for good treatment experience and high repeatability, the demand for minimally invasive treatment methods is increasing, which leads to more and more methods for managing scars.

In recent years, there have been many innovations in the treatment of scars, such as topical retinoic acid, trichloroacetic acid, fractional laser, chemical peeling, microdermabrasion (microneeding), laser resurfacing, toxins, silicone gels, collagen or cortisone injection, and other combined treatments, but all the above treatment options have some problems, such as extra scar formation, hyperpigmentation, high cost, long treatment interval, etc. [1–7].

Among them, as an emerging treatment, PRP has the characteristics of secreting a variety of growth factors, which makes this treatment method show the characteristics of promoting wound healing and improving the appearance of scars compared with other treatments. This led to the great interest of researchers in scar treatment. PRP was known to cable release platelet-derived growth factors (PDGF), vascular endothelial growth factor (VEGF), epidermal growth factor (EGF), transforming growth factors (TGF), insulin-like growth factor (IGF), and interleukin (IL)-1 after activation.

How does the PRP benefit scar treatment? Nam hypothesized there is a negative feedback mechanism of the transforming growth factor (TGF)-β1 signaling pathway that can activate platelet-rich plasma (PRP) release to reduce connective tissue growth factor (CTGF) production and expression of CTGF mRNA in vitro and then improve hypertrophic scars [6].

Currently, there is insufficient evidence to demonstrate the efficacy of PRP in the therapeutic effect of keloid treatment and its ameliorating effect on keloid recurrence. However, a retrospective case study found that postoperative use of PRP combined with radiotherapy can effectively reduce the rate of scar recurrence, but the reliability of the conclusion is low due to the short follow-up time and combined various treatment methods. Large-scale randomized controlled trials are warranted to comprehensively assess the efficacy of PRP therapy and its inverse association with keloid recurrence [7].

Most of the current researches involving PRP in the treatment of scars has focused on adjunctive use in the treatment of atrophic acne scars. Most of the current researches involving PRP in the treatment of scars has focused on adjunctive use in the treatment of atrophic acne scars. Studies have shown that transforming growth factor-beta (TGF-beta) plays an enormous role in scarring. TGF-β1 and TGF-β2 promote collagen synthesis in scars, and TGF-β3 appears to have the ability to promote scarless wound healing. Microneedling or laser can lead to an initial significant upregulation of TGF-β1 and TGF-β2 within a few weeks of treatment, followed by a strong downregulation following. Based on these researches, microneedling and lasers have the potential to be recommended treatment options for scars by

M. Pang
Department of Burn and Plastic Surgery, The Affiliated Hospital of Guizhou Medical University, Guiyang, Guizhou, China

B. Cheng (✉)
Department of Burn & Plastic Surgery, General Hospital of Southern Theater Command, Guangzhou, China

B. Cheng, X. Fu (eds.), *Platelet-Rich Plasma in Tissue Repair and Regeneration*, https://doi.org/10.1007/978-981-99-3193-4_5

improving skin appearance and quality by reducing or preventing atrophic scars through the strong upregulation of TGF-β3 [8].

Striae distensae (SD), known as stretch marks too, usually appears after pregnancy, obesity, or rapid muscle growth causing rapid skin stretching and appearing as localized multiple atrophic scars. Initially, SD presents as striae rubra (SR) and is often accompanied by localized inflammation, elastic tissue degeneration, and mast cell degranulation. Over a period of time, the SR gradually faded and manifested as striae alba (SA) with histopathological findings resembling scarring. Extracellular matrix remodeling and stratum corneum cell stimulation through microneedling with PRP are thought to have a significant improvement in collagen deposition, increasing epidermal proliferative activity and decreasing epidermal apoptotic activity after the treatment of SD.

Several studies have shown that combining PRP with some traditional treatments can treat atrophic scars more effectively and obtain better final treatment results and patient satisfaction.

5.1 Application of PRP and Microneedle in Atrophic Scar

Microneedling (MN) is a minimally invasive technique that uses fine needles to penetrate the skin and is currently widely used in the cosmetic field. Microneedling is a common treatment method to treat scars, wrinkles, and skin aging. Microneedle treatment can be used alone and achieve satisfactory results in some scar patients. The main principle of microneedling treatment of scars is to initiate collagen synthesis, break up the parallel collagen bundles of the superficial layer of the dermis in scars and induce neocollagenesis in an organized, and stimulate the body to initiate the healing process by illuminating some small injuries that are invisible to the naked eye [2]. The general remodeling process will last from 5 weeks to 1 year. However, some patients will have post-inflammatory pigmentation and scars after treatment [3]. In recent years, some researchers have begun to combine microneedle with PRP to treat scars and have achieved good results.

Asif et al. found that microneedling combined with PRP treatment can effectively improve the appearance of scars compared to microneedling treatment alone through a placebo-controlled, split-face study [9]. Meanwhile, Ibrahim et al. designed a randomized controlled experiment to compare microneedle therapy alone (treatment once every 2 weeks), PRP therapy alone (treatment once every 2 weeks), and alternate use of microneedle and PRP intermittent therapy every 2 weeks. Six cycles of treatment were performed to evaluate the therapeutic effects of PRP and microneedling on various types of scars. The results showed that PRP combined with microneedling has the best effect, followed by the PRP treatment group alone and finally the microneedling treatment group alone. And he also conducted a prospective half-face controlled clinical trial to treat moderate to severe scars. Thirty-five patients were treated every 3 weeks for a total of four treatments. All patients got microneedling treatment on the right half of the face and microneedling combined with PRP treatment on the left side. After 3 months, the patient and two blinded doctors evaluated the scar treatment on both sides of each patient and obtained satisfactory results ($p < 0.01$); however, the erythema and swelling on the combined treatment side were relatively lighter ($p < 0.01$) [8, 10]. Chawla found that for patients with severe scars (the right half of the face was treated with microneedles combined with PRP, and the left half of the face was treated with microneedles combined with 15% vitamin C), the combined treatment side obtained higher patient satisfaction ($p = 0.01$) [11]. Randomized controlled experiments conducted by Ibrahim, El-Domyat, Chawla, and others have found that the treatment of microneedles combined with PRP can significantly improve scars and obtain higher patient satisfaction and the combination of microneedles and PRP can significantly relieve erythema and edema caused by microneedling treatment [8, 10, 12].

5.2 Application of PRP and Laser in Atrophic Scar

Faghih, Abdel, Zhu, and others have conducted studies on the fractional ablative laser treatment alone, and combined with PRP intradermal injection, the studies found that PRP intradermal injection combined with fractional ablative laser achieved better treatment effects ($p > 0.05$), compared with the sterile saline subcutaneous injection treatment group (combined with fractional ablative laser) and the single laser treatment group, and the patients in the PRP combination treatment group were more satisfied, the transient erythema after treatment subsided was faster, and the swelling was lighter [13–15]. We observe the efficacy of autologous platelet-rich plasma (PRP) combined with erbium fractional laser therapy for facial acne or acne scars (Figs. 5.1, 5.2, 5.3, and 5.4). After three times of treatment, 90.9% of the patients showed a significant improvement and were satisfied; there is no acne inflammation observed. We believe that PRP combined with erbium fractional laser therapy is an effective and safe approach for treating acne scars or acne, with minimal side effects, and it would simultaneously enhance the recovery of the laser-damaged skin.

Many other studies have also obtained the same results. The PRP combined treatment side not only has better skin texture after treatment but also significantly improves the

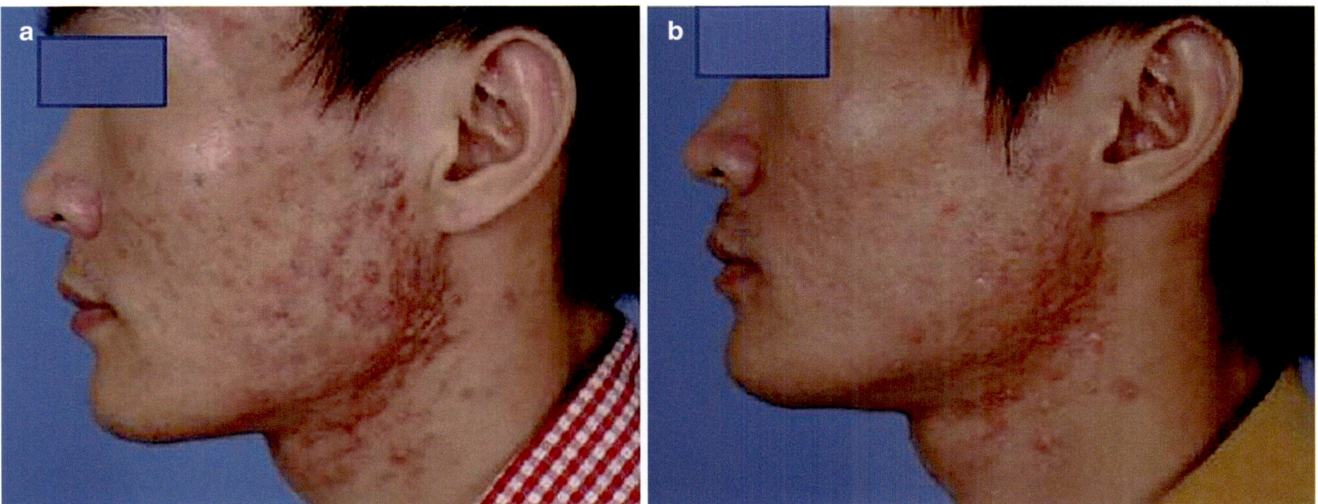

Fig. 5.1 PRP treats acne marks. (**a**) Before treatment. (**b**) Twelve weeks after PRP treatment

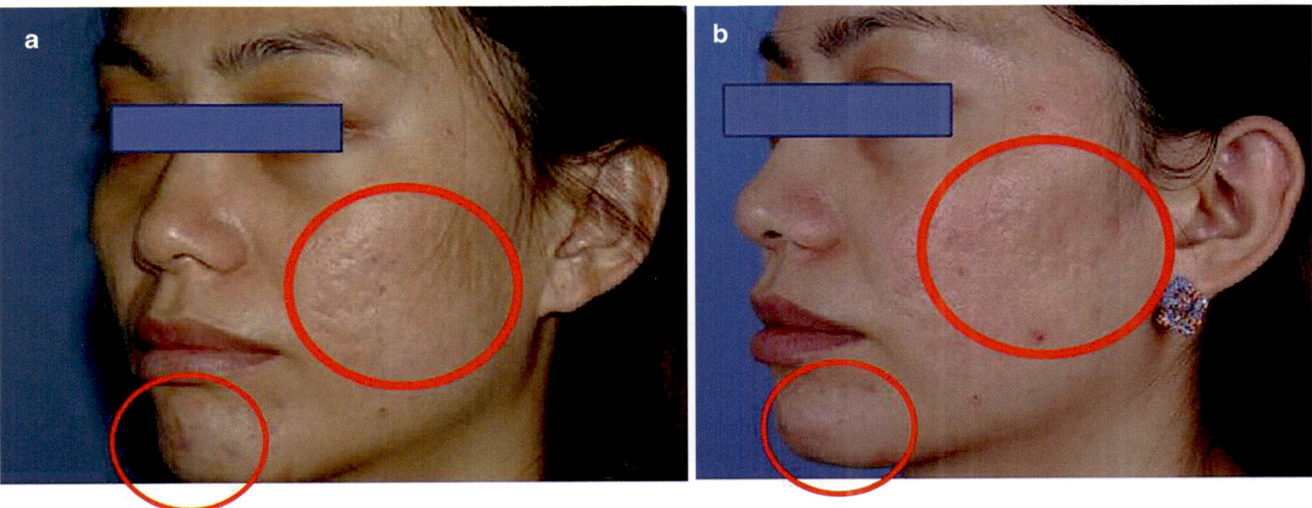

Fig. 5.2 PRP treats acne pits. (**a**) Before treatment. (**b**) Eight weeks after PRP treatment

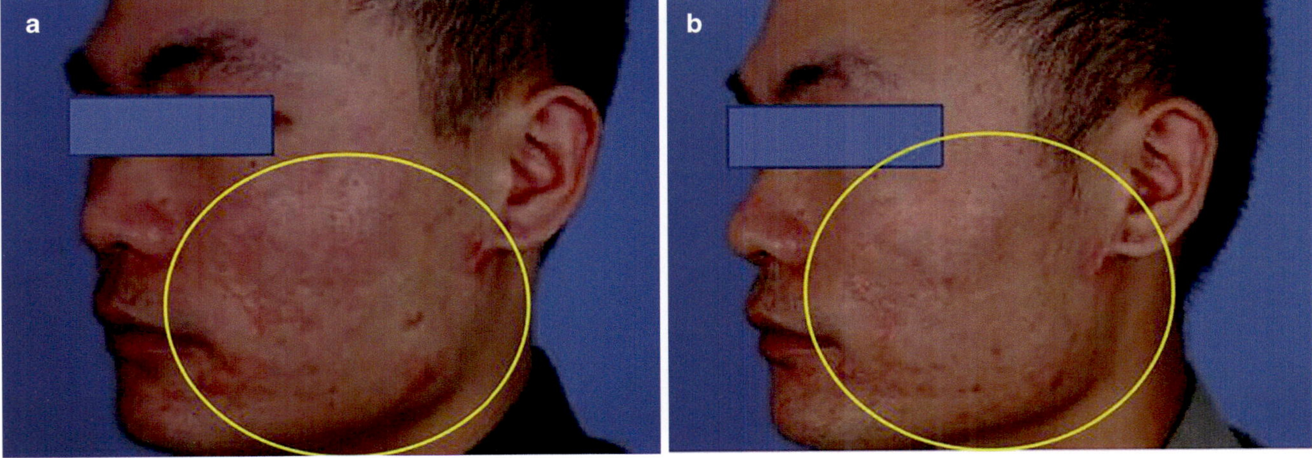

Fig. 5.3 PRP treats acne marks. (**a**) Before treatment. (**b**) Eight weeks after PRP treatment

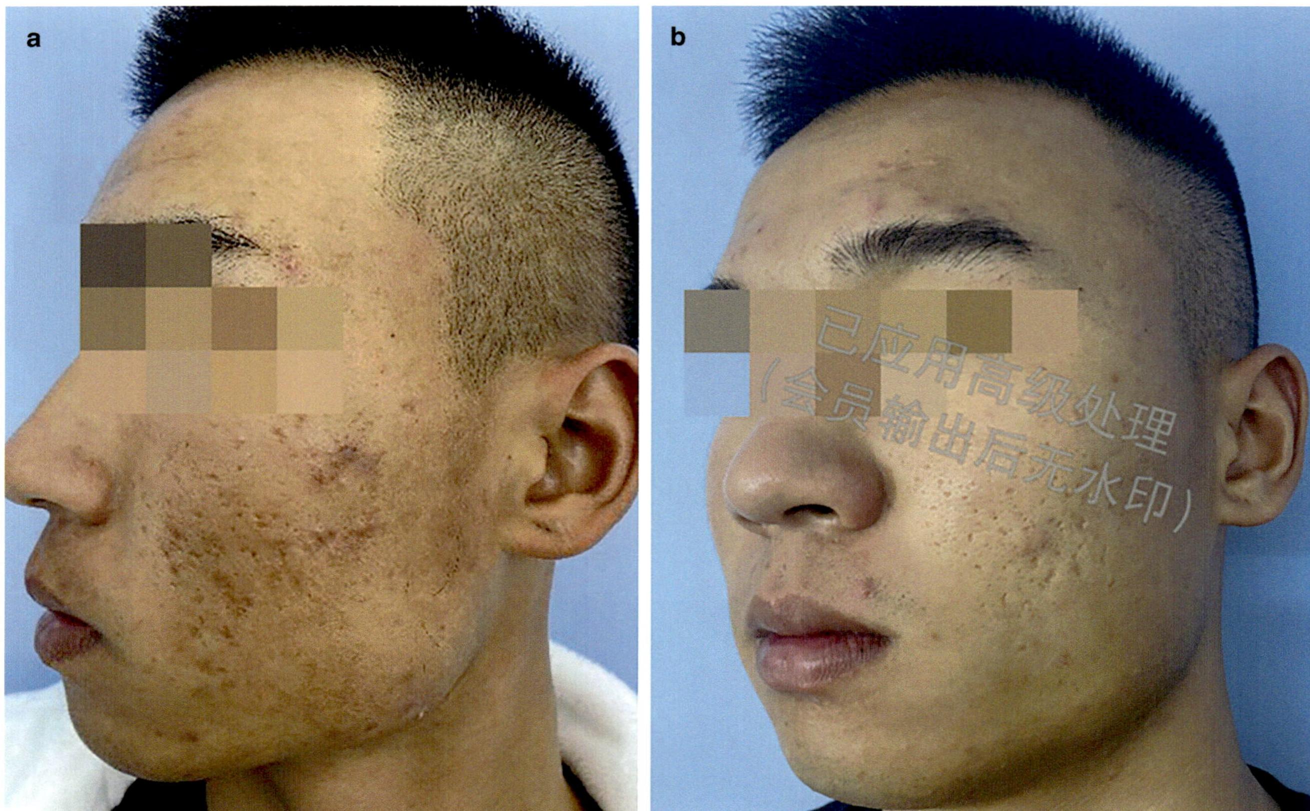

Fig. 5.4 PRP + CO_2 dot array laser treats inflammatory acne + sunken scar. (**a**) 2021.01.02 preoperative; (**b**) 2021.07.18 three times after treatment

appearance of scars, and early erythema, swelling, and scabs after treatment can all disappear earlier [16, 17]. However, there is no significant difference between different PRP-related products in scar treatment, and the use of PRP alone has not achieved obvious therapeutic effects. This may be related to the tight texture of the scar and limited PRP infiltration and limited diffusion after subcutaneous injection. However, the patients showed the redness, pain, and swelling after combined PRP treatments are all less than that of laser treatment alone. Patient satisfaction in the PRP treatment group is generally higher [11, 18], although Nofal et al. showed that activated PRP, pure/neutrophil-containing PRP, and related platelet-rich plasma products have obvious therapeutic effects in treating scars through randomized double-blind controlled experiments. There is no statistical difference in the treatment effect between the various PRP products [19]. It was indicated that PRP can accelerate the skin epithelialization process after treatment and PDGF (platelet-derived growth factors) can improve dermal regeneration and act locally to promote protein and collagen synthesis; it will help endothelial migration or angiogenesis and induces the expression of TGF-beta.

PRP is used as adjuvant therapy for laser and microneedle, and both have achieved good therapeutic effects. Most studies about microneedle combined with PRP treatments have shown significantly improved appearance of scars, and some literature reports that scars are not improved significantly and higher patient satisfaction has been obtained in the combination group. This may be related to the relatively insignificant erythema and edema after treatment in the combined treatment.

Even some studies have shown that treating with L-PRP may lead to the pro-inflammation environment through decreasing IκBα and increasing p-NFκB/NFκB ratio, IL-1β, and TNF-α [20, 21]. The commonly used laser types for treatment are fractional ablative CO_2 laser and erbium laser, combined with AA-L-PRP (activated, leukocyte-, and platelet-rich plasma), which will achieve good scar improvement effects and less related erythema, edema, and light symptoms such as pain. That means we should pay attention to the different effects of L-PRP and AA-L-PRP in the induction of the pro-inflammation environment and the possible influence of the laser combination therapy on the induction of the inflammation environment. Gawdat believes that local and intradermal injections of L-PRP after laser treatment have achieved the same obvious improvement effect [17]. The use of the fractional laser can promote the penetration of PRP, thereby obtaining better results. Conversely, Kar found that the ablative laser combined with inactive L-PRP treatment did not show a significant effect. However, the additional topical application of PRP can significantly alleviate the side effects after treatment and at the same time can avoid the pain during injection and simplify the treatment process, and the patient's treatment tolerance is better [18].

5.3 Hyperplastic Scar: Keloid

Platelet-rich plasma (PRP) has been reported to improve scar collagen structural organization and help decrease pain or functional disabilities related to scar tissue deposition. The mutigrowth factors will release when platelets are activated and promote wound healing, angiogenesis, collagen remodeling, and tissue restoration. Nowadays, PRP is believed to be effective in anti-inflammatory, healing, and cosmetic purposes.

For patients who have suffered from scars for a long time after burns, the bad appearance, the prone to repeated infection, and unbearable itching symptoms, contracture deformities, it has been found that an effective treatment for scars is urgent. Malek et al. [22] found that platelet-rich plasma (PRP) intralesional injection can improve the appearance, pigmentation, itching, and pliability of scar but had a poor effect on scar thickness. PRP treatment of scars improves the above problems significantly better than silicone products; it is very exciting. Even though the author has acknowledged that there are limitations of this study, which contain too small sample size, the operator may have insufficient clinical experience and insufficient evidence of relevant treatment data, but we are still rejoicing that this may be the dawn of scar healing.

Majani et al. [23] evaluated fat grafting in 28 patients for the treatment of different types of scars including burns, trauma, and postoperative scars. Eleven of these patients (group 1) received fat grafting only, and another 11 patients (group 2) received PRP treatment before fat grafting; in the final 6 patients (group 3) with multiple scars (both left and right), the left scar was treated with simple fat grafting, and the right side was treated with PRP combined with fat grafting. The authors indicated that the combination of PRP and lipografting can lead to more durable corrections, particularly in situations where vascularization is more impaired. The following picture is the simulation of the PRP injection scar effect (Fig. 5.5).

At the same time, Cheng's research group has achieved good results in the treatment of various scars with PRP alone clinically. When PRP was applied to the treatment of lip scars, the researchers found that the lip scars gradually receded and approached the color of the surrounding skin (Fig. 5.6). In addition, PRP is also used in the treatment of depression scars, nodular scars, and/or acne. Results showed that PRP treatments significantly improved inflammatory acne and post-

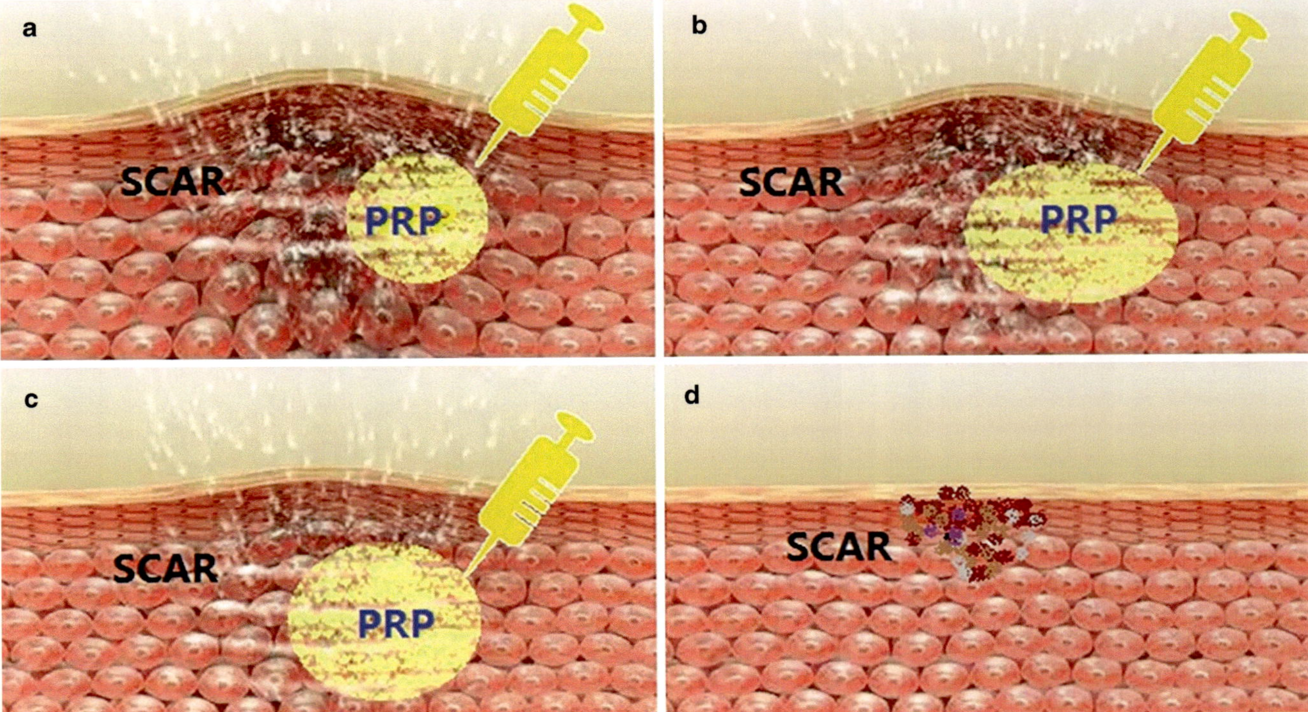

Fig. 5.5 PRP injection in scar: (**a**) first time, (**b**) second time (after 1 month), and (**c**) third time (after 2 months), and (**d**) treatment after 3 months

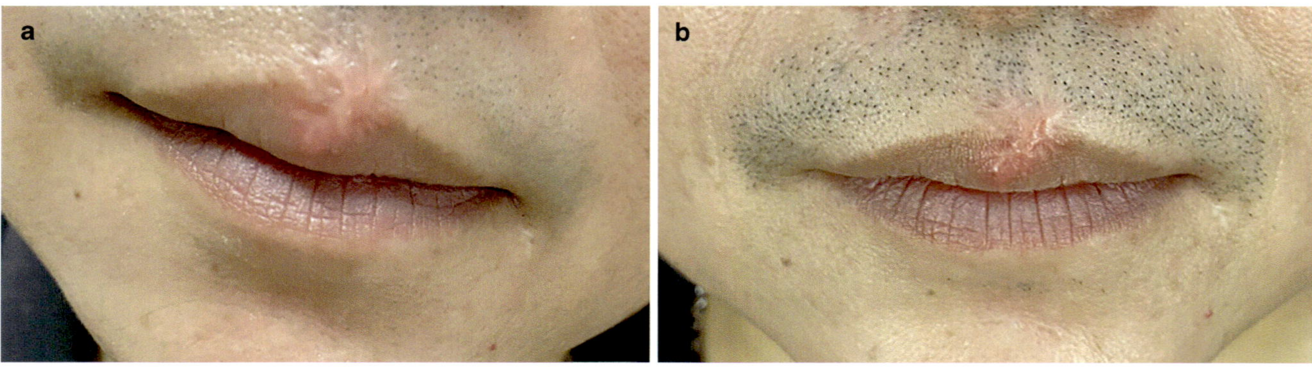

Fig. 5.6 PRP injection in lip scars: (**a**) Before the treatment and (**b**) 25 days after treatment

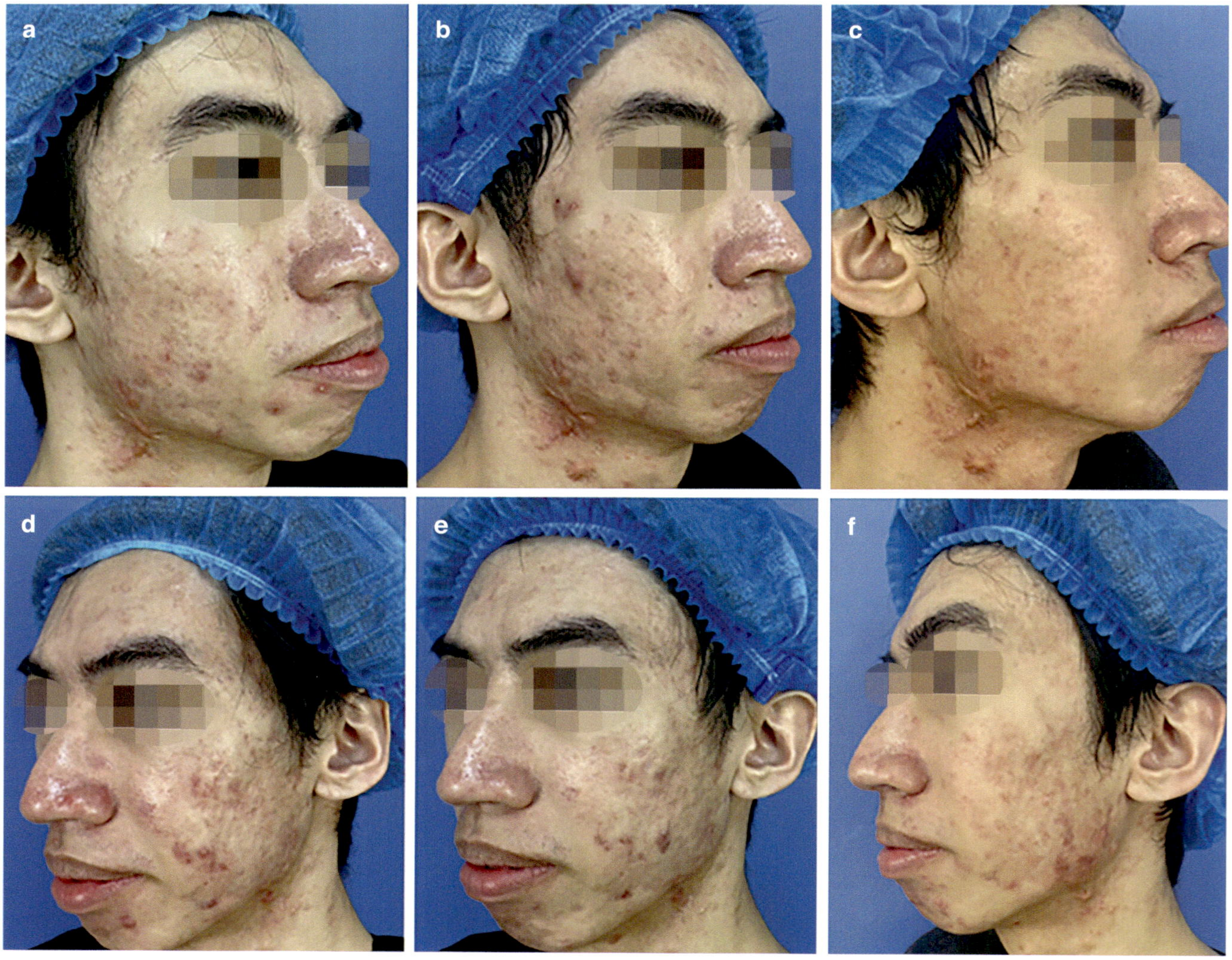

Fig. 5.7 PRP injection in depression and nodular scars left by facial acne: (**a**) right side, before the first operation; (**b**) right side, 20 days after the first operation before the second operation; and (**c**) eight side, 77 days after the second operation. (**d**) Left side: Before the first operation; (**e**) left side, 20 days after the first operation before the second operation; and (**f**) left side, 77 days after the second operation

acne depressions and/or nodular scars. All these results suggest that PRP plays an important role in regulating the skin immune barrier/skin function remodeling (Fig. 5.7).

Many studies found an improvement in wound healing with less keloid recurrences after PRP injection after keloid excision.

The treatment of keloids has the characteristics of complicated, high treatment difficulty, long treatment period, and easy recurrence, and there is no effective optimal treatment plan at this stage. The common treatment options now include surgery, intralesional steroid injections, compressed silicone pads, botulinum toxin, and radiation therapy which have been used, and intralesional bleomycin, interferon, and 5-fluorouracil (5-fluorouracil) injection have also been used. Although previous studies have shown positive effects of PRP as a treatment for anti-scarring, there is still some skepticism about the treatment of PRP because there is no clear conclusion about PRP in the treatment of keloids. Albalat observed the therapeutic effect of several intra-scar injection drugs, including corticosteroids, verapamil, platelet-rich plasma, and 5-FU, and the authors noted that verapamil had the best therapeutic effect, showing that rich platelet plasma is effective, triamcinolone acetonide has no serious side effects in the treatment, and 5-fluorouracil is less effective in the treatment of keloids [24]. Keloid surgical excision has a high recurrence, which is why combining other treatment options is necessary. Azzam combined surgical excision with cryosurgery and platelet-rich plasma (PRP) for auricular keloids. The results showed that this combination therapy type was effectively leading to a low recurrence rate and a favorable cosmetic outcome. And it was well tolerated and had no significant side effects [25].

Jones excised all complete lesions under either intravenous sedation or local anesthesia. After adequate subcutaneous dissociation, the surrounding tissue is dissociated for minimal skin tension and sutured. An appropriate amount of PRP is then applied to the wound bed and under the skin flap. Drainage tubes were routinely placed postoperatively. Postoperatively, PRP was applied to the skin surface and surgical wound, and Dermabond (2-octyl cyanoacrylate; Ethicon, Somerville, New Jersey) was applied after drying. Then within 72 h of excision, superficial photon X-ray radiation was used. It was reported that PRP can decrease inflammation and collagen deposition, leading organized collagen structures in injured vocal cords. Jones found that PRP could improve wound healing with lower keloid recurrence [26, 27]. Hersant also verified that platelet-rich plasma intralesional injection is an effective and safe method for keloid scar treatment [28].

5.4 Promotes Healing and Prevents/Reduces Scarring

Since the 1970s, PRP has received great attention from researchers in tissue repair and regeneration. In the past few years, due to the improvement of economic level and living standards, more and more people have paid more attention to external aesthetics, and surgical or postoperative scars have also received special attention. A few studies have investigated the effect of PRP in optimizing final scar quality.

Tehranian et al. [29] conducted a RCT involving 140 patients undergoing elective cesarean delivery. They were randomized into two groups; the intervention group received PRP treatment, it was used in subcutaneous tissue of the wound before closing the wound, whereas the control group received the usual care (i.e., irrigation of the wound with saline before closure). The authors found that the quality of scarring was significantly improved in patients treated with topical PRP. However, the author noted the limitations of the short follow-up period, which did not extend into the remodeling phase of scar maturation. This will lead to a significant reduction in the reliability of the conclusions.

Cheng's group [30] observed and evaluated the efficacy of autologous platelet-rich plasma on wound healing after cosmetic operation. Six female patients undergo plastic and cosmetic surgery, such as face lifting, reduction mammaplasty, etc. All wounds on one side of the body were treated with autologous platelet-rich plasma on top of standard wound care, and those on the other side were treated with standard care to serve as controls. The quality of wound healing was assessed after 1–2 years of follow-up; the healing of the wounds treated by autologous platelet-rich plasma was significantly better with reduced scars, compared to the control wounds. The survival of the injected fat was better as compared to the control. This observation showed that autologous platelet-rich plasma can significantly improve wound healing and help to prevent or reduce scarring.

At present, limitations of all studies mainly include short follow-up time, nonstandardized treatment regimen, and the variable use of triamcinolone; these factors make it difficult to provide an objective and effective assessment of the effect of PRP on wound treatment and eventual recurrence rate. It was speculated that PRP regulates the secretion and recruitment of inflammatory cells such as monocytes and leukocytes at the site of injury. Therefore, PRP-mediated therapeutic effects and tissue regeneration processes appear to result from the control of local inflammatory processes. Subsequently, the healing process is adjusted to reduce scarring under PRP intervention microenvironmental conditions.

References

1. Harris DW, Buckley CC, Ostlere LS, Rustin MH. Topical retinoic acid in the treatment of fine acne scarring. Br J Dermatol. 1991;125:81–2. https://doi.org/10.1111/j.1365-2133.1991.tb06048.x.
2. Dogra S, Yadav S, Sarangal R. Microneedling for acne scars in Asian skin type: an effective low cost treatment modality. J Cosmet Dermatol. 2014;13:180–7. https://doi.org/10.1111/jocd.12095.

3. Lee JB, Chung WG, Kwahck H, Lee KH. Focal treatment of acne scars with trichloroacetic acid: chemical reconstruction of skin scars method. Dermatol Surg. 2002;28:1017–21; discussion 1021. https://doi.org/10.1046/j.1524-4725.2002.02095.x.
4. Walia S, Alster TS. Prolonged clinical and histologic effects from CO2 laser resurfacing of atrophic acne scars. Dermatol Surg. 1999;25:926–30. https://doi.org/10.1046/j.1524-4725.1999.99115.x.
5. Joseph JH, Shamban A, Eaton L, Lehman A, Cohen S, Spencer J, Bruce S, Grimes P, Tedaldi R, Callender V, Werschler P. Polymethylmethacrylate collagen gel-injectable dermal filler for full face atrophic acne scar correction. Dermatol Surg. 2019;45:1558–66. https://doi.org/10.1097/DSS.0000000000001863.
6. Nam SM, Kim YB. The effects of platelet-rich plasma on hypertrophic scars fibroblasts. Int Wound J. 2018;15:547–54. https://doi.org/10.1111/iwj.12896.
7. Jones ME, Hardy C, Ridgway J. Keloid management: a retrospective case review on a new approach using surgical excision, platelet-rich plasma, and in-office superficial photon X-ray radiation therapy. Adv Skin Wound Care. 2016;29(7):303–7.
8. Ibrahim ZA, El-Ashmawy AA, Shora OA. Therapeutic effect of microneedling and autologous platelet-rich plasma in the treatment of atrophic scars: a randomized study. J Cosmet Dermatol. 2017;16:388–99. https://doi.org/10.1111/jocd.12356.
9. Asif M, Kanodia S, Singh K. Combined autologous platelet-rich plasma with microneedling verses microneedling with distilled water in the treatment of atrophic acne scars: a concurrent split-face study. J Cosmet Dermatol. 2016;15:434–43. https://doi.org/10.1111/jocd.12207.
10. Ibrahim MK, Ibrahim SM, Salem AM. Skin microneedling plus platelet-rich plasma versus skin microneedling alone in the treatment of atrophic post acne scars: a split face comparative study. J Dermatolog Treat. 2018;29:281–6. https://doi.org/10.1080/09546634.2017.1365111.
11. Chawla S. Split face comparative study of microneedling with PRP versus microneedling with vitamin C in treating atrophic post acne scars. J Cutan Aesthet Surg. 2014;7:209–12. https://doi.org/10.4103/0974-2077.150742.
12. Microneedling combined with platelet-rich plasma or trichloroacetic acid peeling for management of acne scarring: A split-face clinical and histologic comparison. n.d.. https://pubmed.ncbi.nlm.nih.gov/29226630/. Accessed 8 Nov 2020.
13. Faghihi G, Keyvan S, Asilian A, Nouraei S, Behfar S, Nilforoushzadeh MA. Efficacy of autologous platelet-rich plasma combined with fractional ablative carbon dioxide resurfacing laser in treatment of facial atrophic acne scars: a split-face randomized clinical trial. Indian J Dermatol Venereol Leprol. 2016;82:162–8. https://doi.org/10.4103/0378-6323.174378.
14. Abdel Aal AM, Ibrahim IM, Sami NA, Abdel Kareem IM. Evaluation of autologous platelet-rich plasma plus ablative carbon dioxide fractional laser in the treatment of acne scars. J Cosmet Laser Ther. 2018;20:106–13. https://doi.org/10.1080/14764172.2017.1368667.
15. Zhu J-T, Xuan M, Zhang Y-N, Liu H-W, Cai J-H, Wu Y-H, Xiang X-F, Shan G-Q, Cheng B. The efficacy of autologous platelet-rich plasma combined with erbium fractional laser therapy for facial acne scars or acne. Mol Med Rep. 2013;8:233–7. https://doi.org/10.3892/mmr.2013.1455.
16. The efficacy of autologous platelet rich plasma combined with ablative carbon dioxide fractional resurfacing for acne scars: a simultaneous split-face trial. n.d.. https://pubmed.ncbi.nlm.nih.gov/21635618/. Accessed 8 Nov 2020.
17. Autologous platelet rich plasma: topical versus intradermal after fractional ablative carbon dioxide laser treatment of atrophic acne scars. n.d.. https://pubmed.ncbi.nlm.nih.gov/24354616/. Accessed 8 Nov 2020.
18. Kar BR, Raj C. Fractional CO2 laser vs fractional CO2 with topical platelet-rich plasma in the treatment of acne scars: a split-face comparison trial. J Cutan Aesthet Surg. 2017;10:136–44. https://doi.org/10.4103/JCAS.JCAS_99_17.
19. Nofal E, Helmy A, Nofal A, Alakad R, Nasr M. Platelet-rich plasma versus CROSS technique with 100% trichloroacetic acid versus combined skin needling and platelet rich plasma in the treatment of atrophic acne scars: a comparative study. Dermatol Surg. 2014;40:864–73. https://doi.org/10.1111/dsu.0000000000000091.
20. Leukocyte inclusion within a platelet rich plasma-derived fibrin scaffold stimulates a more pro-inflammatory environment and alters fibrin properties. n.d.. https://pubmed.ncbi.nlm.nih.gov/25823008/. Accessed 8 Nov 2020.
21. Anitua E, Zalduendo MM, Prado R, Alkhraisat MH, Orive G. Morphogen and proinflammatory cytokine release kinetics from PRGF-Endoret fibrin scaffolds: evaluation of the effect of leukocyte inclusion. J Biomed Mater Res A. 2015;103:1011–20. https://doi.org/10.1002/jbm.a.35244.
22. Malek E, Mohamed AM, Amr M, Omar SE. Evaluation of the effect of platelet-rich plasma on post-burn scars. Open Access J Surg. 2017;5(1):555660. https://doi.org/10.19080/OAJS.2017.05.555660.
23. Majani U, Majani A. Correction of scars by autologous fat graft and platelet rich plasma (PRP). Acta Med Mediterr. 2012;28:99–100.
24. Albalat W, Nabil S, Khattab F. Assessment of various intralesional injections in keloid: comparative analysis. J Dermatolog Treat. 2021;13:1–30.
25. Azzam EZ, Omar SS. Treatment of auricular keloids by triple combination therapy: surgical excision, platelet-rich plasma, and cryosurgery. J Cosmet Dermatol. 2018;17(3):502–10.
26. Jones ME, Hardy C, Ridgway J. Keloid management: a retrospective case review on a new approach using surgical excision, platelet-rich plasma, and in-office superficial photon X-ray radiation therapy. J Adv Skin Wound Care. 2016;29:303–7.
27. Jones ME, McLane J, Adenegan R, et al. Advancing keloid treatment: a novel multimodal approach to ear keloids. Dermatol Surg. 2017;43:1164–9.
28. Hersant B, SidAhmed-Mezi M, Picard F, et al. Efficacy of autologous platelet concentrates as adjuvant therapy to surgical excision in the treatment of keloid scars refractory to conventional treatments: a pilot prospective study. Ann Plast Surg. 2018;81:170–5.
29. Tehranian A, Esfehani-Mehr B, Pirjani R, et al. Application of autologous platelet-rich plasma (PRP) on wound healing after caesarean section in high-risk patients. Iran Red Crescent Med J. 2016;18(7):e34449.
30. Cheng B, Liu HW, Tang JB, et al. Effect of autologous platelet-rich plasma on the wound healing of cosmetic surgery. Chin J Blood Transfus. 2011;24(4):282–4.

6 Platelet-Rich Plasma and Hair Regeneration

Linlin Li, Meishu Zhu, and Sha Yuan

Mammalian hair is used to keep warm and help to complete metabolism. But in modern society, the primary function of human hair is decoration. Alopecia is a chronic inflammatory disease of hair follicles caused by autoimmunity, which can irritate the skin. Although hair loss is not a life-threatening or painful disease, it can cause serious psychological problems, like serious anxiety and depression. Research is currently showing that platelet-rich plasma (PRP) therapy is a promising treatment for certain types of baldness.

Hair cycling is the rhythmic change of the hair follicle through phases of growth (anagen), regression (catagen), and rest (telogen). The human scalp, eyebrows, and lashes consist of long, thick, medullated, and pigmented terminal hair shafts, whereas the body is covered with short, thin, and often unpigmented vellus hairs. Each of us displays an estimated total number of five million hair follicles, of which 80,000–150,000 are located on the scalp. The hair length is defined by the duration of anagen, which lasts for 2–6 years. Catagen lasts only for a few weeks, followed by the telogen phase, which lasts 2–4 months [1].

L. Li (✉)
Department of Plastic Surgery, Dermatology Hospital of Fuzhou, Fuzhou, Fujian, China

M. Zhu
Department of Burn and Plastic Surgery, Shenzhen Institute of Translational Medicine, Shenzhen Second People's Hospital, The First Affiliated Hospital of Shenzhen University Health Science Center, Shenzhen, Guangdong, China

Department of Wound Repair, Shenzhen Institute of Translational Medicine, Shenzhen Second People's Hospital, The First Affiliated Hospital of Shenzhen University Health Science Center, Shenzhen, Guangdong, China

S. Yuan
Dermatological Department, Hangzhou Meilai Medical Hospital, Hangzhou, Zhejiang, China

6.1 Physiological Structure of Hair Follicle

Hair can be divided into two parts: the shaft, which is exposed outside the skin, and the root, which is buried inside the skin. The root of the hair is wrapped by the hair follicle; the end of the hair follicle is enlarged into a ball, called the bulb. The structure of the hair follicle from deep layer to surface layer is mainly divided into four parts: bulb, superior bulb region, isthmus, and infundibulum.

6.1.1 Hair Bulb

They are usually found in fat and include the mother material cells and the dermal papilla, which is a mesenchymal structure derived from the dermis and located in the depression of the bulb of the hair follicle.

6.1.2 Superior Bulb Region

The hair bulb reaches the part where the trichodermis is embedded in the root sheath of the hair follicle, and the structure of each layer of the hair follicle begins to differentiate during the growth stage.

6.1.3 Isthmus

Down to the place where the arrector pili muscle is embedded in the fibrous sheath of the hair follicle, up to the opening of the sebaceous duct in the hair follicle passage.

6.1.4 Infundibulum

The shallowest part of the hair follicle, with the sebaceous gland opening as the lower margin.

B. Cheng, X. Fu (eds.), *Platelet-Rich Plasma in Tissue Repair and Regeneration*, https://doi.org/10.1007/978-981-99-3193-4_6

Hair follicles have eight complex concentric sheaths, each with different functions and properties, from the center of the hair follicle to the outer layer: (1) hair medulla; (2) hair stem intermediate layer (HS medulla); (3) hair stem cortex (HS cortex); (4) HS cuticle; (5) inner root sheath, Huxley layer; (6) Henle layer of inner root sheath; (7) companion layer; and (8) outer root sheath (ORS) [2].

6.2 The Growth Cycle of Hair Follicles

Hair follicles are characterized by periodic growth throughout life, including resting period, growing period, and regression period. For rodents, (1) hair follicles enter telogen, which is a relatively static stage of proliferation and biochemical activity. The hair follicle remains at this stage until it is reactivated by signals both inside and outside the hair follicle. At this point, uncolored bar hair usually remains in the roots. (2) Anagen is a rapid growth phase in which stem cells in the carina produce hair matrix, which is activated to proliferate and differentiate to form inner root sheath and hair shaft. (3) During catagen, hair follicles undergo a highly controlled process of degeneration. During this stage, programmed death of most keratinocytes occurs, melanin production stops, and some melanocytes die. Dermal papillae coagulates and move upward, resting below the carina.

6.3 Hair Follicle Signaling Pathway

The Wnt/β-catenin signal pathway is the main signal pathway that controls hair growth. Dermal papilla cells (DPCs) are responsible for receiving and transmitting signals through the Wnt/β-catenin signal pathway to control proliferation and differentiation of hair follicle stem cells. In a regularly cycling hair follicle, activation of Wnt in the DP cells leads to accumulation of b-catenin in the cytoplasm. β-Catenin then translocates to the nucleus and in combination with T-cell factor/lymphoid enhancer-binding factor (TCF/LEF) family members. In this way, the DP cells secrete proteins to stimulate differentiation and hair follicle formation in stem cells as part of their paracrine interactions. Consequently, transition from telogen to anagen is encouraged, leading to the next cycle of hair growth, while GSK-3β regulate negatively the growth of hair by targeting β-catenin phosphorylation.

6.4 Basic Study on PRP and Hair Follicle Regeneration

PRP supply growth factors exogenously, which affect DPC attachment, proliferation, and differentiation, promote the accumulation of extracellular matrix, and change the growth cycle of hair. PRP growth factors including PDGF, TGF-β, VEGF, EGF, and FGF promote proliferation of DPCs in the bulge area of the hair follicle through increasing accumulation of FGF-7 and β-catenin [3], activating ERK signaling as well as promoting transition from telogen to anagen. Insulin-like growth factor 1/factor 2, FGF-7, and PDGF have been implicated in the increase in hair growth and the lengthening of anagen. Duration of anagen is increased through the prevention of catagen phase and activation of anti-apoptosis signaling pathways. Binding of growth factors to their cell surface receptors results in a signaling cascade activating antiapoptotic regulators, such as Bcl-2 and Akt. Through phosphorylation of proapoptotic inhibitors, Bcl-2-associated death promoter (BAD), and GSK-3b, AKt prevents Bcl-2 inhibition and β-catenin degradation, respectively [3–5].

In 2006, the Uebel [6] team first tried preconditioning hair follicle units for transplantation with PRP. The authors observed that prP-treated hair transplant areas survived 18.7 hair follicle units per cm^2 compared with 16.4 hair follicle units per cm^2 in the control area of the scalp, a 15.1% increase in density. They suspect that growth factors released from platelets may act on stem cells in hair follicle protuberance, stimulating stem cell differentiation and promoting the formation of new blood vessels. In 2011, Takikawa et al. [7] compared AGA (androgenetic alopecia) patients by subcutaneous injection of normal saline, PRP, and heparin-protamine particles combined with PRP (D-P PRP) and found that the cross-sectional area of hair in PRP group and D-P PRP group significantly increased; the proliferation of collagen fibers and fibroblasts in hair follicles and hyperplasia of blood vessels around the hair follicle was observed under microscope. In 2012, Li et al. [3] observed the effect of activated PRP on the proliferation of DPCs and injected activated PRP subcutaneously into mice. Comparison with the control group showed that activated PRP increased proliferation of DPCs, stimulated extracellular signal transduction kinases ERK and Akt, and upregulated fibroblast growth factor 7 (FGF-7) and β-catenin in DPC. Mice injected with activated PRP induced a more rapid transition from resting to growing period than the control group. Since then, PRP has been considered as a potential tool to promote hair growth, and researchers have continuously applied PRP in the treatment of AGA patients.

Based on the clinical application of PRP in AGA treatment, ideal results were obtained, due to the lack of effective gold standards and testing methods in clinical studies and lack of research on the mechanism of PRP effect on hair follicles. Our research group has confirmed the effectiveness of PRP in treating AGA in clinical work. In addition, the effectiveness of PRP in promoting hair follicle development was verified in animal experiments. Finally, the effects of PRP on hair follicle stem cells and hair follicle growth and its mechanism were discussed through cell and animal experiments, so as to provide theoretical and methodological basis for clinical application of PRP in treating AGA [6, 7].

In order to confirm the promotion effect of PRP on hair growth, we used neonatal C57BL/6 suckling mice as an animal model and found that PRP can promote hair follicle development and maturation [8].

Forty newborn C57BL/6 suckling mice were randomly divided into PRP experimental group and normal saline control group, with 20 mice in each group. The experimental group was injected with 0.05 mL PRP intradermal injection, while the control group was injected with normal saline. At day 3, day 5, day 7, and day 10, five mice in each group were selected for general observation, and Image J software was used to measure skin gray value. The whole layer of skin tissue was cut and embedded in paraffin for routine HE (hematoxylin and eosin) staining. The tissue sections were taken for histological observation and shooting, and the indexes of hair follicle staging and number were observed. The data were analyzed using SPSS (Statistical Package for the Social Sciences) statistical software.

The results showed that skin color change of mice in PRP group occurred earlier than that in control group on days 3, 5, and 7, and the results were consistent with the statistical results of gray value detection ($p \leq 0.01$). At the same time, the hair density of PRP group was significantly higher than that of saline group on day 10. HE staining results showed that the number of hair follicles in PRP group and the development of hair follicles in the same day were significantly better than those in the control group (Fig. 6.1).

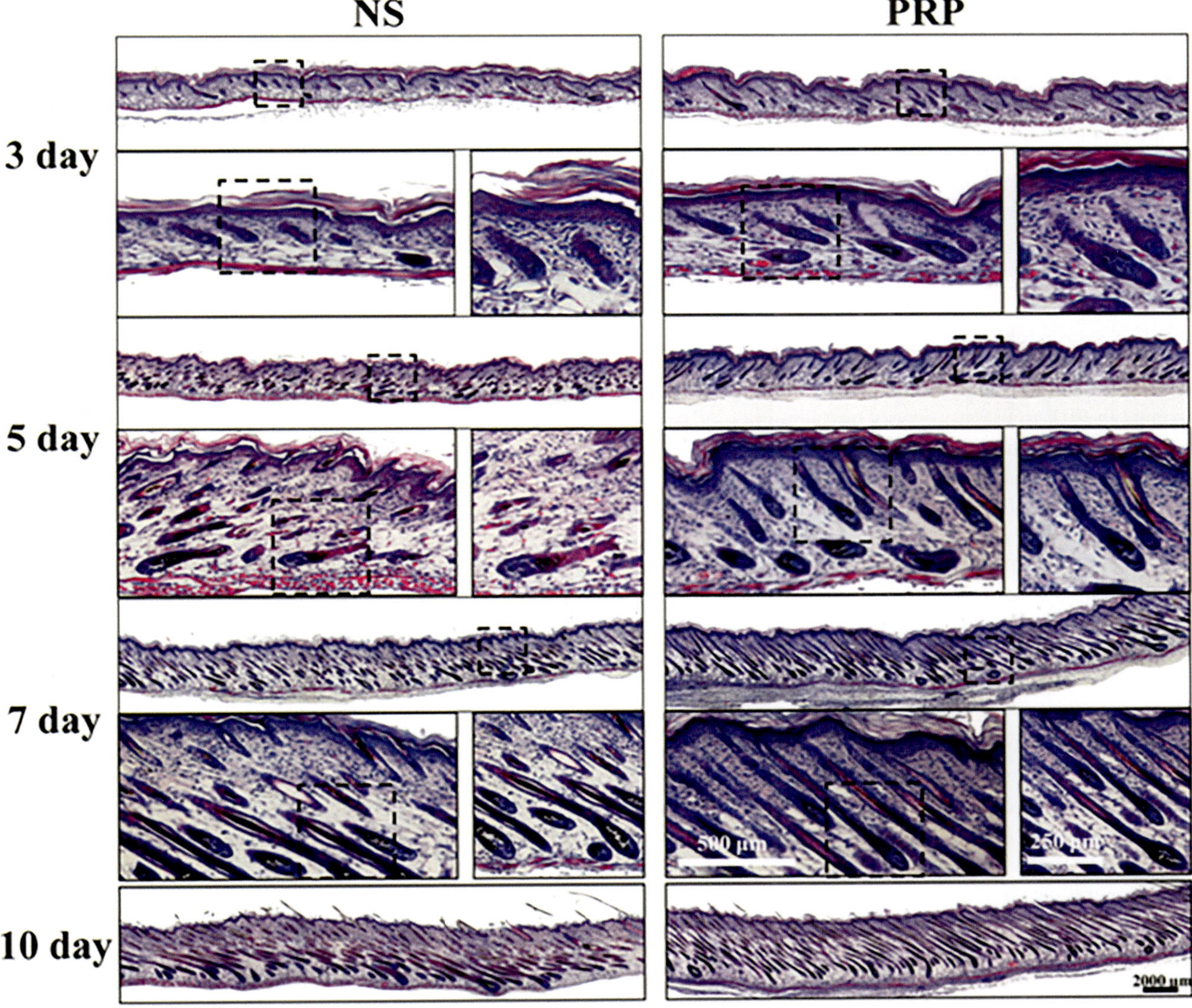

Fig. 6.1 Histological staining of skin hair follicles in C57BL/6 suckling rats after birth; bar: 250 μm, 500 μm, and 2000 μm

In PRP injection of the group, the hair follicle development speed was significantly accelerated, the hair bulb increased, the outer root sheath and inner root sheath differentiated and formed, the hair follicle went deep into the subcutaneous tissue, and most of the hair follicle developments was in the fifth stage. On day 5, histological observation in the PRP group showed that the papilla was thin and surrounded by hair parent material. Most hair follicles are in stage 6 of development, which is significantly better than the development of the control group. On day 7, the hair follicles in PRP group were deeper, and part of the hair stem grew out of the epidermis through the hair tubules, and the hair follicles developed and differentiated into stages 7–8. In the control group, more than half of the hair follicles were in stage 6 and some were in stage 7.

PRP promotes the formation of new hair follicles in newborn rats, increasing the number of new hair follicles, and regeneration of hair follicle development (stage 8) has obvious promoting effect and makes new hair follicles to mature faster development of hair follicles, thus speeding up the newborn rats by reddish skin color into a gray; gray process gradually turned into a black phenomenon.

Therefore, in-depth characterization and observation of PRP on the development of hair follicles proved that PRP can promote the development of early hair follicles in suckling mice, providing a theoretical basis and guiding significance for skin tissue injury repair and skin hair follicle regeneration research.

However, the underlying cellular and molecular mechanisms along with their effect on hair follicle stem cells are poorly understood. In another study, we designed to induce platelets in PRP to release factors by calcium chloride (PC) or by sonication where platelet lysates (PS) or the supernatants of platelet lysate (PSS) were used to evaluate their effect on the hair follicle activation and regeneration. We found that PSS and PS exhibited a superior effect in activating telogen hair follicles than PC. In addition, PSS injection into the skin activated quiescent hair follicles and induced K15+ hair follicle stem cell proliferation in K14-H2B-GFP mice. Moreover, PSS promoted skin-derived precursor (SKP) survival in vitro and enhanced hair follicle formation in vivo. In consistence, protein array analysis of different PRP preparations revealed that PSS contained higher levels of 16 growth factors (out of 41 factors analyzed) than PC, many of them have been known to promote hair follicle regeneration. Thus, our data indicate that sonicated PRP promotes hair follicle stem cell activation and de novo hair follicle regeneration.

To examine the effect of various PRP preparations on hair follicle activation, 7-week-old C57 mice (hair follicles in telogen phase) received intra-cutaneous injection of saline (NS), calcium-activated PRP (PC), PRP sonicate (PS), or the supernatant of PS (PSS). After 14 days, hair regrowth was observed at the injection sites of PS and PSS, while sparse hair regrowth was found at the injection sites of NS and PC. Quantitation of the hair regrowth areas showed that PSS induced enhanced hair regrowth compared to NS and PC. Thirty days after the injection, the skin tissue of the injection site was excised and subjected to AP stain; more AP-positive hair follicles in anagen phase were detected in the skin receiving PS injection. These results indicate that PRP sonicates have enhanced effect in inducing hair follicle telogen-anagen transition (TAT).

To investigate the mechanisms underlying PRP-induced hair follicle TAT, K14-H2B-GFP mice (7 weeks old) whose K14+ cells expressed high-level GFP in the nuclei received skin injection of PSS or saline. Five days after injection, confocal microscopy showed a dramatic increase in the number of K14-GFP-positive cells in the hair follicle at the injection site of PSS, compared to the saline injection site. In consistence, Ki67 stain showed increased numbers of proliferating K14-GFP cells in the hair follicle after PSS injection. To examine alterations of HFSCs after the treatments, we performed dual immunofluorescence stain for K15+ cells and Ki67 and observed a significant increase in the number of K15+ cells in the hair follicle after PSS treatment compared to saline treatment, which was associated with an increase in the number of dividing K15+ cells which expressed Ki67. These results indicate that factors released from platelets activate quiescent HFSCs and promote their proliferation, resulting in hair follicle TAT.

To examine the effect of PRP on skin cells, we supplemented PRP preparations to human keratinocyte (HaCaT) and mouse dermal stem cell (SKP) cultures. Both PC and PSS significantly promoted the proliferation of keratinocytes. In the absence of regular supplement, SKPs formed small cell aggregates in basal medium. Notably, supplementation of PC to basal medium resulted in the formation of large cell aggregates, but a considerable fraction of cells died after 2 days; when PSS was added to the culture, however, SKPs formed large aggregates with healthy morphology ($93 \pm 2.9\%$ cell viability, $p < 0.001$). The results indicated that PSS exhibited enhanced effect in promoting SKP survival.

To examine the effect of PRP in hair follicle formation, we performed hair follicle reconstitution assay. One hundred six epidermal cells and 2×10^6 dermal cells (per wound) derived from neonatal K14-H2B-GFPmice in 20% PSS or equal volume of saline were implanted into 2.5 mm excisional wounds. Three weeks after transplantation, sites of grafts containing PSS generated more hairs than sites of grafts containing control saline. In addition, two-photon microscopy showed that the PSS-supplemented grafts generated larger hair follicles than saline-supplemented grafts. These results indicate that PRP sonicates enhance de novo hair regeneration and hair growth.

6.5 Clinical Application of PRP in Treatment of Hair Regeneration

6.5.1 PRP Treatment for Androgenetic Alopecia

In order to observe the effect of PRP on androgenic alopecia, we collected 12 patients suffering from androgen alopecia from January 2016 to December 2019 in our hospital who were received PRP injections. All patients were given injections on the affected area of alopecia every 1–2 months. Eleven patients completed 2–3 injections, and the clinical effect was observed, while only 1 patient was treated once. A 40 ml venous blood was extracted during each treatment and 5 ml PRP was obtained after two centrifugations. The platelet enrichment multiple of PRP obtained by this method was 5.1 ± 1.3 times of the baseline value. After 2–3 times of treatment, 11 patients presented clinical improvement in the hair counts, hair thickness, hair texture, and hair color(Figs. 6.2, 6.3, 6.4, and 6.5). Patient's satisfaction rate is 91.6%. We found that PRP is a safe, economical, and feasible treatment for androgenic alopecia with no obvious adverse effects.

Around 40–60 ml of venous blood was extracted from the median cubital vein into an EDTA (ethylenediamine tetraacetic acid) anticoagulant tube. Autogenous PRP was prepared by a two-step centrifugation: the anticoagulant tube was centrifuged at 660 × *g* (1500 rpm) per minute for 10 min in a centrifuge. After centrifugation, the blood was divided into three layers from top to bottom, the upper layer was plasma, the middle layer was white membrane layer, and the lower layer was red blood cell layer. To obtain the upper plasma layer and white film layer with a syringe (avoid the red blood cells) and transfer it to a sterile centrifuge tube. Centrifuge the tube at 1500 × g (3000 RPM) for 20 minutes, then extract the supernatant for platelet-poor plasma and leave the platelet-rich plasma at the bottom of the tube. This is the method for preparing PRP.

The concentration was (5.1 ± 1.3) times the baseline value, due to a slight deviation in operator proficiency. Thrombin freeze-dried powder and calcium gluconate injection were prepared with 100 U/mL thrombin solution, and PRP was added in a 10:1 ratio. PRP was heated in a water bath at 37 °C for 1 h to obtain platelet lysate (PL). Treatment: Inform patients of side effects and obtain informed consent prior to treatment. The scalp of the treatment area was anesthetized with compound lidocaine cream. After the effect of anesthetics, normal saline was cleaned and iodine plates was disinfected.

The "5D" method (dose-direction-depth-densely-deliver injection method) was firstly proposed by the Pro. Cheng [6]: attention is paid to the dose, direction, depth, density, and method of administration. 1 ml syringe, insulin needle, and 30G needle can be used for injection therapy. 0.1 ml/cm^2 dermal injection is performed at an angle of about 45–90° (consistent with the direction of the scalp from the head), with a depth of about 0.5–2 mm and a distance of 0.25–0.5 cm. The needle angle can be adjusted along the hair growth direction so that the tip of the needle can reach the root of the hair follicle. At the same time, the treatment can be supplemented by microneedles, with 1–1.5 mm microneedles rolling in different directions on the scalp surface. According to the treatment frequency of 1–2 months, 1–3 times of treatment were completed, and the general picture was taken before each treatment to evaluate the improvement of symptoms.

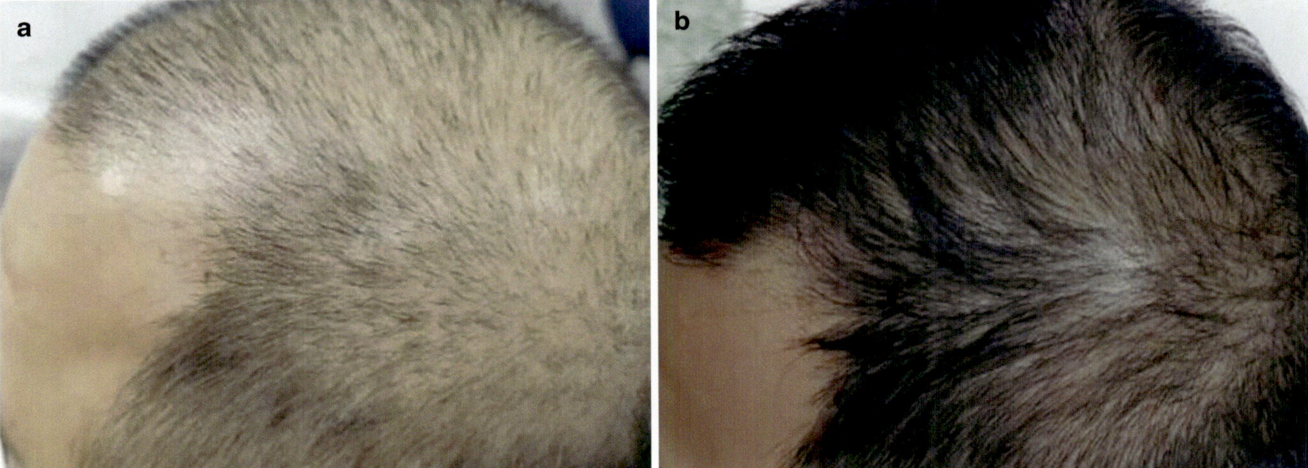

Fig. 6.2 Comparison of efficacy in male patients (BASP typing: M2V1): (**a**) general photos before treatment and (**b**) general photos of RP after a 3-month treatment

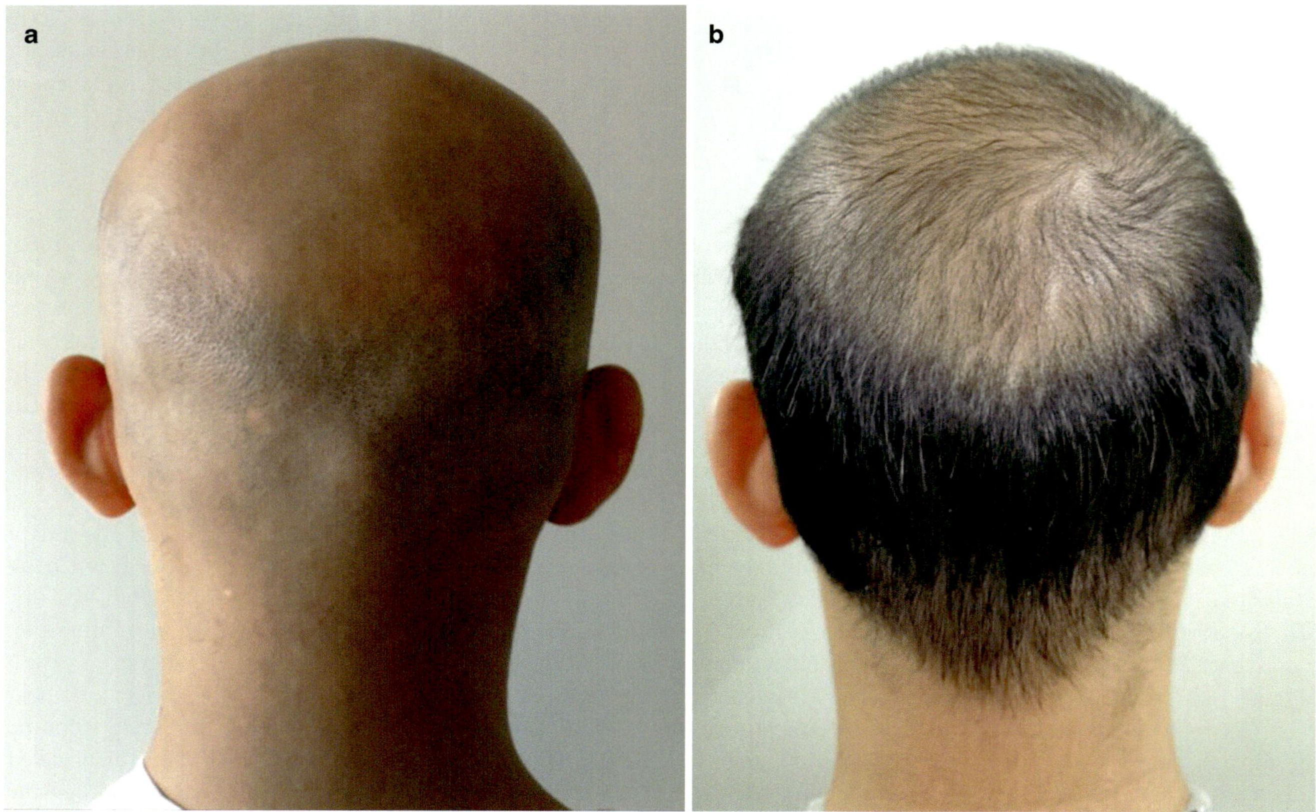

Fig. 6.3 Comparison of efficacy in male patients: (**a**) general photos before treatment and (**b**) general photos of RP after a 3-month treatment

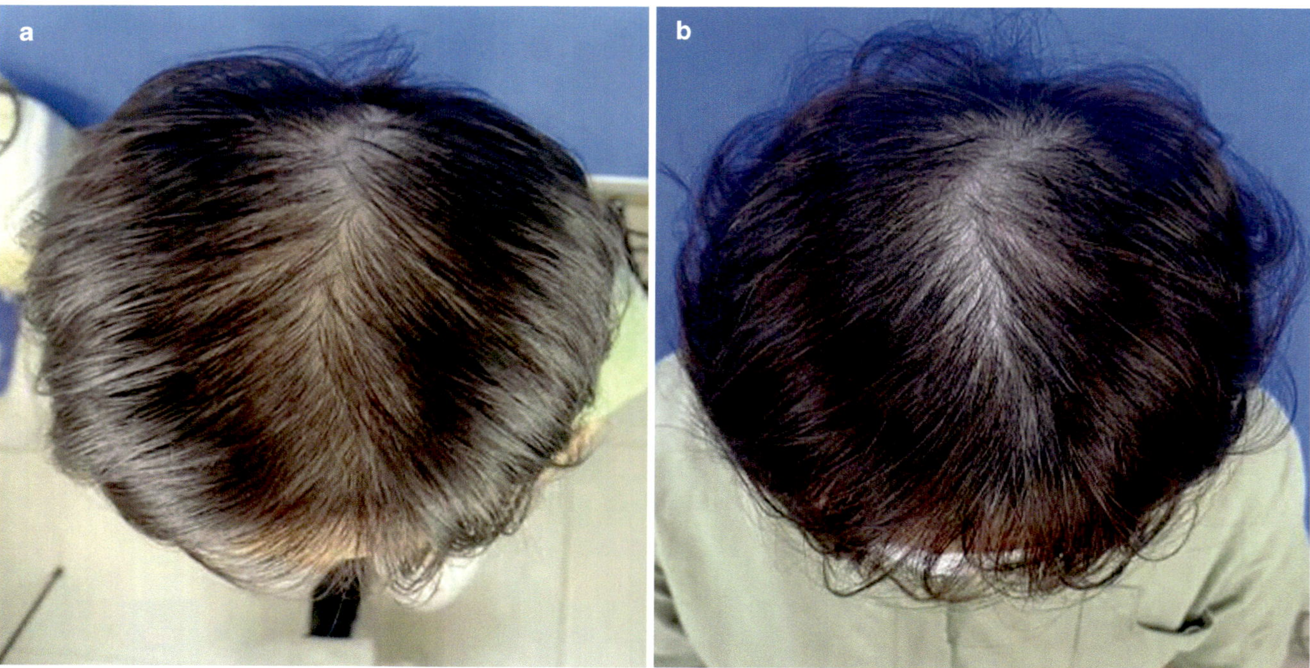

Fig. 6.4 Comparison of efficacy of female patients (BASP typing: C0F1): (**a**) general photos before treatment and (**b**) general photos of RP after a 3-month treatment

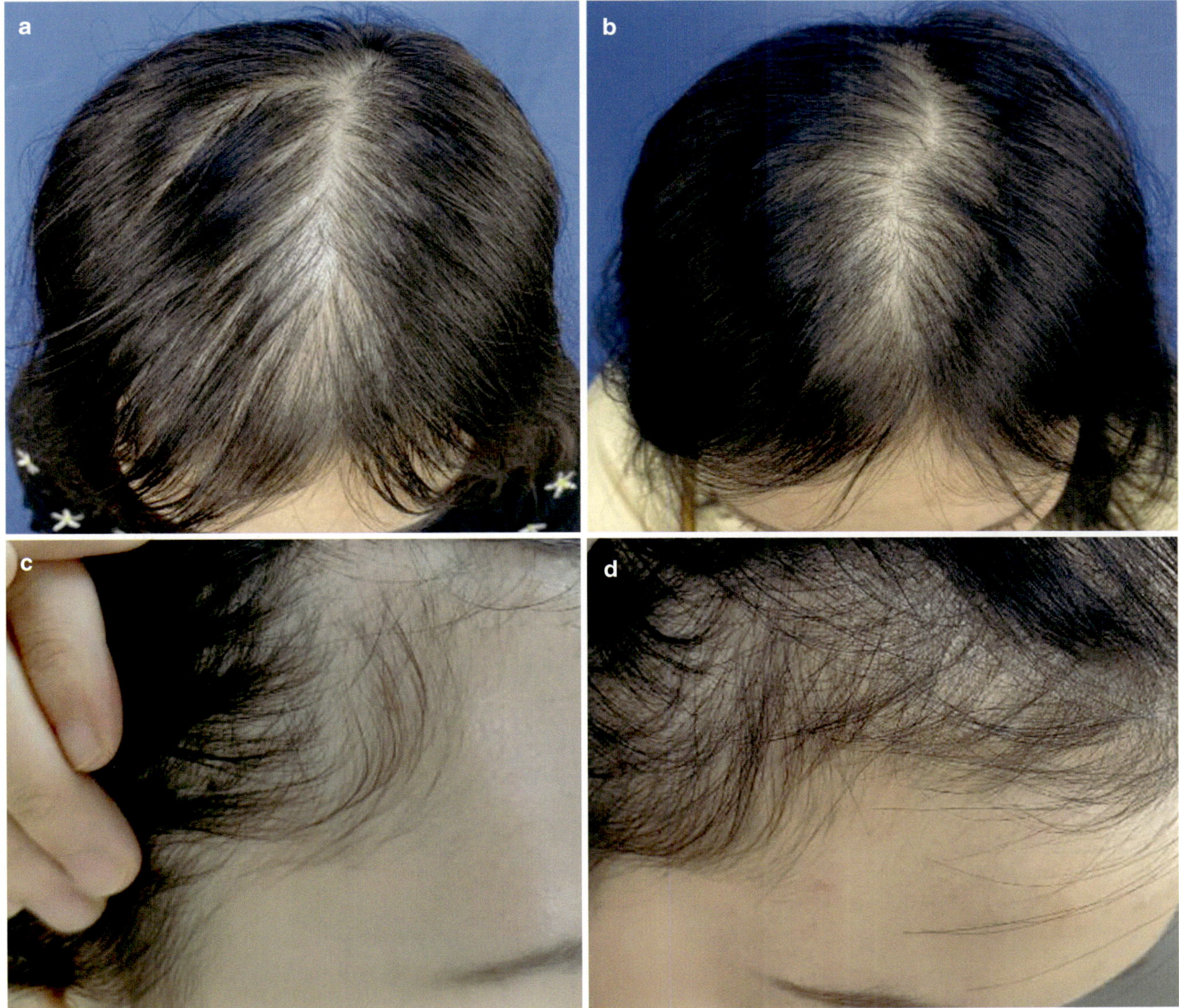

Fig. 6.5 Hairline and scalp hair regeneration after treatments of PRP: (**a**) 2021.10.09 Before first-time treatment, (**b**) 2021.11.11 Scalp hair regeneration after twice treatment, (**c**) 2021.10.09 Before first-time treatment, (**d**) 2021.11.11 Hairline condition after twice treatment

6.5.2 PRP Treatment for Patients with Alopecia Areata

Alopecia armata (AA) is a common clinical chronic inflammatory disease, which often presents as localized hair loss, bringing great psychological pressure to patients. The pathogenesis of AA is still unclear, but it is generally believed that the immune immunity of hair follicles is destroyed, and CD8+NKG2D+T lymphocytes release a large number of inflammatory factors, which leads to the impaired function of hair follicles and the early degeneration stage and then causes hair loss. Most of the existing treatments for AA have uncertain efficacy, and the most commonly used glucocorticoids have adverse reactions such as skin atrophy, telangiectasia, and weight gain. Platelet-rich plasma can promote the proliferation and differentiation of hair follicle stem cells and improve the surrounding environment of hair follicle, thus promoting hair growth, and has the potential to treat AA.

Trink et al. [9] conducted the first double-blind controlled study of PRP in the treatment of AA. In this study, 45 patients with multifocal AA with a course of disease over 2 years were randomly divided into PRP group, triamcinolone acetonide group and placebo group, and only half of the scalp was injected with the drug every month. The proportion was only 26.6% in the trianonide group, much lower than that in the PRP group. In addition, PRP group had more colored hair and improved ki-67 level in scalp;

pramcinolone acetonide group had better itching and burning sensation. The recurrence rate and the number of hair with malnutrition were lower than that of triamcinolone acetonide group. Sinahl's [10] 20 AA patients with a disease course of more than 2 years received PRP injection every month. After six treatments, all patients showed significant hair regeneration, and only one patient relapsed after 1 year of follow-up. In EI Taieb et al.'s study [11], 90 patients were randomly divided into three groups, group 1 5% minoxidil topical two times per day, 2 set of PRP injection once a month, the first. Three for the placebo group, 3 months after treatment the PRP group 70% type single stove or multifocal AA patients and 30% bald patients experienced significant hair regeneration, and minoxidil treatment group has no obvious difference, but PRP group had faster onset and more colored hair under dermoscopic observation, while improvement of nutritive hair, short vellus hair, and yellow spot sign was more obvious. In addition, this study found that PRP had a good effect only on single or multiple foci AA, a limited effect on alopecia generalis, and almost no effect on total alopecia. In Albalat et al.'s study [12], in order to compare the efficacy of PRP-wan glucocorticoid on AA, 80 patients were randomly divided into Yanaid group and PRP group, which received local injection once every 2 weeks. After 3–5 times of treatment, it was found that 72.5% of patients in PRP group achieved more than 70% hair regeneration, while 65% of patients in triamcinolone group achieved hair regeneration. There was no statistical difference between the increase in the number of hairs and the decrease in the number of hairs with malnutrition. After 6 months of follow-up, the recurrence rate was only 5% in the PRP group, compared with 25% in the triamcinolone acetonide group. These experimental results proved the effectiveness of PRP combined with drugs in the treatment of alopecia areata.

References

1. Sperling LC, Lupton GP. Histopathology of non-scarring alopecia. J Cutan Pathol. 2010;22(2):97.
2. Schneider MR, Schmidt-Ullrich R, Paus R. The hair follicle as a dynamic miniorgan. Curr Biol. 2009;19(3):R132–42.
3. Li ZJ, Choi H, Choi D, et al. Autologous platelet-rich plasma: a potential therapeutic tool for promoting hair growth. Dermatol Surg. 2012;38(7 Pt 1):1040–6.
4. Gupta AK, Carviel J. A mechanistic model of platelet-rich plasma treatment for androgenetic alopecia. Dermatol Surg. 2016;42(12):1335–9.
5. Gkini MA, Kouskoukis AE, Tripsianis G, et al. Study of platelet-rich plasma injections in the treatment of androgenetic alopecia through an one-year period. J Cutan Aesthet Surg. 2014;7(4):213–9.
6. Li L, Dong Y, Xu P, et al. Clinical observation of platelet-rich plasma in the treatment of androgenic alopecia. Chin J Aesthet Med. 2020;286(10):24–6.
7. Zhu M, Kong D, Tian R, et al. Platelet sonicates activate hair follicle stem cells and mediate enhanced hair follicle regeneration. J Cell Mol Med. 2020;24(2):1786.
8. Yuan S, Zhang L, Tang J, et al. Effect of platelet-rich plasma on the skin and follicle development of neonatal mice. Chin J Exp Surg. 2018;35(7):3.
9. Trink A, Sorbellini E, Bezzola P, et al. A randomized, double-blind, placebo-and active-controlled, half-head study to evaluate the effects of platelet-rich plasma on alopecia areata. Br J Dermatol. 2013;169(3):690–4.
10. Singh S. Role of platelet-rich plasma in chronic alopecia areata: our centre experience. Indian J Plast Surg. 2015;48(1):57–9.
11. EI Taieb MA, Ibrahim H, Nada EA, et al. Platelets rich plasma versus minoxidil 5% in treatment of alopecia areata: a trichoscopic evaluation. Dermatol Ther. 2017;30(1):e12437.
12. Albalat W, Ebrahim HM. Evaluation of platelet-rich plasma vs intralesional steroid in treatment of alopecia areata. J Cosmet Dermatol. 2019;18:1456. https://doi.org/10.1111/iocd.12858.

7 The Application of Platelet-Rich Plasma in Facial Rejuvenation

Xiaoxuan Lei, Liuhanghang Cheng, and Yu Yang

7.1 Introduction

The treatment of facial rejuvenation has been popularized among the general public. Facial aging is a common and complex biological process, influenced by intrinsic aging and external environmental factors such as ultraviolet radiation (UVR) and reactive oxygen species (ROS). The main signs of aging manifested are wrinkles, the atrophy of the epidermis and dermis, rough texture, telangiectasia, the loss of fat volume, and skin sagging.

The therapies of facial aging consist of injection of exogenous fillers and invasive surgery [1–3]. These injectables may have disadvantages such as persistent swelling and infections. At present, the most common form of platelet concentration and its derivatives in clinical application is platelet-rich plasma (PRP), while other forms include platelet concentration, platelet gel (PG), platelet-rich gel (PRG), platelet-rich fibrin (PRF), plasma rich in growth factors, concentrated growth factors and platelet lysates, etc. PRP, platelet concentrates obtained from autologous whole blood, composed of platelets, fibrin, and leukocytes [4]. Platelet activation and degranulation can release a host of growth factors such as transforming growth factor-β (TGF-β), platelet-derived growth factor (PDGF), vascular endothelial growth factor (VEGF), cytokines, microRNAs (miRNA), and other bioactive proteins to facilitate the repair and regeneration of tissue. The molecular and cellular mechanisms of PRP include the following:

1. These bioactive substances can target on a variety of skin cells to promote cell proliferation, matrix synthesis, and collagen deposition, thereby promoting tissue repair. In addition, several bioactive substances, such as serotonin, histamine, dopamine, calcium, and adenosine, are involved in multiple responses to tissue repair (Fig. 7.1) [5].
2. Platelet concentrate contains anti-inflammatory cytokines, which play a regulatory role in the inflammatory response of the body.
3. Platelet concentrate also contains adhesion factors such as fibrin, fibronectin, and hypolenin. They can locally construct three-dimensional structures required for tissue repair, wrap platelets, and white blood cells, prevent their loss, and provide scaffolds for the migration of repair cells, which is conducive to wound repair.
4. Platelet concentrate can induce the release of local growth/cytokines or other active substances (including microRNA) through autocrine, paracrine, and other ways to continuously promote wound healing.
5. Platelet activation releases chemokine, histamine, adenosine, Ig, and other bioactive substances, which can directly induce platelet aggregation or indirectly play a bactericidal role by chemotactic leukocytes. In recent years, PRP has been widely applied to treat facial aging and achieved excellent clinical outcomes.

X. Lei
Department of Burn and Plastic Surgery, General Hospital of Southern Theater Command, PLA, Guangzhou, Guangdong, China

L. Cheng
Department of Burn and Plastic Surgery, PLA General Hospital, Beijing, China

Y. Yang (✉)
Department of Plastic Surgery, The Third Affiliated Hospital of Guangzhou Medical University, Guangzhou, Guangdong, China

B. Cheng, X. Fu (eds.), *Platelet-Rich Plasma in Tissue Repair and Regeneration*, https://doi.org/10.1007/978-981-99-3193-4_7

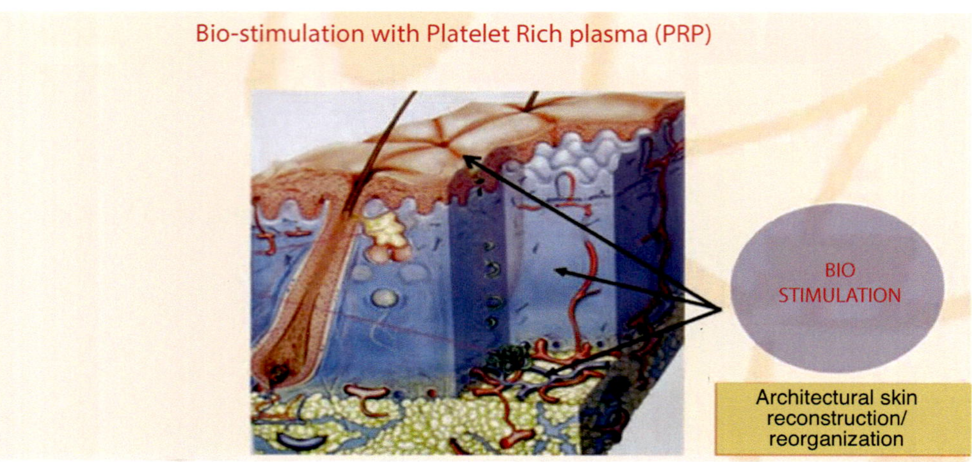

Fig. 7.1 Bio-stimulation with platelet-rich plasma

7.2 The Functional Mechanisms of PRP on Facial Rejuvenation

7.2.1 Platelet Concentrate Can Directly Promote Skin Renewal and Collagen Deposition

Platelet concentrate contains concentrated platelets, growth factors, leukocyte, fibrinogen/fibrin, and a host of proteins and electrolytes in blood, which have an excellent promotion effect on skin repair involved in accelerating granulation tissue formation, angiogenesis, and collagen deposition, preventing and reducing scar formation, and promoting re-epithelialization. In addition, it also has anti-inflammatory and antibacterial effects. Studies have shown that platelet concentrate can improve the quality of skin repair by activating proliferation of dermal fibroblasts and mesenchymal stem cells (MSCs) and promoting the secretion of endogenous hyaluronic acid (HA) and type I collagen. At the same time, it can adjust the proportion of type I and type III collagen, which plays a positive role in preventing and alleviating scar formation.

Platelet concentrate can increase the expression of MMP-1, MMP-3, and MMP-9 in matrix metalloproteinases protein (MMP) and then participate in the antiaging process by degrading collagen and other ECM and promote dermal regeneration, which promote new collagen deposition. Therefore, concentrated platelets, on the basis of clear light damage to the ECM, induce fibroblast synthesis of new collagen and reconstruct the ECM. Fibroblasts, in turn, proliferate through their stimulation, a virtuous cycle that improves the color, texture, and volume of the skin.

7.2.2 Platelet Concentrate Can Promote Neovascularization and Tissue Regeneration

Platelet can promote chemotaxis, cell adhesion, mitosis, proliferation, and angiogenesis. Neovascularization plays an important role in development, wound healing, and tissue and organ regeneration. The proportion of various angiogenic factors is crucial in the formation of new blood vessels. Platelet concentrates are rich in VEGF, thrombospondin-1 (Tsp-1), angiopoetin (Ang), and other angiogenic factors, which can stimulate the growth and migration of vascular endothelial cells, thereby inducing angiogenesis and promoting the formation of vascular sample tubular structure. Those events play a direct or key role in promoting angiogenesis and re-epithelialization.

7.2.3 Platelet Concentrates Release Bioactive Substances to Regulate Inflammatory Response

The microparticles released by platelets during activation contain some bioactive molecules, such as 5-hydroxytryptamine (5-HT), histamine, dopamine, calcium ions, and adrenaline, which can increase membrane permeability and regulate inflammatory response. Platelet concentrates contain a host of platelet-derived antibacterial peptides (PDAPs) such as platelet microbicidal protein-1 (TPMP-1) and platelet factor 4 (PF4), which have bacteriostatic and analgesic effects. In addition, leukocyte in platelet concentrate also plays a positive role in bacteriostatic/antibacterial and prevention and treatment of infectious lesions, but its role is controversial. At the same time, a variety

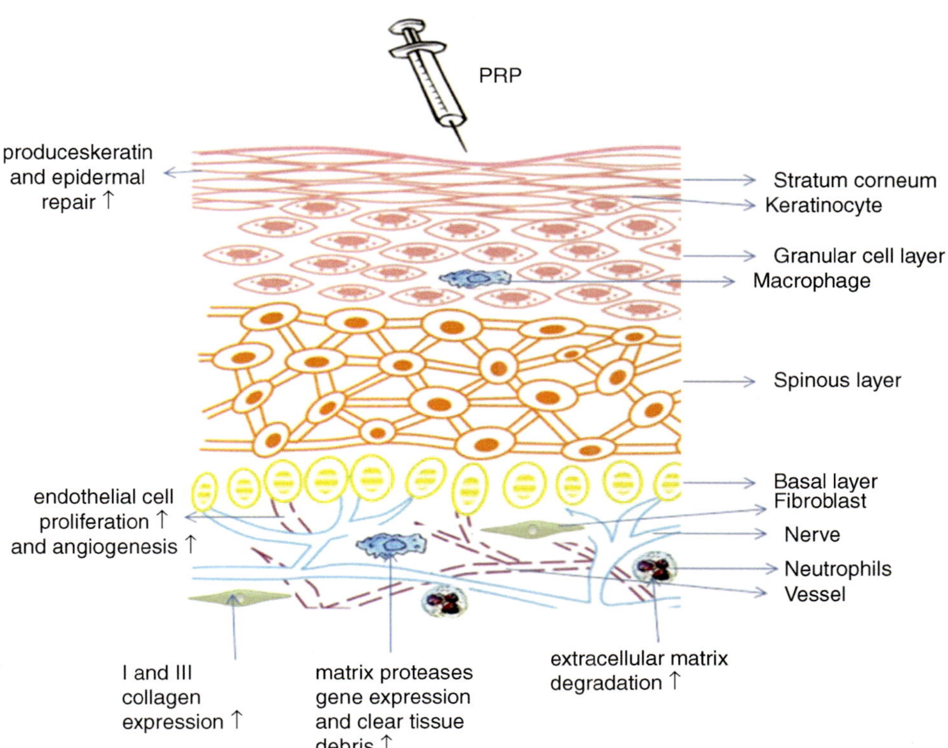

Fig. 7.2 The mechanisms of PRP on facial rejuvenation

of anti-inflammatory factors in platelet concentrate play an important role in the regulation of skin inflammatory reaction, contributing to reduce the noninfectious inflammatory reaction so as to reduce erythema, edema, and other effects (Fig. 7.2).

7.3 The Application of Facial Rejuvenation with PRP

7.3.1 The Treatment of PRP Alone on Facial Aging

Female adults underwent facial therapy by autologous PRP. All patients were taken three treatments every 4 weeks and were followed up for 3 months. The facial aging signs (turgor, smoothness, hydration, overall vitality) in PRP treatment group showed a significant improvement. Furthermore, PRP showed a sustained efficacy on the improvement of periorbital wrinkles (Figs. 7.3 and 7.4).

In another relevant study, patients were injected with PRP to treat facial wrinkles such as nasolabial folds and marionette lines and fill facial depression part such as supraorbital grooves and mid-cheek grooves. The results showed that patient's satisfaction was high. The mean time for treatment effects to appear was 2 months. PPR treatment improves the wrinkle severity grading (Figs. 7.5, 7.6, 7.7, 7.8, 7.9, 7.10, and 7.11).

In our previous study, an adult female with lip wrinkles and an adult male with sunburn were chosen to receive the treatment of PRP. After PRP treatment, the appearance of lip wrinkles, smoothness, and luminosity improved significantly. Furthermore, the male patients injected with PRP improved couperose skin and pigmentation (Fig. 7.12).

7.3.2 The Treatment of PRP with Adipose Tissue on Facial Aging

A systematic evaluation was conducted by Frautschi et al. [6] (n = 10) to compare the effect between PRP + fat transplantation and fat transplantation alone. The ratio of PRP and fat was 2:1. The results showed that PRP + fat transplantation had a better maintenance rate of facial contour than fat transplantation alone after 1 year. Another RCT (n = 49) observation showed that the mixture ratio of fat and PRP was 4:1. After 1 year, there was a significant difference between the PRP + fat transplantation group and the fat transplantation group.

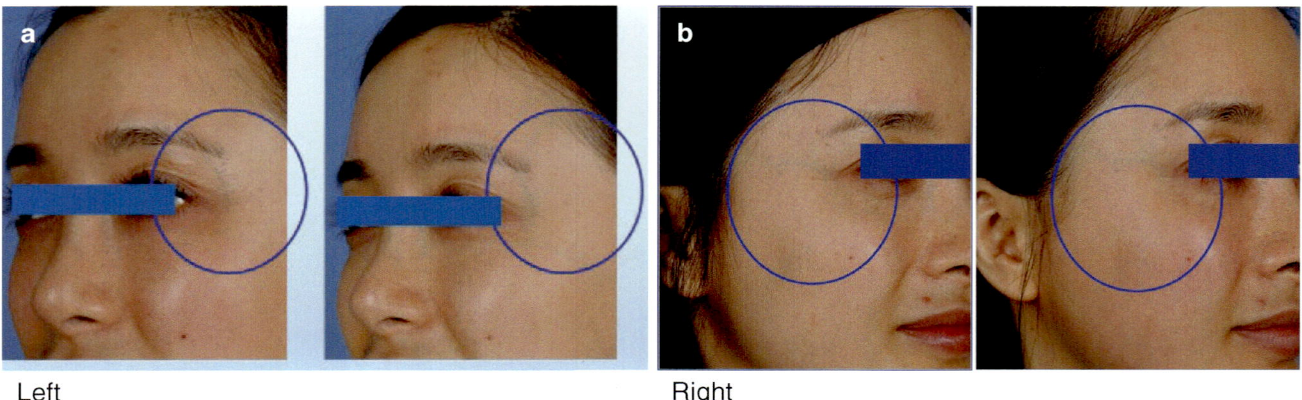

Fig. 7.3 A 30-year-old woman who was taken with the last treatment of PRP for 3 months showed a significant improvement of periorbital wrinkle. (**a**) Left, (**b**) right

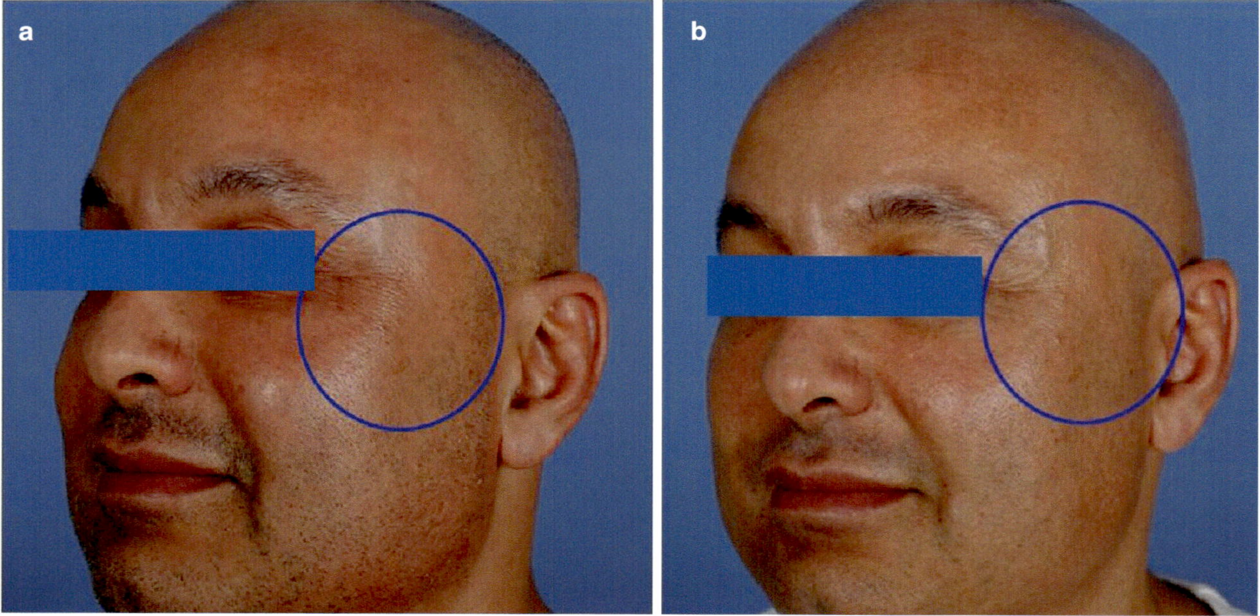

Fig. 7.4 A 45-year-old man who was taken with the last treatment of PRP for 3 months showed a significant improvement of periorbital wrinkle. (**a**) Before (left). (**b**) After (left)

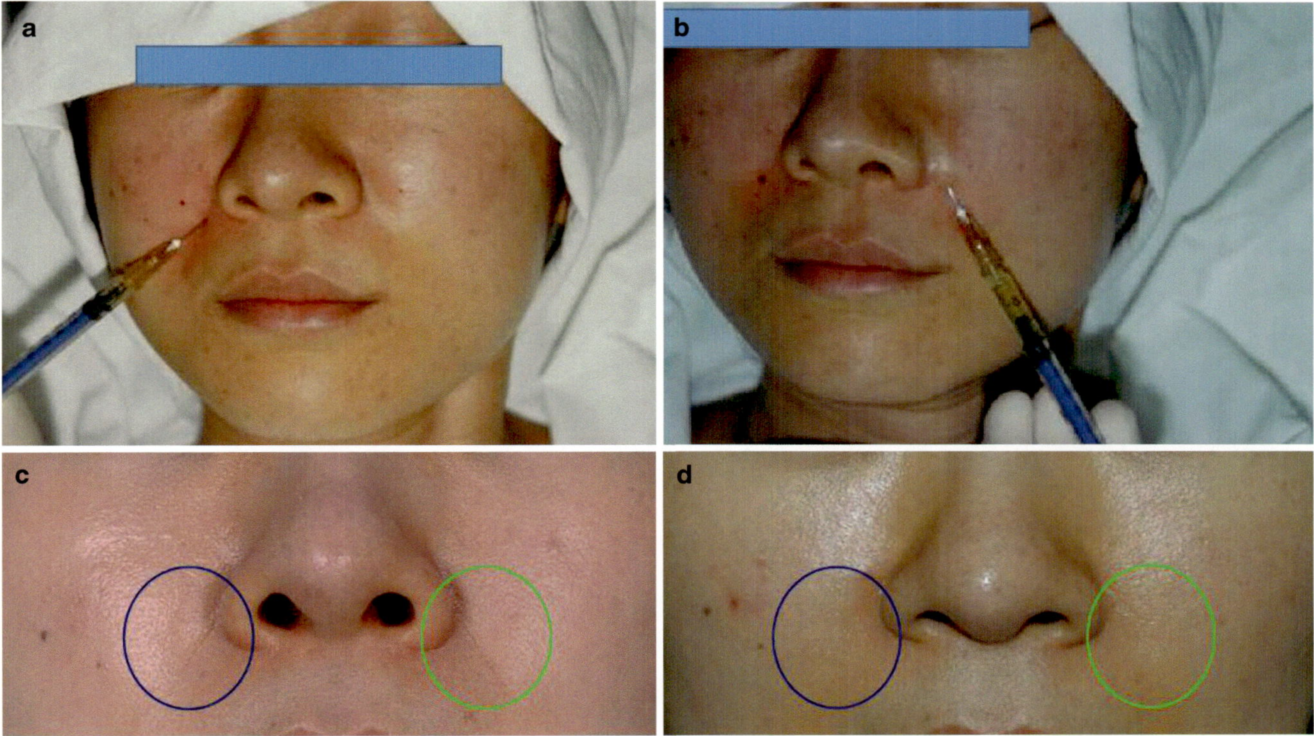

Fig. 7.5 Female adults were injected with 1 mL PRP into the nasolabial folds each side of the face. (**a**, **c**) Before treatment. (**b**, **d**) Two months after the first treatment. The nasolabial fold of patients showed a significant improvement by PRP treatment

In 2018, Motosko et al. [7] evaluated the efficacy of PRP + fat transplantation in facial rejuvenation (n = 437). The results showed that the optimal ratio of fat and PRP mixture was 2:1–10:1. Meanwhile, the results also confirmed that adding PRP into transplanted fat could contribute to maintain facial volume.

7.3.3 The Treatment of PRP with Other Photoelectric Therapies on Facial Aging

In 2015, a systematic evaluation was conducted by Sclafani and Azzi [8] using a RCT study (n = 22) to compare the efficacy of PRP combined with fractional laser and fractional laser alone in facial rejuvenation. The study found that PRP combined with fractional laser could improve patients' satisfaction and skin elasticity and reduce erythema index.

In 2017, Ulusal [9] conducted eight times of PRP treatment for patients. After treatment, general appearance, skin laxity, and skin texture are significantly improved. The degree of cosmetic improvement and patients' satisfaction were directly correlated with the number of treatments, while the average score of skin pigmentation improvement was not directly correlated with the number of treatments. Adverse reactions included transient mild edema, ecchymosis more than 10 days in 8% patients, and no obvious or persistent adverse reactions.

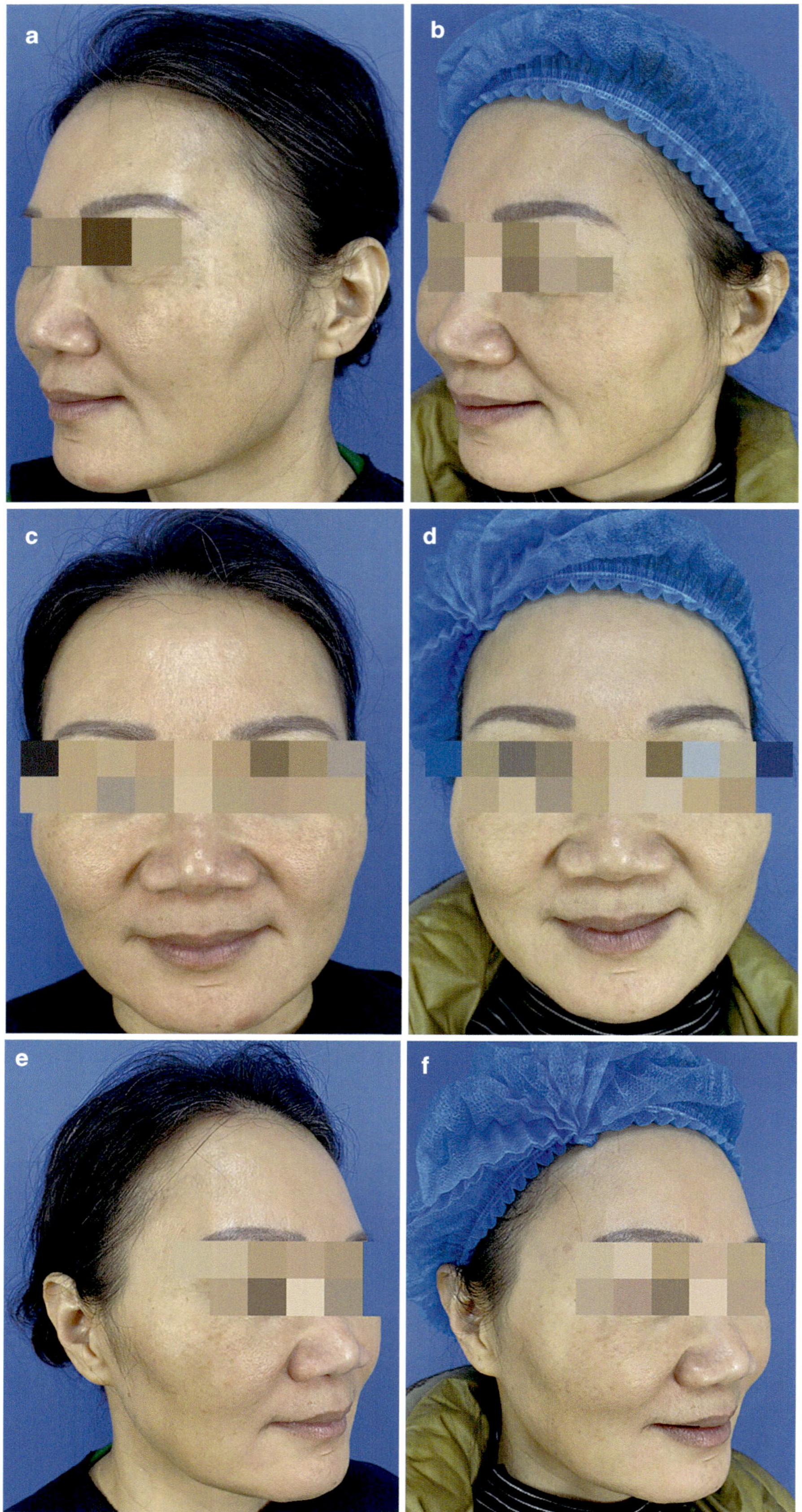

Fig. 7.6 The application of PRP in facial rejuvenation. (**a**, **c**, **e**) 2021.11.02 Before the treatment. (**b**, **d**, **f**) 2021.12.31 After the treatment. (**g–i**) Visia comparison

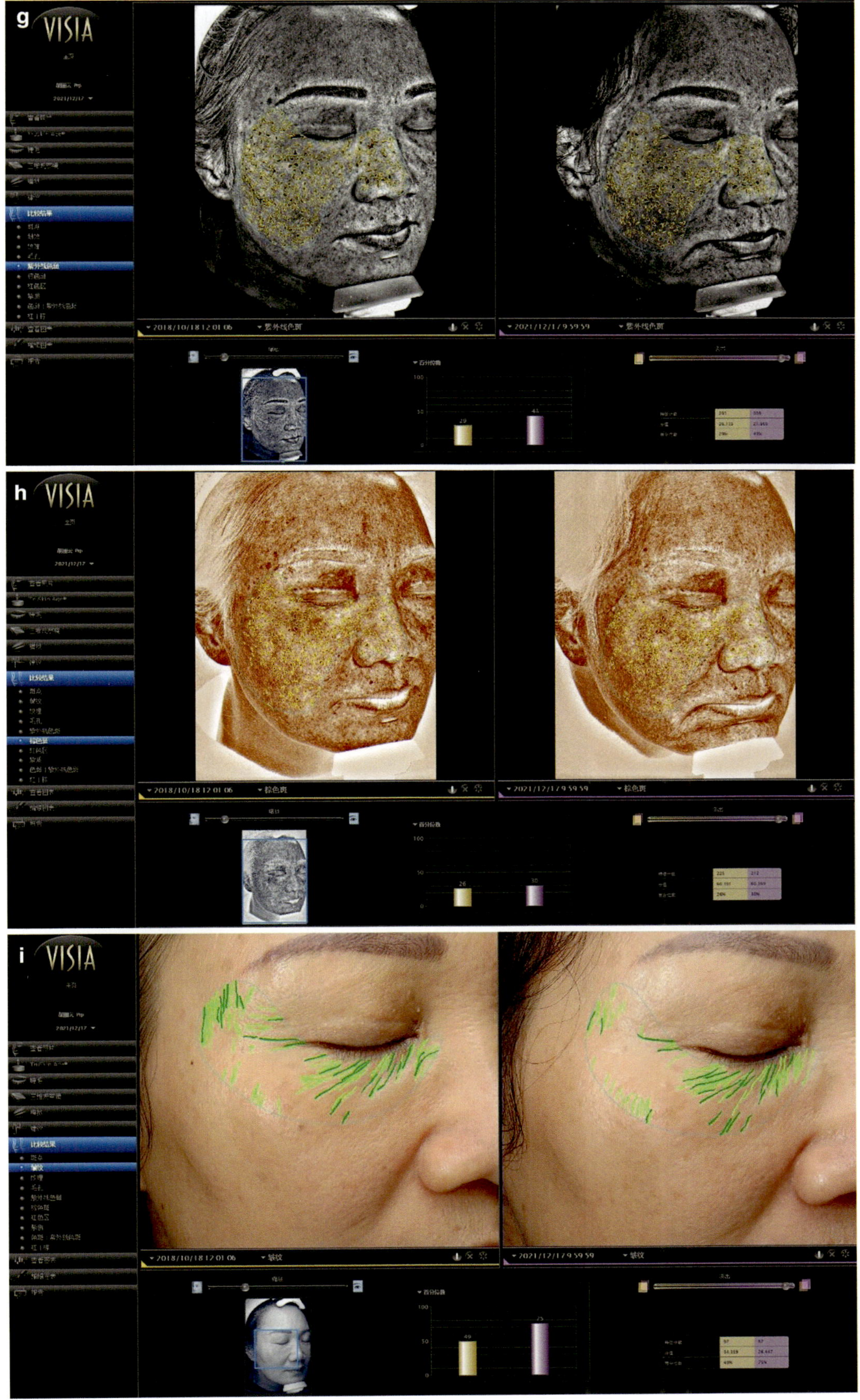

Fig. 7.6 (continued)

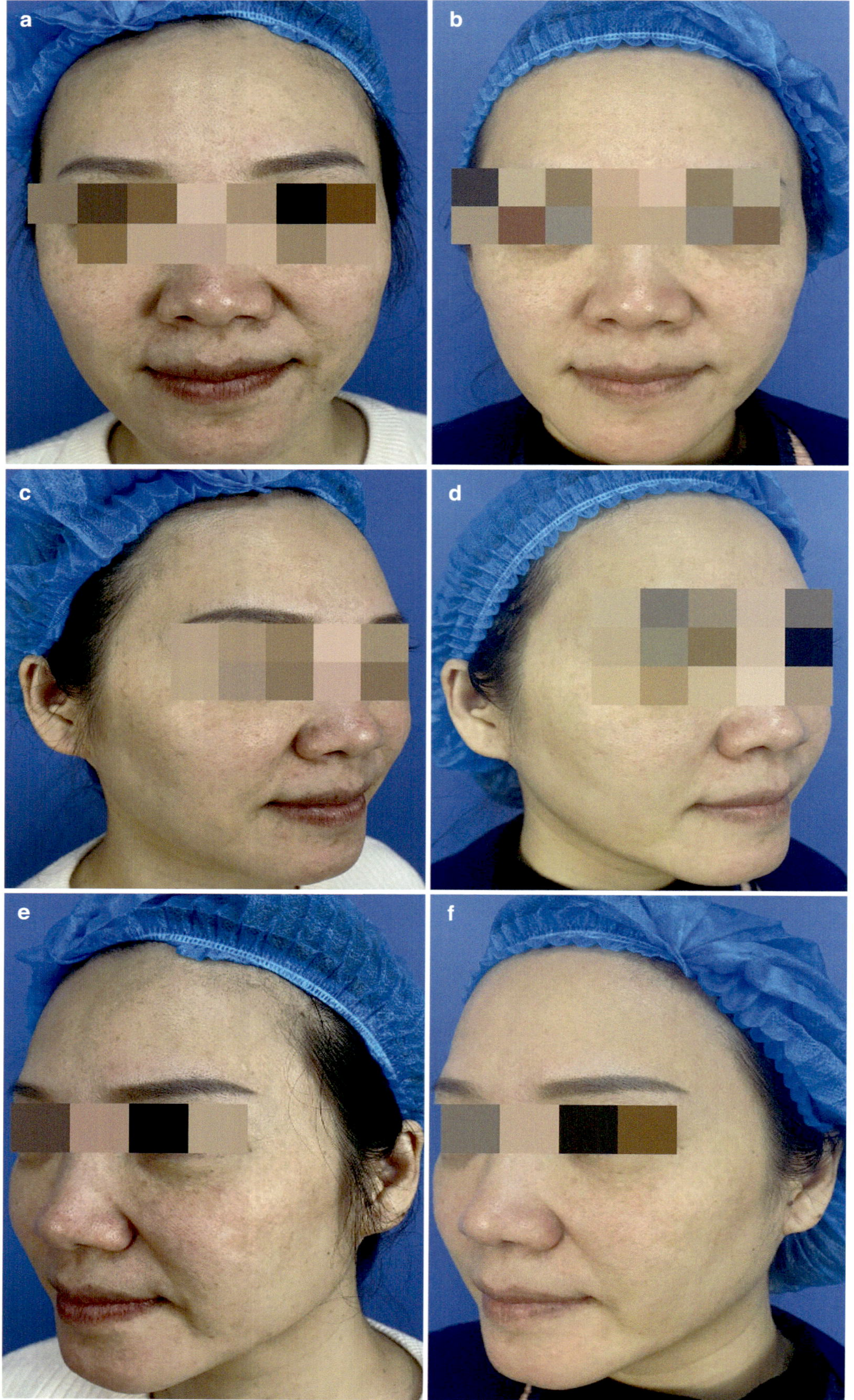

Fig. 7.7 The application of PRP in facial rejuvenation. (**a**, **c**, **e**) 2021.11.15 Before the treatment. (**b**, **d**, **f**) 2021.12.07 After the treatment

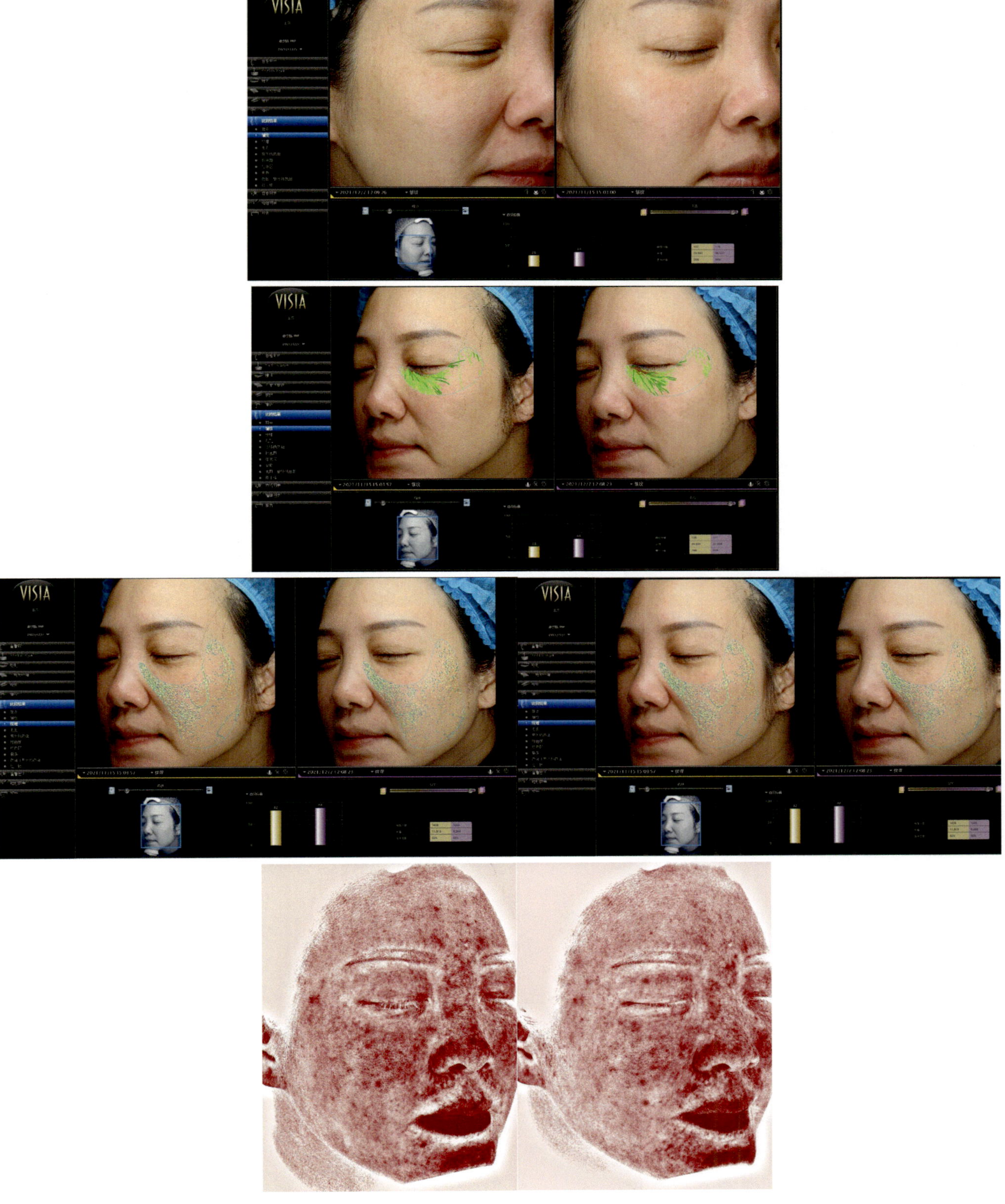

Fig. 7.8 One month after the treatment of PRP showing a significant improvement of peri-orbit wrinkles, pore bulky

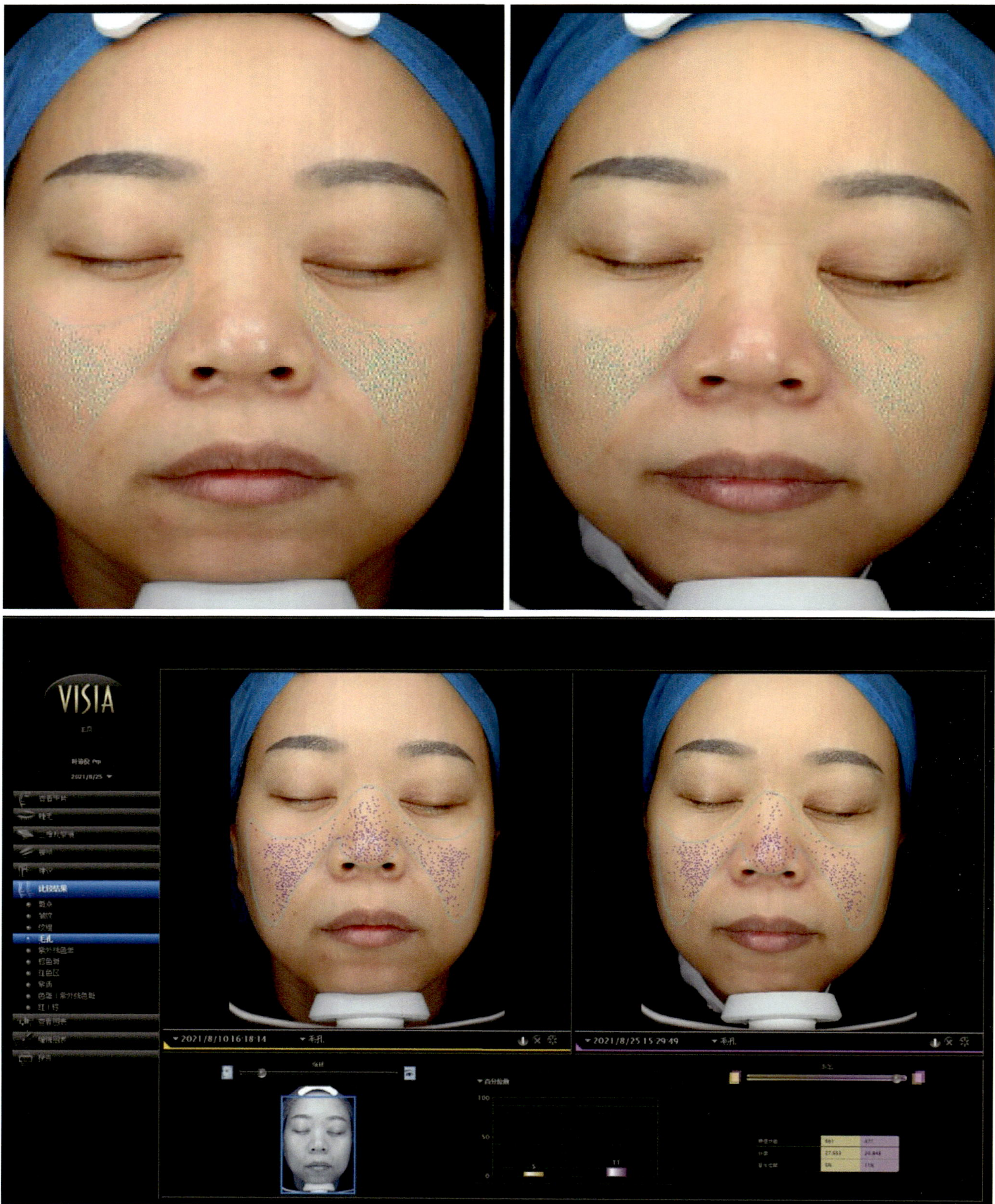

Fig. 7.9 One month after the treatment of PRP showing a significant improvement of peri-orbit wrinkles, pore bulky

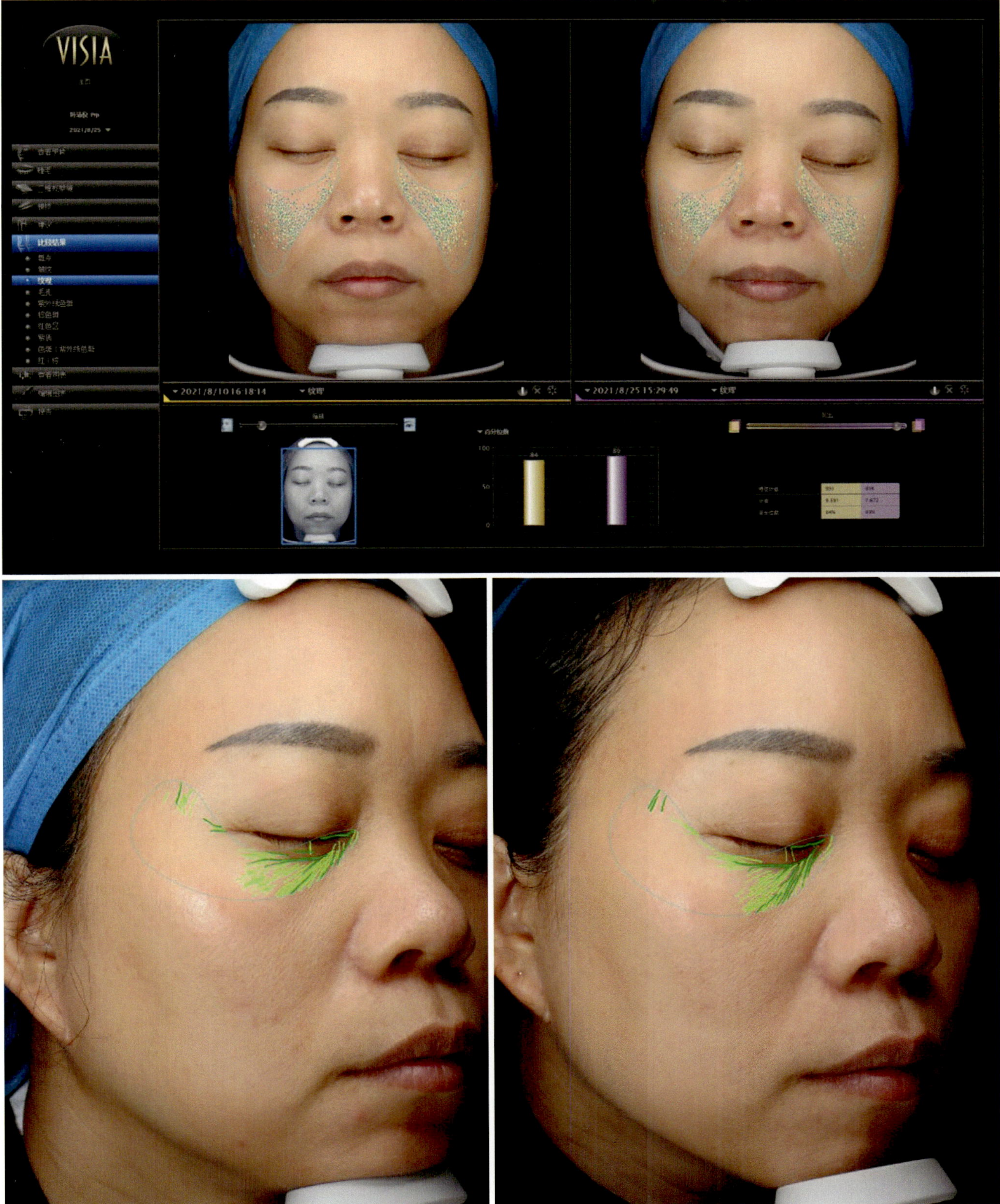

Fig. 7.9 (continued)

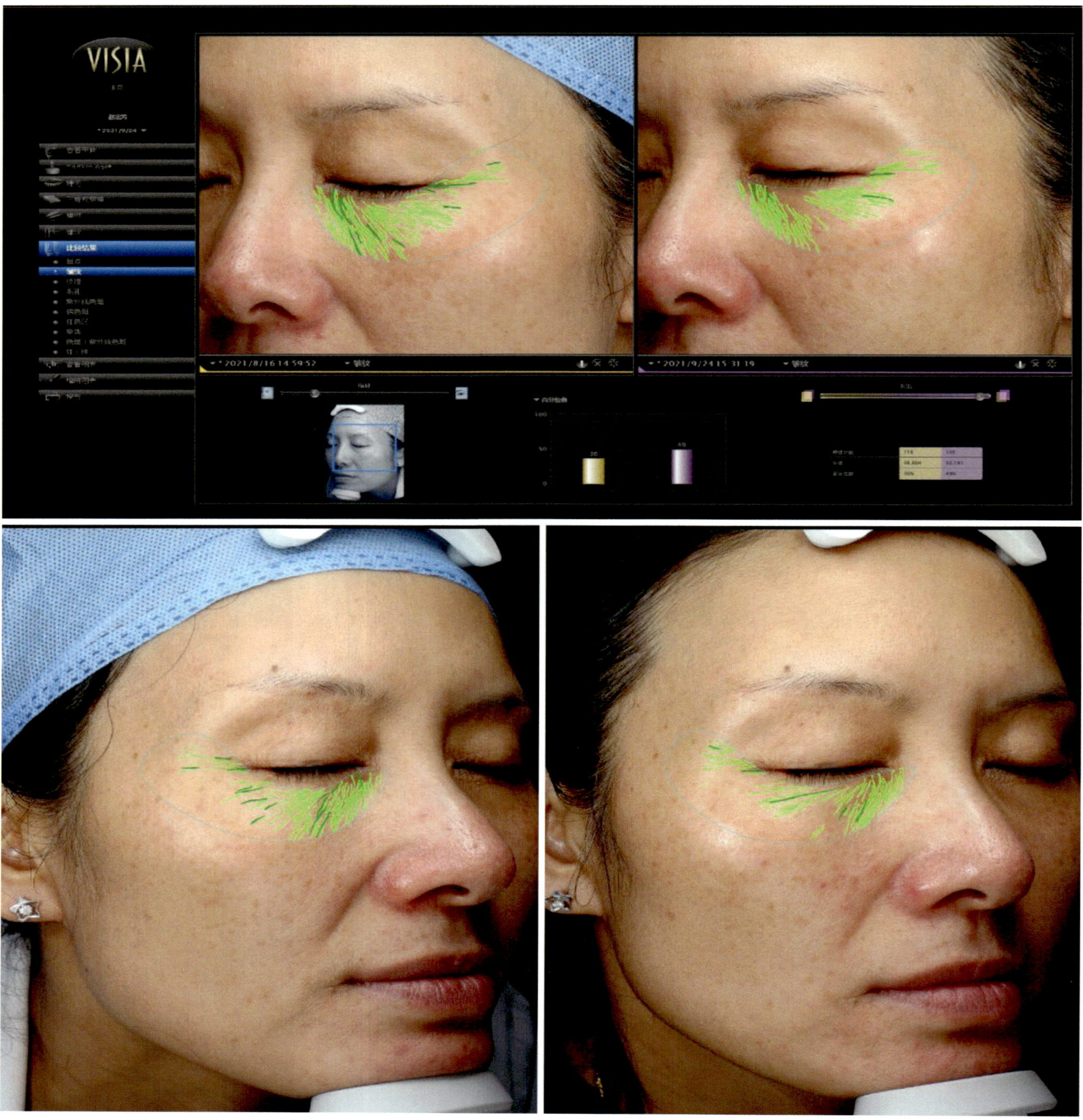

Fig. 7.10 After the treatment of PRP showing a significant improvement of peri-orbit wrinkles, pore bulky

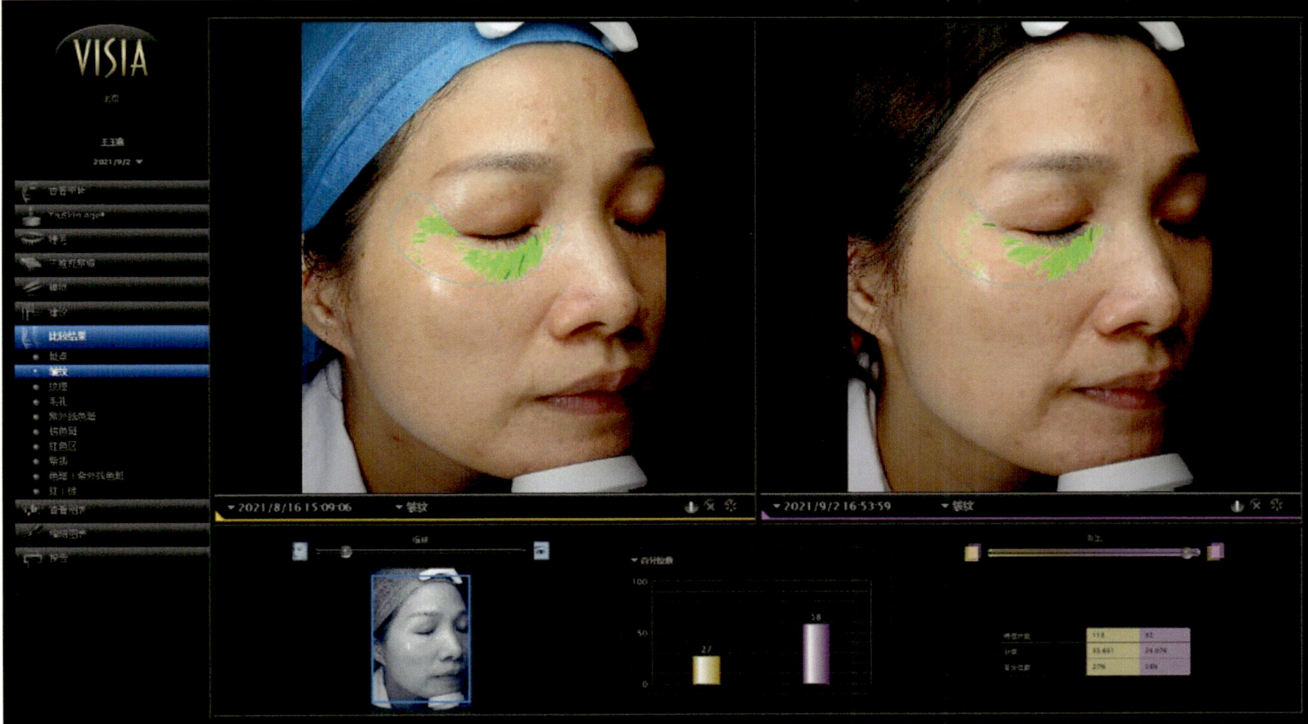

Fig. 7.10 (continued)

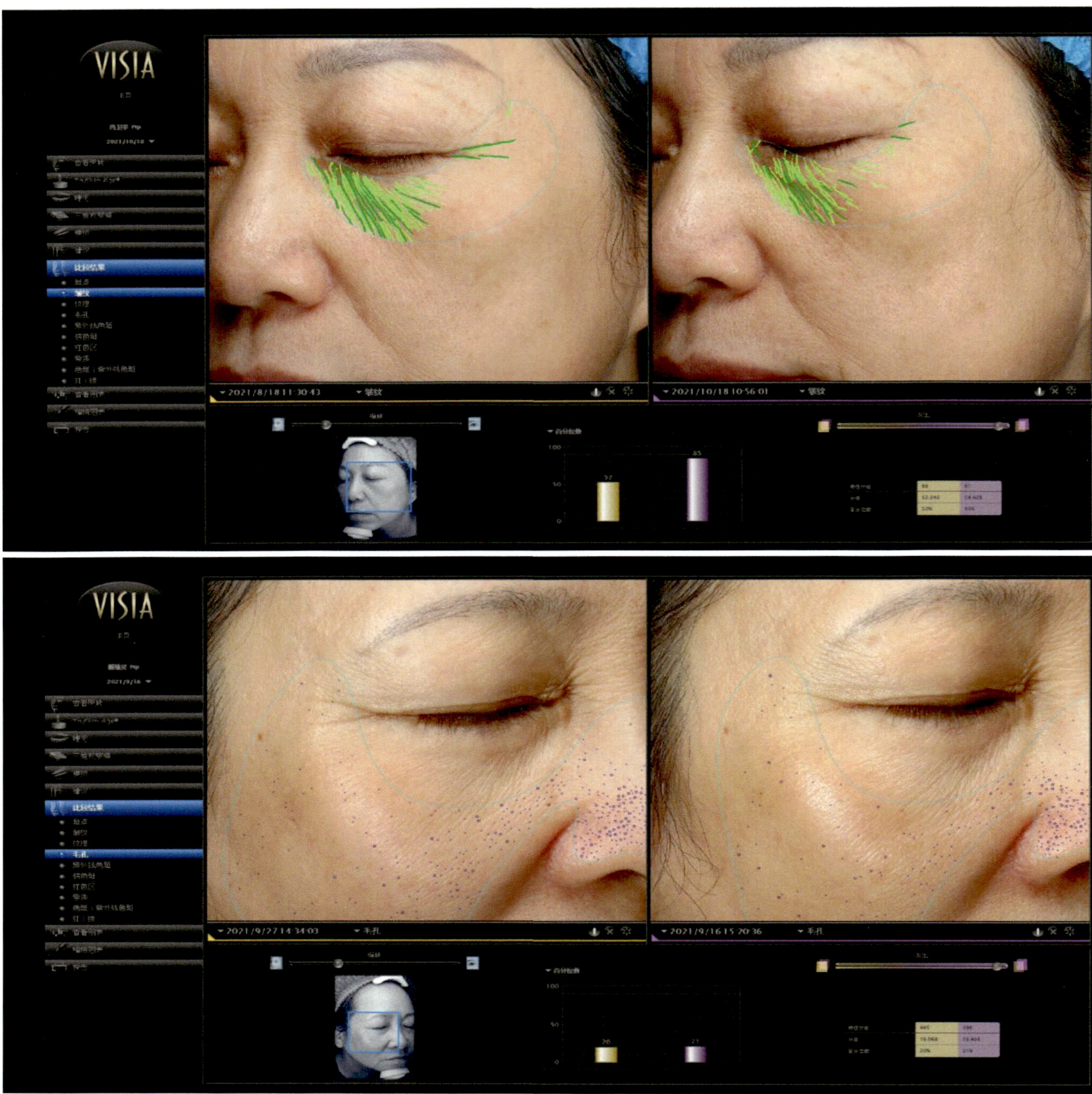

Fig. 7.11 After the treatment of PRP showing a significant improvement of peri-orbit wrinkles, pore bulky

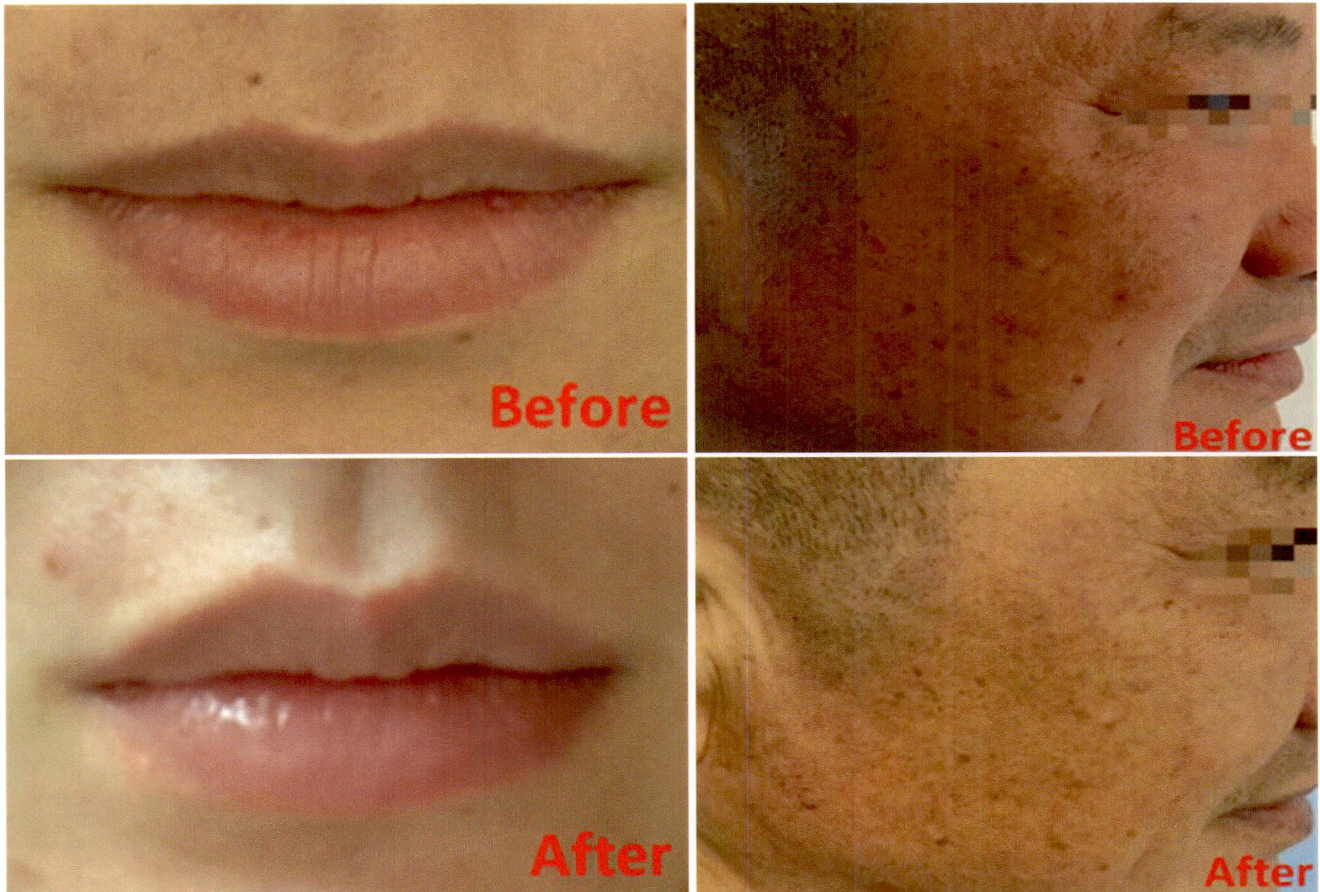

Fig. 7.12 Treatment of PRP for facial rejuvenation. (**a**) Front view of a 28-year-old woman; 1 month after the treatment of PRP showing a significant improvement of lip wrinkles (left). (**b**) Right view of a 55-year-old man; 1 month after the treatment of PRP showing a significant improvement of couperose skin and pigmentation (right)

7.4 The Treatment and Notes of PRP

7.4.1 Assessment of Facial Problems, Preoperative Photographing Method, and Informed Consent

Experts suggest: Related matters should be communicated with the patients and their families. The possible outcomes should be informed and informed consent should be signed. Preoperative multi-angle photography is required to collect data.

7.4.2 Control of Systemic State

Albumin >30 g/L, hemoglobin >60 g/L, white blood cell <300 × 10^9/L, postprandial blood glucose <11 mmol/L, correct hypoxemia, maintained normal thyroxine level, correct electrolyte, and acid-base imbalance.

Experts suggest: In general, it is not recommended to inject with autologous concentrated blood for facial rejuvenation only if several indexes are below the lower limit of normal values.

7.4.3 Control of Local Condition

Preoperative facial cleansing must be performed routinely. Iodophor or 75% ethanol is used for disinfection. Surface anesthesia (e.g., 5% lidocaine cream) should be performed at the injection area, and the time of anesthesia should be held flexibly according to the drug instructions and skin sensitivity. Block anesthesia of the main facial nerves (supraorbital, infraorbital, and mental nerves) may also be used.

Experts suggest: Before the application of platelet concentrate products, the facial treatment area should be as clean as possible, and appropriate anesthesia should be adopted.

7.4.4 Collect Blood and Preparation Technology

The blood is collected from the anterior cubital vein, and appropriate blood can be taken according to the treatment needs, usually 10–50 mL. The platelet concentrates are generally 1/10–1/8 of the blood collected.

Experts suggest: It is necessary to set the corresponding preparation parameters according to different centrifugal equipment; platelets in venous blood and PRP should be detected before and after preparation to ensure that qualified PRP, PRF, CGF, and platelet lysates are obtained. The concentration of platelet concentrate products is recommended to be above 1000 × 10^9/L.

7.4.5 The Method of PRP Therapy

After disinfection, skin surface anesthesia is performed. Active or inactive PRP is extracted into 1 mL syringe with 30G fine needle. Then, the needle was injected into the dermis or subcutaneous tissue at an angle of 45° along the direction of wrinkles. The optimal concentration of PRP is 3–8 times to the whole blood. After treatment, ice compress for 15–20 min. The treatment of facial rejuvenation can achieve a significantly therapeutic effect after 1–3 injections, and alopecia needs to be treated with 3–6 injections.

The following conditions are not suitable for this treatment

1. Platelet dysfunction syndrome
2. Severe hypokalemia
3. Systemic sepsis
4. Facial infection
5. Those who are unwilling to accept the risk of treatment of blood products
6. Anticoagulant allergy
7. Those who suffer from mental illness or have too high expectation for treatment

Notes after treatment:

1. Do not get water on the treatment site within 24 h after injection.
2. Mild bruising at the injection site is normal.
3. If the injection site has redness, swelling, heat, and pain, consult with the doctor immediately.
4. Avoid taking the spicy foods for 1 week after treatment.
5. Avoid taking aspirin for 1 week after treatment.
6. Pay attention to sunscreen at the treatment site.

References

1. Innocenti M, Ramoni S, Doria C, Antropoli C, Garbagna N, Grossi E, Veraldi S. Treatment of periocular wrinkles with topical nifedipine. J Dermatolog Treat. 2010;21:282–5.
2. Gold MH, Biron JA, Sensing W. Facial skin rejuvenation by combination treatment of IPL followed by continuous and fractional radiofrequency. J Cosmet Laser Ther. 2016;18:2–6.
3. Beeson W, Woods E, Agha R. Tissue engineering, regenerative medicine, and rejuvenation in 2010: the role of adipose-derived stem cells. Facial Plast Surg. 2011;27:378–87.
4. Harrison P, Cramer EM. Platelet alpha-granules. Blood Rev. 1993;7:52–62.
5. Alsousou J, Thompson M, Hulley P, Noble A, Willett K. The biology of platelet-rich plasma and its application in trauma and orthopaedic surgery: a review of the literature. J Bone Joint Surg Br. 2009;91:987–96.

6. Frautschi RS, Hashem AM, Halasa B, et al. Current evidence for clinical efficacy of platelet rich plasma in aesthetic surgery: a systematic review. Aesthet Surg J. 2017;37(3):353–60.
7. Motosko CC, Khouri KS, Poudrier G, et al. Evaluating platelet-rich therapy for facial aesthetics and alopecia: a critical review of the literature. Plast Reconstr Surg. 2018;141(5):1115–23.
8. Sclafani AP, Azzi J. Platelet preparations for use in facial rejuvenation and wound healing: a critical review of current literature. Aesthet Plast Surg. 2015;39(4):495–505.
9. Ulusal BG. Platelet-rich plasma and hyaluronic acid an efficient biostimulation method for face rejuvenation. J Cosmet Dermatol. 2017;16(1):112–9.

8 Platelet-Rich Plasma and Skin Pigmentation

Weidong Zhu and Yu Yang

Whether hyperpigmentation or hypopigmentation, abnormal skin pigmentation has become a common disease. Ultraviolet irradiation is the main cause of various skin pigmentation diseases, often leading to skin tanning, melasma, and other excessive pigmentations, but can also lead to skin pigmentation loss (such as vitiligo). Therefore, skin pigmentation is a complex, changeable, and highly responsive pathological process to changes in the microenvironment.

Epidermal melanin is synthesized by melanocytes that provide melanin to keratinocytes in the proximal basal layer of the epidermis to resist ultraviolet irradiation. Melanocytes originate from the neural crest and contain the organelle that synthesizes melanin, the melanosome. Melanosomes contain a large number of proteins and enzymes associated with melanogenesis. For example, microphthalmia-associated transcription factor (MITF) is a key transcription factor in melanosomes that regulates melanin formation and activates transcription of tyrosinase. Tyrosinase (TYR) is a key rate-limiting enzyme for melanogenesis in melanosomes, which is translated in the endoplasmic reticulum and glycosylated in the Golgi apparatus [1], and its activity is limited to melanosome. Melanosomes also contain proteins associated with TYR activity, such as tyrosine-associated protein 1 (TYRP1) and tyrosine-associated protein 2 (TYRP2).

Melanosomes mature and synthesize melanin over four periods. Stage I melanosomes are composed of intraluminal vesicles and irregular PMEL protein fibrils, which become stage II melanosomes when irregular fibrils are transformed into ordered stripes along the long axis of the melanosome. After transporting enzymes such as TYR and TYRP1, melanin is synthesized and deposited on PMEL fibers, producing dense streaks with stage III melanosome characteristics. Melanin further accumulates in the organelles until stage IV melanosomes are reached, that is, fully colored mature melanosomes. The maturation capacity of melanosomes determines the degree of epidermal pigmentation. The maturation ability of melanosomes has obvious racial differences, and the melanosomes of most white races only stay in stage II melanosomes [2]. Studies have shown that melanosomes in dark skin are larger, more pigmented, and transferred more to keratinocytes than white skin [3]. In addition to genetic heterogeneity, the function of melanocytes is affected by a variety of stimuli, such as ultraviolet irradiation, inflammatory stimulation, estrogen, etc.; abnormal melanocytes can lead to hyperpigmentation (such as melasma) or hypopigmentation (such as vitiligo).

Studies have shown no significant difference in the number of melanocytes in the epidermis of different human races. Therefore, except for melanocytosis (blue nevus, mongolian spot, nevus of ota, and melanocytoma, etc.) or melanocytopenia diseases (vitiligo), most pigmentation disorders such as melasma, skin tanning, etc. are related to changes in the ability of melanocytes to synthesize melanin, and there is no significant change in the number of melanocytes. Therefore, whitening products should avoid containing melanocyte toxic ingredients to avoid irreversible hypopigmentation or depigmentation. And in whitening products, gentle, controllable, and physiological are the primary factors that beauty seekers should consider.

Platelets are closely related to pigmentation. From the genetic view, platelets and the genes that regulate pigment are located on the same chromosome; Swank et al. [4] found that the mouse gunmetal pigment mutant has obvious thrombocytopenia and platelet dysfunction, while the autosomal recessive genetic disease unique to humans, Hermansky-Pudlak syndrome [1] (commonly known as albinism-platelet disease), also shows albinism of the eyes and skin and platelet defects caused by hemorrhagic diathesis. At the organelle level, the melanocytes that determine pigment synthesis are the same as the medium-dense particles and α particles of platelets belonging to lysosomal-associated organelles

W. Zhu (✉)
Department of Burn and Plastic Surgery, General Hospital of Southern Theater Command, PLA, Guangzhou, Guangdong, China

Y. Yang
Department of Plastic Surgery, The Third Affiliated Hospital of Guangzhou Medical University, Guangzhou, Guangdong, China

B. Cheng, X. Fu (eds.), *Platelet-Rich Plasma in Tissue Repair and Regeneration*, https://doi.org/10.1007/978-981-99-3193-4_8

(LRO), and the genes that control the biogenesis or regulation of platelet-dense granules also play a role in melanocyte formation [5]. A more intuitive understanding of our clinicians is the treatment of melasma by tranexamic acid, as well as the antiplatelet and anti-pigment properties of tretinoin, the combination of "hemostasis" and "reduced pigmentation."

The melanogenesis capacity of melanocytes is highly responsive to changes in the microenvironment, in which the microenvironment redox disorder is the key. Redox imbalance in the skin microenvironment affects the pigment synthesis function of melanocytes in both directions. Platelets, because of their small size, travel in various microcirculations. When the tissue microenvironment changes, platelets can respond quickly and produce factors that regulate the local conditions. Therefore, tiny platelets are not simply responsible for the body's hemostasis function.

PRP is a derivative of autologous whole blood, and its role is mainly exerted by the large number of active ingredients released by the enriched platelets after activation. These include a variety of growth factors such as PDGF (platelet-derived growth factor), VEGF (vascular endothelial growth factor), TGF-β (transforming growth factor), bFGF (basic fibroblast growth factor), etc., as well as active ingredients such as lipids and small RNA or extracellular vesicles with membrane structure. Studies have found that these growth factors are associated with pigment metabolism in the skin.

This chapter focuses on the operability and potential possibilities of PRP when applying skin pigment diseases.

8.1 PRP and Skin Hyperpigmentation

Long-term exposure of the skin to ultraviolet irradiation (mainly UVB) leads to an increase in melanocyte pigment synthesis, which is, in effect, a self-protective function of the skin to ensure that keratinocytes are protected from DNA damage caused by ultraviolet rays. However, excessive pigment synthesis and exceeding the metabolic capacity of the epidermis will cause pigmentation such as melasma, skin tanning (photoaging), and so on.

TGF-β is a growth factor with a wide range of cell targets, involved in the growth and functional regulation of various types of cells. At present, a large number of studies have confirmed that TGF-β is involved in the regulation of pigment synthesis of melanocytes. Klar et al. [6] found that adipose-derived mesenchymal stem cells secrete TGF-β1 to inhibit melanogenesis in melanoma cells and reduce skin pigmentation. TGF-β1 is one of the main growth factors released after platelet activation (especially in extracellular vesicles released by platelets). Hofng et al. [7] found that patients with melasma had significantly reduced pigmentation after PRP treatment and that TGF-β in lesions were widely expressed in various layers of skin tissue. Therefore, TGF-β1 may be one of the main components of PRP regulating melanocyte pigment synthesis.

Studies have shown that long-term ultraviolet irradiation can cause melanocytes to senescence, and senescent melanocytes will show a state of high melanin synthesis [8]. The occurrence of cellular senescence is greatly related to the excessive oxidative stress of the microenvironment, and PRP is rich in various growth factors and active ingredients that regulate the cell cycle, which can regulate cell senescence, alleviate the oxidative stress state of cells, and then reduce the stress of the endoplasmic reticulum in cells. Cui et al. [9] (Cheng Biao's team) did the corresponding basic research and found that melanocytes after PRP intervention showed stronger antioxidant capacity to combat cellular DNA damage and oxidative stress caused by UVB and alleviate the increase in melanin synthesis caused by excessive oxidative stress of melanocytes, and the molecular mechanism exploration found that the PI3K/AKT/GSK3β signaling pathway plays an important role in it. The discovery of this mechanism gives us more evidence to support our previous suspicion that PRP regulates exogenous skin pigmentation by regulating the oxidative stress state of the microenvironment, including radiant pigmentation (photoaging, melasma, etc.). The chief editor team has applied PRP to treat multiple melasma patients and achieved significant improvements. In addition, clinical reports of PRP in the treatment of melasma have also been reported [10, 11]. However, a high-quality clinical study did not find an effect of PRP on pigment changes in facial photoaging [12]. Therefore, the mechanism of PRP for the treatment of exogenous pigmentation may be more complex than we think, and what may be more important is the adaptive selectivity of different microenvironments.

The most common disease of skin pigmentation caused by ultraviolet irradiation is melasma. Melasma is common in female patients with Fitzpatrick skin grades III–V, in which the epidermal melanocytes mostly have fully functional melanosomes (stages III and IV), so once stimulated, it may lead to increased melanosome function. Recent studies have found that the triggers for melasma include an increase in stem cell factors and nerve and vascular growth factors. In addition, basic research has found that platelet-derived growth factor (PDGF) and basic fibroblast growth factor (bFGF) can promote the proliferation of melanocytes and melanin synthesis [13–17]. PRP rich in these growth factors has been reported by several clinical studies to reduce the pigmentation of melasma; also the chief editor's own team also tried to apply PRP in the treatment of melasma and found that it can achieve the effect of reducing pigmentation. However, clinical cases have been reported in which no effect of PRP on the pigmentation of chloasma was observed. Therefore, we speculate that PRP treatment of melasma is not simply regulated by growth factors; we think it also involves complex microenvironment regulation and platelet component selection (component selection of extracellular vesicles). It is well known that platelet lysis is a way of releasing all the components of platelets and is also a way of activating PRP. Cheng Biao's team treated the cultured primary human epidermal melanocytes (PHEMC) by applying platelet lysate to find that this platelet-full component activation fluid produced significant morphological changes to melanocytes, making the melanocyte cell body hypertrophied and the pseudopod shortened but increasing (Fig. 8.1). We speculate that this morphological change may imply that PRP breaks down the distribution form of epidermal melanocytes. Although further research found that this all-component activating fluid (PL) reduced the proliferative capacity of melanocytes, it increased its melanin content (Fig. 8.2). Therefore, platelets may have ingredients that promote pigment synthesis (e.g., PDGF, bFGF) and inappropriate activation patterns, or PRP that has not been screened for ingredients may not be suitable for the treatment of exogenous pigmentation.

However, the one-sided increase in melanocyte melanin content test does not indicate that PRP promotes pigmentation, because the increase in pigmentation depends not only on the pigment synthesis ability of melanocytes but also on the ability of melanocytes to deliver melanin. Mutations encoding melanocyte transport-related molecular genes such as myosin Va, RAB27A, and SLAC-2A have been found to cause human pigment diseases, known as Griscelli syndrome, which is characterized by dilution of skin and hair color [18, 19]. Melanosome biogenesis begins in the perinuclear region, is transferred through microtubules to the end of the dendrite, and is transferred from actin filaments to nearby keratin-forming cells [20, 21]. Studies have shown that after interrupting melanosome movement, melanin accumulates around the nucleus and the pseudopodia shortens [22]. This phenomenon is similar to that found by Cheng Biao's team, that is, after PRP treatment, the melanocyte cell body becomes larger (possibly caused by melanosome aggregation) and the pseudopod shortens (melanosome transport is restricted). Therefore, we speculate that PRP may have the ability to interrupt the movement of melanosomes, causing melanin to accumulate in melanocytes, leading to an increase in melanin content test. But in what way is this accumulation of melanin in melanocytes metabolized?

Autophagy may be one of its metabolic methods. Ramkumar et al. [23] confirmed that in melanocytes, LC3B is involved in assembling the microtubule transporter complex on the melanosome, mediating the transfer of melanosomes from the cell center to the end of the dendrite on the microtubules. LC3B is one of the important autophagy-related regulators involved in the occurrence and development of autophagy. A large number of basic studies have confirmed that increased autophagy in melanocytes can degrade melanocytes, thereby reducing the pigment synthesis capacity of melanocytes [22, 24, 25]. Moreover, studies

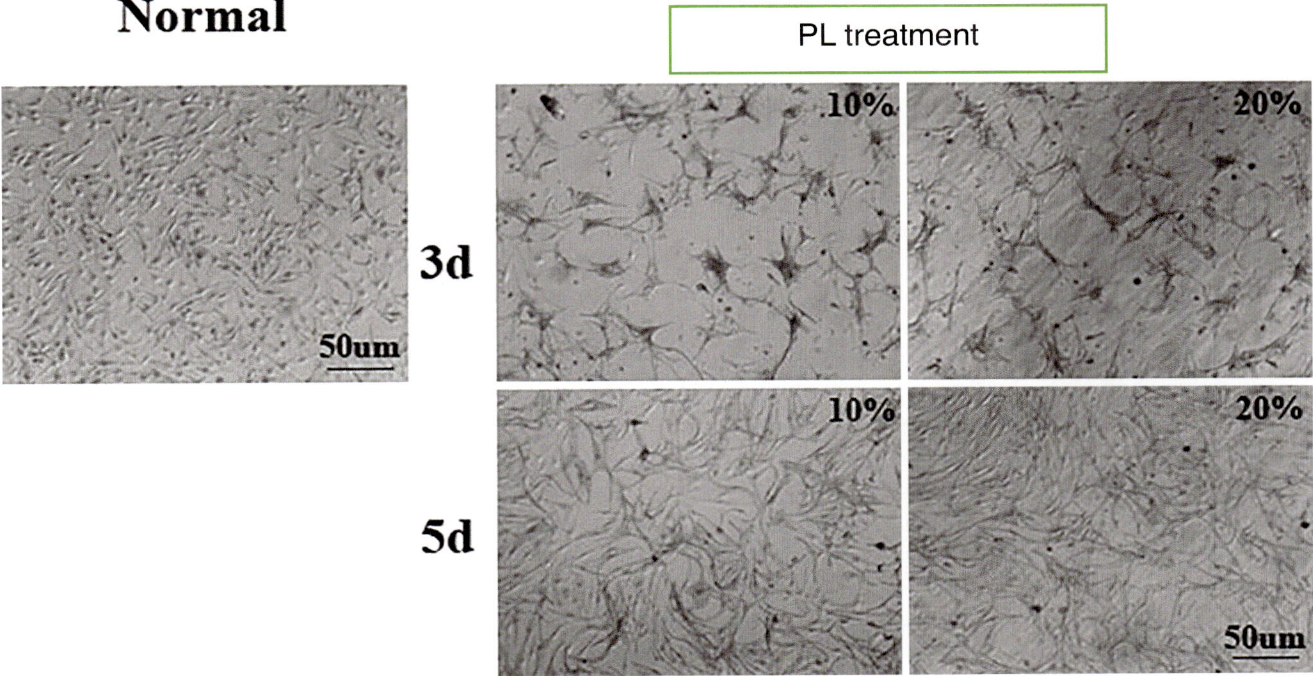

Fig. 8.1 The morphological changes of PHEMC after PL treatment

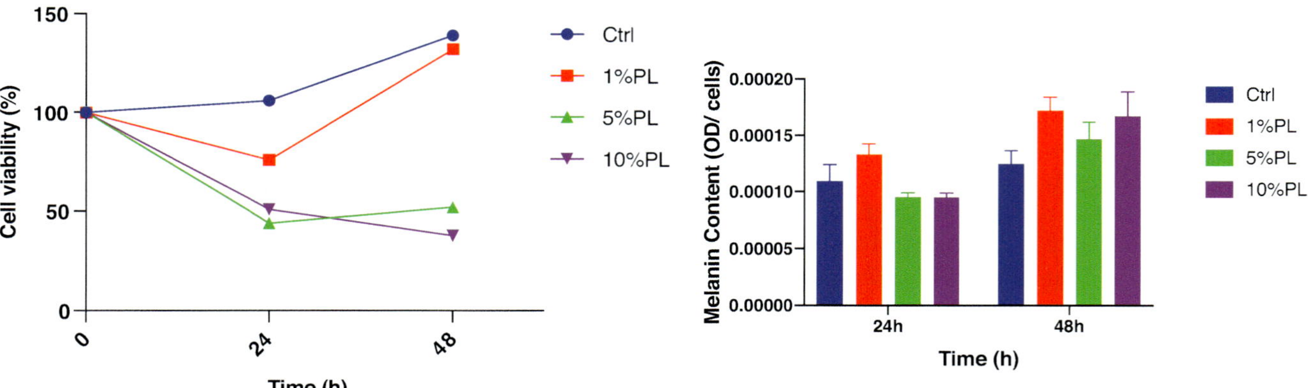

Fig. 8.2 Left: PHEMC cell viability after PL treatment was detected by CCK8. Right: The melanin content after PL treatment was detected by NaOH lysis

have shown that arginase 2 inhibits the autophagic degradation of melanocytes and enhances the pigmentation of melasma [26]. Other studies have shown that autophagic degradation melanosomes are also present in keratinocytes [27], the process may be regulated by arginase 2 (miR-1299 as a target), and there are ethnic differences in autophagy activity, and degradation activity is high in the Caucasian race [28]. PRP also has the ability to regulate autophagy, so we hypothesized whether PRP could block melanin excretion within melanocytes and enhance intracellular metabolic capacity (autophagy?) to achieve the effect of reducing pigmentation, which requires further research and exploration.

The current understanding of melasma is not limited to pigment changes in the epidermis, and the pathological changes of melasma also involve damage to the basement membrane and dermis. Most patients with melasma have a history of long-term UV exposure, so pathological damage to their skin also includes the dermis' solar elastin fiber damage as well as damage to the skin basement membrane [29]. Pathological damage to these dermal layers puts the skin in a microenvironmental inflammatory state; among them, the destruction of the basement membrane leads to the easier penetration of inflammatory cells and inflammatory substances into the epidermis, leaving melanocytes in a state of redox imbalance. PRP, which has a strong ability to promote tissue repair, may improve the pigmentation of melasma by repairing broken basement membranes and elastic fibers, improving the redox state of skin tissues. Therefore, before PRP treats melasma, it may be necessary to perform rigorous indication screening and refine dermatological examinations to determine whether dermal combined melasma or epidermal melasma may be determined and avoid using calcium-activated PRP or physically activated PRP (which produces a large number of nonselective platelet components).

All types of inflammatory skin disorders can eventually lead to post-inflammatory hyperpigmentation (PIH), including pigmentation after wound healing or laser treatment, which is common in plastic surgery. Dark-skinned people (Fitzpatrick skin grading III–VI) are more likely to develop PIH. Increased melanocyte melanin synthesis due to inflammation is associated with redox dysregulation. PRP regulates the oxidative stress state of cells and improves the oxidative stress of cells at the site of inflammation. Therefore, PRP may reduce melanin synthesis by reducing the oxidative stress of melanocytes in an inflammatory environment.

Periorbital hyperpigmentation (POH) refers to increased skin pigmentation of the lower eyelid, which occurs in people of all ages and worsens with age, which may suggest that POH is a structural disorder (due to skin aging). POH can be divided into pigmented, vascular, structural, and mixed types. The criteria for classification are specifically whether the pigmentation of the epidermis increases, whether the thickness of the dermis changes, the exposure of muscle and blood vessels, and other structural changes. Aggravating factors may be associated with increased pigmentation, thinning of the periorbital skin, sagging, tear troughs, or age-related tear grooves. Corresponding literature has been reported to have a good therapeutic effect of PRP on POH [30]. The chief editor's team also had a corresponding treatment case and found that PRP can reduce periorbital pigmentation (Figs. 8.3 and 8.4). The treatment mechanism of PRP for POH is currently inconclusive, and we speculate that the mechanism may be derived from PRP's strong tissue repair ability (antiaging), which can rebuild the continuity of skin tissue structure, make the subcutaneous structure tighter, reduce the bulge of orbital lipids, increase the thickness of the dermis, and reduce the exposure of subcutaneous muscle vessels. Therefore, PRP has also been reported to improve the pigmentation homogeneity of POH but has not significantly reduced melanin content [31].

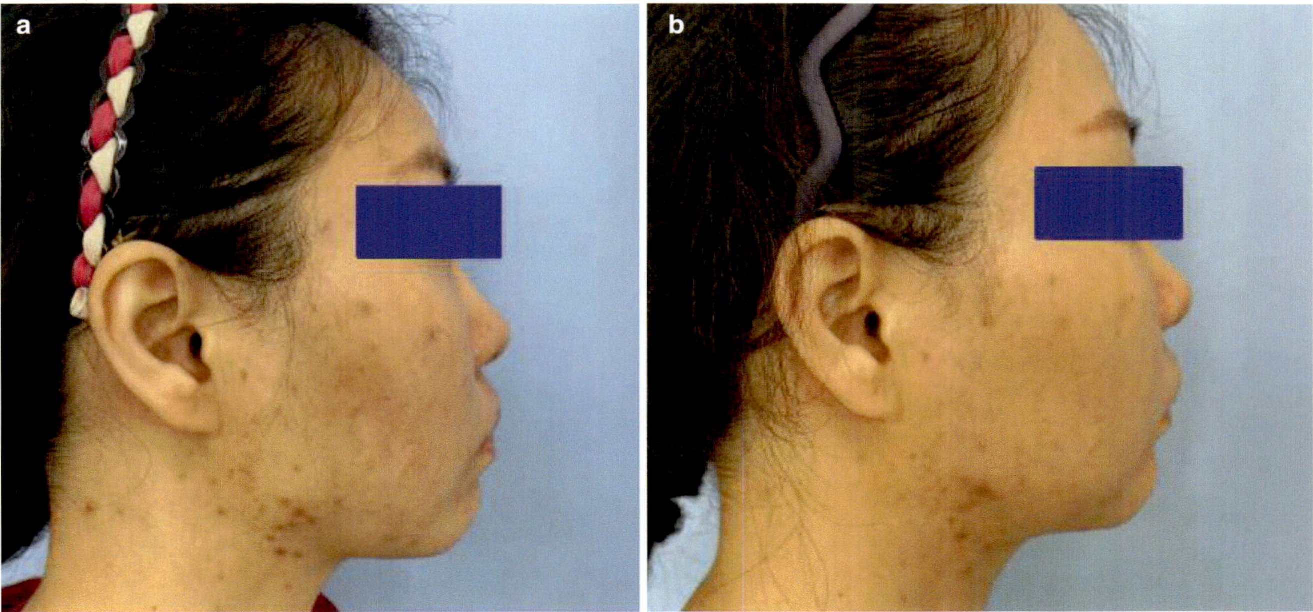

Fig. 8.3 Effect of PRP on skin pigment. (**a**) Preoperative; (**b**) 1 month after PRP treatment

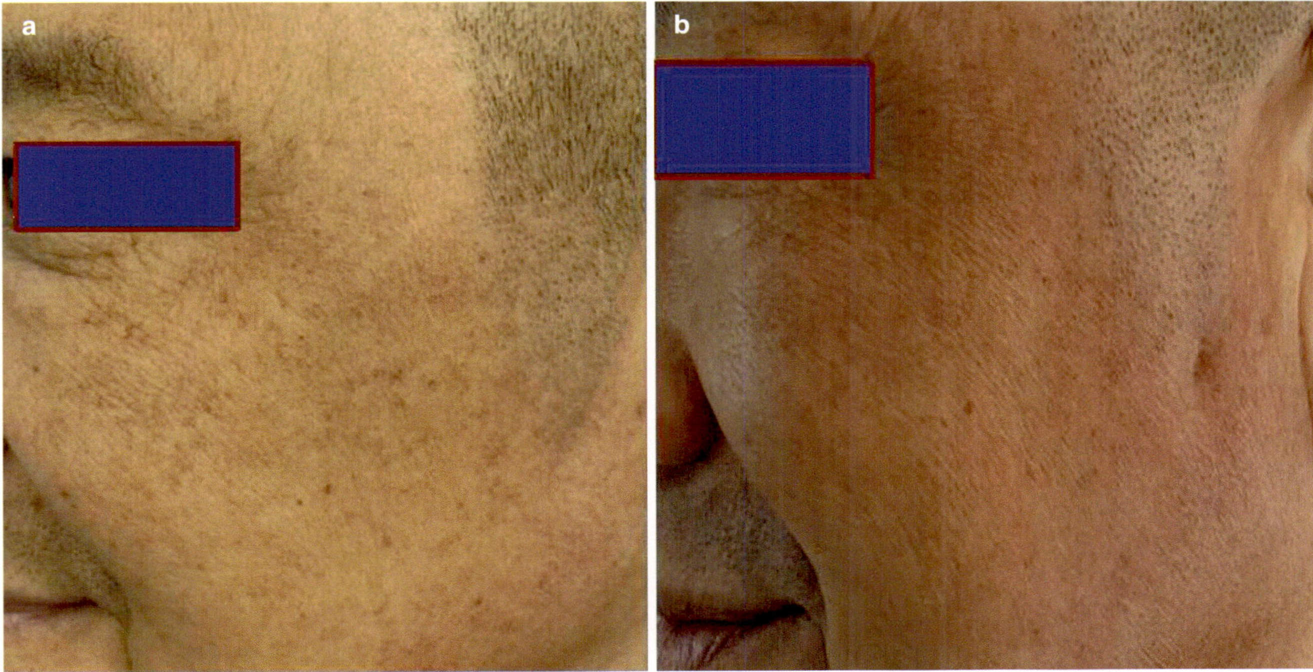

Fig. 8.4 Effect of PRP on skin pigment. (**a**) Preoperative; (**b**) 1 month after PRP treatment

8.2 PRP and Skin Hypopigmentation (Figs. 8.5, 8.6 and 8.7) or Depigmentation

Vitiligo is an acquired pigment skin disease in which melanocyte function in the lesions disappears or even dies, resulting in complete loss of pigment from the mucosal of localized or generalized skin. Studies have found that there is a redox imbalance in vitiligo lesions, and excessive oxidative stress may be the cause of melanocyte function loss or even apoptosis [32]. In addition, autoimmune disorder is also a trigger of vitiligo, such as T cell attack [33]. A large number of active substances in PRP have the ability to regulate oxidative stress. In addition, as mentioned above, PDGF and bFGF

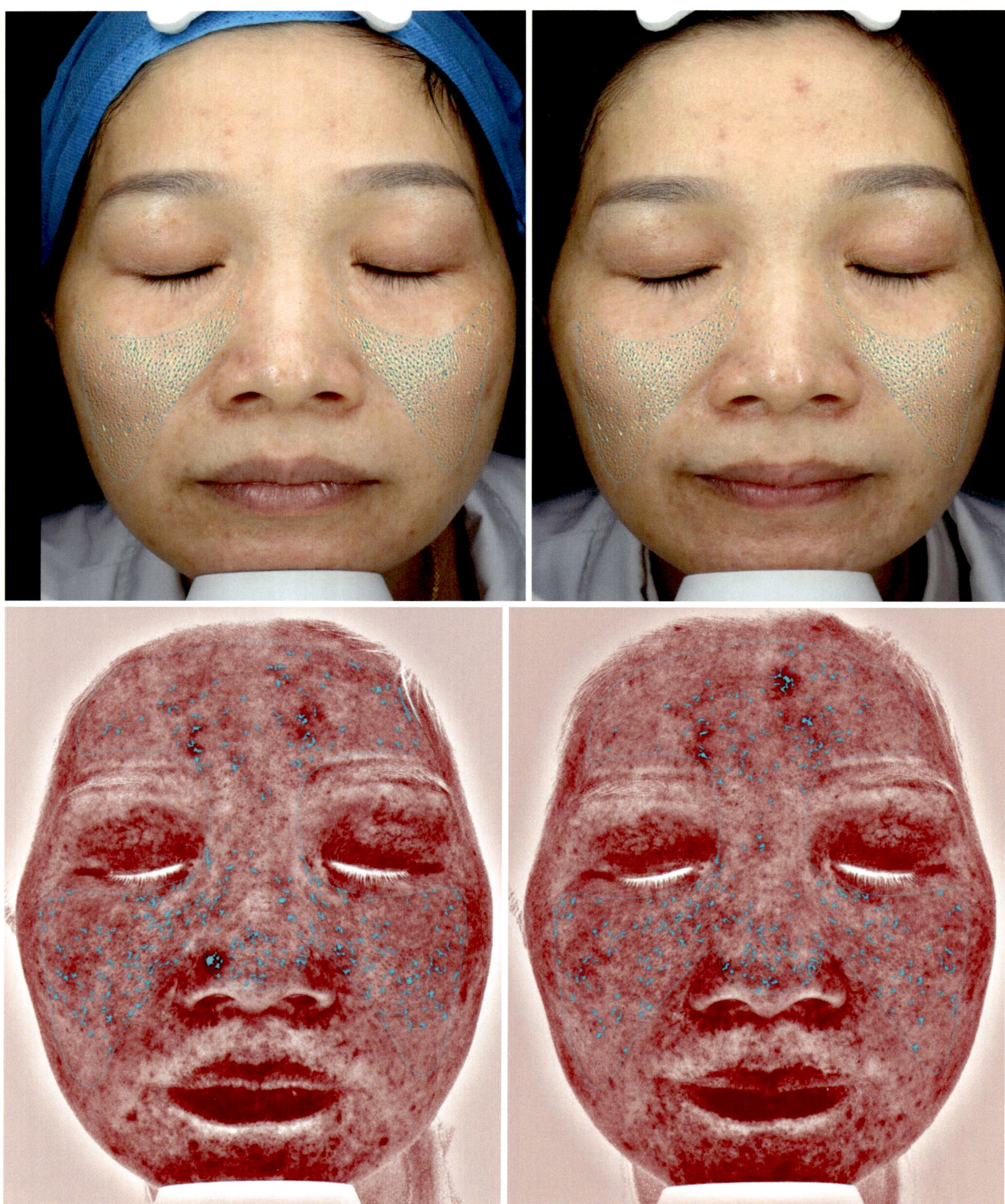

Fig. 8.5 Two months after the treatment of PRP showing a significant improvement of pigmentation

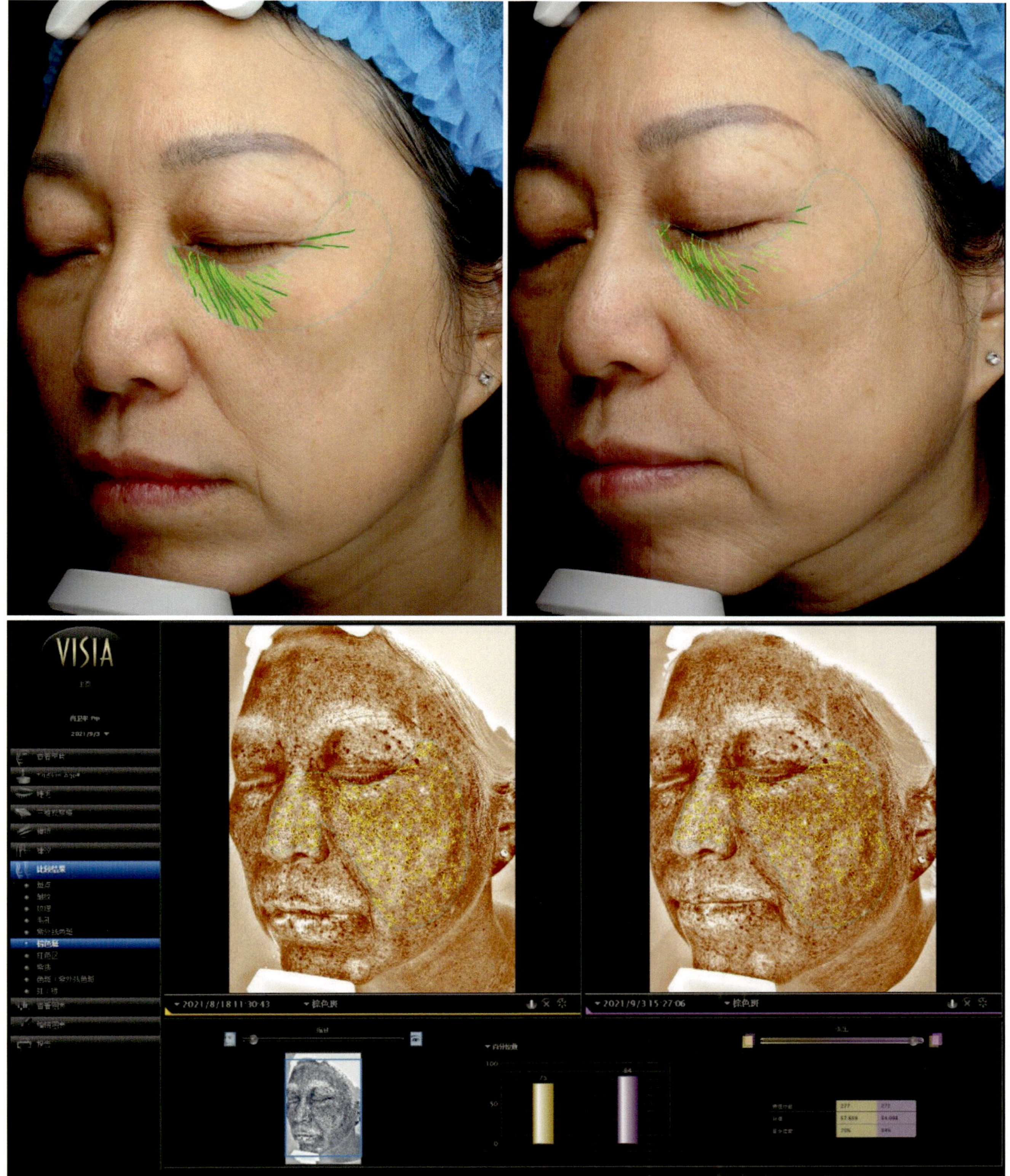

Fig. 8.6 Two months after the treatment of PRP showing a significant improvement of pigmentation

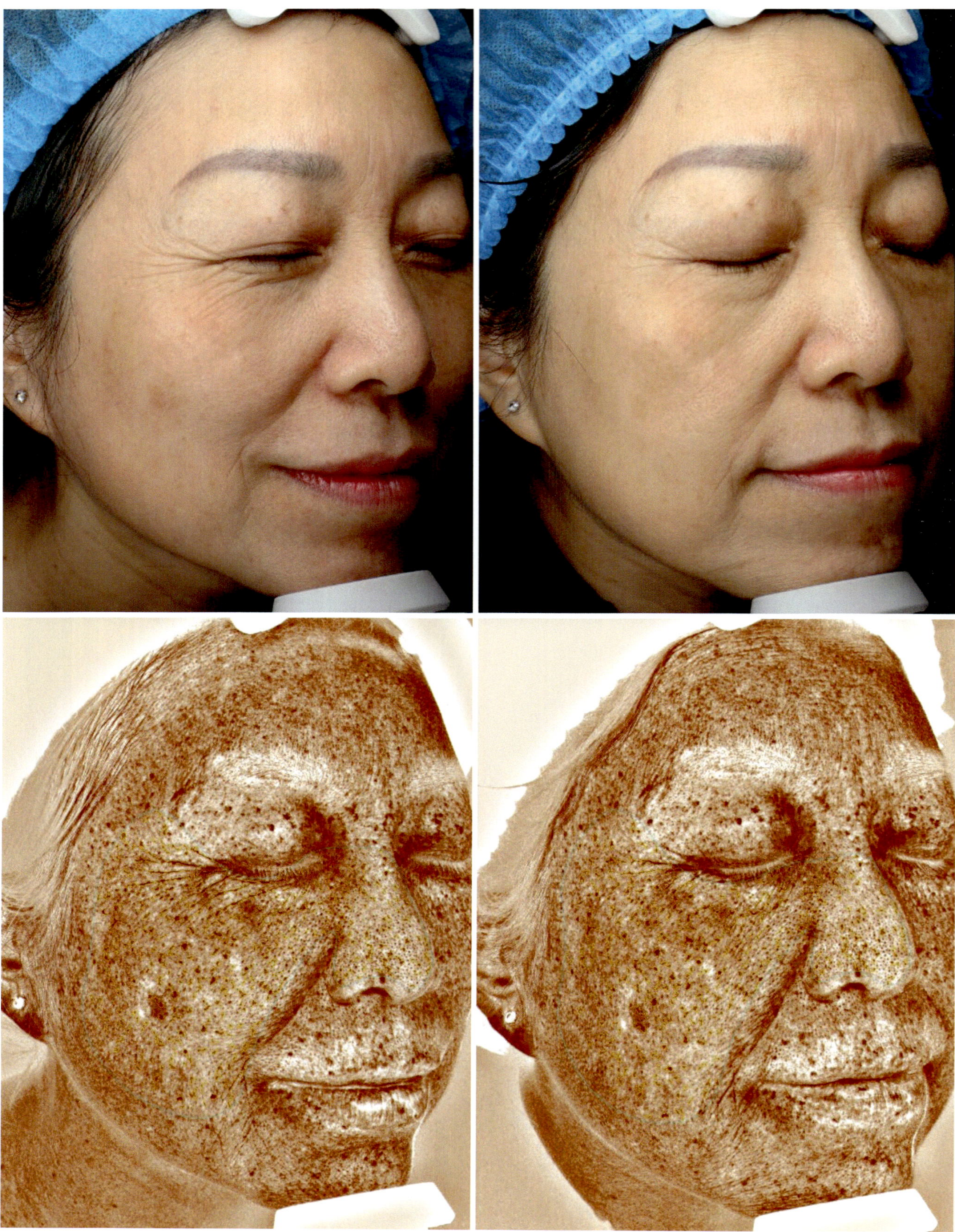

Fig. 8.7 Two months after the treatment of PRP showing a significant improvement of pigmentation

contribute to the proliferation, differentiation, and pigment synthesis of melanocytes. PRP also has the ability of immune regulation [34]. Clinical studies have also found that bFGF can improve the improvement of vitiligo lesions by ultraviolet therapy [35]. At the same time, there are also corresponding clinical studies reporting that PRP combined with ultraviolet therapy can improve the pigmentation loss of vitiligo and promote skin pigment recovery. Although PRP alone is less effective in vitiligo treatment, the effect of vitiligo returning to black is significantly improved when PRP is combined with narrow-wave ultraviolet therapy (NBUVB), laser [36], mini-punch grafting, or non-cultured epidermal cell suspension (NCES) [35, 37, 38].

8.3 Apply PRP Alone or in Combination

PRP can be used alone or in combination with other treatments for pigment diseases. For current clinical studies, the effect of PRP alone is less significant and may be related to the screening of indications. A number of clinical studies have reported that PRP can be used as an adjunctive treatment to treat hyperpigmentation of the skin in combination with laser, chemical peeling, microneedling, etc., and the data effect is much better than that of single treatment [39–42]. This may be related to the fact that after the tissue is injured, PRP can better play its role in regeneration regulation. Therefore, invasive treatments (e.g., lasers, chemical peels, microneedles, etc.), combined with PRP, may be an excellent adjunctive treatment. Na et al. compared fractional carbon dioxide laser combined with PRP therapy to reduce the melanin index after laser damage and reduce the risk of PIH [43].

Ulusal [44] conducted PRP combined with hyaluronic acid to treat facial aging problems such as fine lines, sagging skin, pigmentation, etc. in 94 female patients (ages 53.0 ± 5.6) and found that it could improve the degree of pigmentation and responded earlier and more positively in fair-skinned individuals, with a certain individual specificity, but the degree of improvement was not significantly related to the number of treatments.

PRP can be used as an adjunctive treatment for vitiligo and can achieve satisfactory anti-blackness when combined with narrow-wave ultraviolet therapy (NBUVB), CO_2 lattice laser, mini-punch grafting, or non-cultured epidermal cell suspension (NCES). Abdelghani et al. [36] tested a sequential therapy for vitiligo that combined carbon dioxide fractional laser and PRP (i.e., laser treatment for 1 week, followed by intradermal injection of PRP in the lesions, and repeated this four times) was applied to vitiligo therapy and compared with laser alone or in combination with narrow-wave ultraviolet light therapy; it was found that the melanin recovery index was significantly increased.

Since the effect of PRP on skin pigment is bidirectional, the quality control of PRP should be done when PRP is applied to skin pigment diseases, especially the control of platelet enrichment concentration and activation. No matter PRP is applied to skin hyperpigmentation disease or hypopigmentation disease, platelet concentration is not suitable for too high; Cheng Biao's team conducted relevant basic research and found that too high platelet concentration will inhibit the survival of melanocytes, increase their apoptosis, and may cause increased synthesis of melanin during the damage process.

8.4 Conclusion

There is still insufficient evidence-based medical evidence for the application of PRP to skin pigment diseases, but despite this, PRP's powerful redox modulation ability may be its target for the treatment of pigment diseases. For hyperpigmentation disorders, the current common treatment is still laser or chemical peeling, and these traumatic treatments often lead to local inflammation or redox disorders, and PRP may be a good companion for these traumatic treatments. For depigmentation disorders, PRP may help with pigment recovery through its powerful regenerative ability.

References

1. Merideth MA, et al. Genetic variants associated with Hermansky-Pudlak syndrome. Platelets. 2020;31(4):544–7.
2. Minwalla L, et al. Keratinocytes play a role in regulating distribution patterns of recipient melanosomes in vitro. J Invest Dermatol. 2001;117(2):341–7.
3. Montagna W, Carlisle K. The architecture of black and white facial skin. J Am Acad Dermatol. 1991;24(6 Pt 1):929–37.
4. Swank RT, et al. Inherited abnormalities in platelet organelles and platelet formation and associated altered expression of low molecular weight guanosine triphosphate-binding proteins in the mouse pigment mutant gunmetal. Blood. 1993;81(10):2626–35.
5. Dell'Angelica EC, et al. Lysosome-related organelles. FASEB J. 2000;14(10):1265–78.
6. Klar AS, et al. Human adipose mesenchymal cells inhibit melanocyte differentiation and the pigmentation of human skin via increased expression of TGF-beta1. J Invest Dermatol. 2017;137(12):2560–9.
7. Hofny ERM, et al. Increased expression of TGF-beta protein in the lesional skins of melasma patients following treatment with platelet-rich plasma. J Cosmet Laser Ther. 2019;21(7–8):382–9.
8. Choi SY, et al. Exposure of human melanocytes to UVB twice and subsequent incubation leads to cellular senescence and senescence-associated pigmentation through the prolonged p53 expression. J Dermatol Sci. 2018;90(3):303–12.
9. Ma Y, et al. Platelet-rich plasma protects human melanocytes from oxidative stress and ameliorates melanogenesis induced by UVB irradiation. Biosci Biotechnol Biochem. 2021;85(7):1686–96.
10. Hofny ERM, et al. Platelet-rich plasma is a useful therapeutic option in melasma. J Dermatolog Treat. 2019;30(4):396–401.

11. Sirithanabadeekul P, Dannarongchai A, Suwanchinda A. Platelet-rich plasma treatment for melasma: a pilot study. J Cosmet Dermatol. 2020;19(6):1321–7.
12. Alam M, et al. Effect of platelet-rich plasma injection for rejuvenation of photoaged facial skin: a randomized clinical trial. JAMA Dermatol. 2018;154(12):1447–52.
13. Kwon SH, et al. Heterogeneous pathology of melasma and its clinical implications. Int J Mol Sci. 2016;17(6):824.
14. Kim EH, et al. The vascular characteristics of melasma. J Dermatol Sci. 2007;46(2):111–6.
15. Lee AY. Recent progress in melasma pathogenesis. Pigment Cell Melanoma Res. 2015;28(6):648–60.
16. Hirobe T. Basic fibroblast growth factor stimulates the sustained proliferation of mouse epidermal melanoblasts in a serum-free medium in the presence of dibutyryl cyclic AMP and keratinocytes. Development. 1992;114(2):435–45.
17. Hirobe T, et al. Platelet-derived growth factor regulates the proliferation and differentiation of human melanocytes in a differentiation-stage-specific manner. J Dermatol Sci. 2016;83(3):200–9.
18. Menasche G, et al. Griscelli syndrome restricted to hypopigmentation results from a melanophilin defect (GS3) or a MYO5A F-exon deletion (GS1). J Clin Invest. 2003;112(3):450–6.
19. Van Gele M, Dynoodt P, Lambert J. Griscelli syndrome: a model system to study vesicular trafficking. Pigment Cell Melanoma Res. 2009;22(3):268–82.
20. Marks MS, Seabra MC. The melanosome: membrane dynamics in black and white. Nat Rev Mol Cell Biol. 2001;2(10):738–48.
21. Bouzat S, Levi V, Bruno L. Transport properties of melanosomes along microtubules interpreted by a tug-of-war model with loose mechanical coupling. PLoS One. 2012;7(8):e43599.
22. Katsuyama Y, et al. Disruption of melanosome transport in melanocytes treated with theophylline causes their degradation by autophagy. Biochem Biophys Res Commun. 2017;485(1):126–30.
23. Ramkumar A, et al. Classical autophagy proteins LC3B and ATG4B facilitate melanosome movement on cytoskeletal tracks. Autophagy. 2017;13(8):1331–47.
24. Katsuyama Y, et al. 3-O-Glyceryl-2-O-hexyl ascorbate suppresses melanogenesis through activation of the autophagy system. Biol Pharm Bull. 2018;41(5):824–7.
25. Lee KW, et al. Depigmentation of alpha-melanocyte-stimulating hormone-treated melanoma cells by beta-mangostin is mediated by selective autophagy. Exp Dermatol. 2017;26(7):585–91.
26. Kim NH, et al. Arginase-2, a miR-1299 target, enhances pigmentation in melasma by reducing melanosome degradation via senescence-induced autophagy inhibition. Pigment Cell Melanoma Res. 2017;30(6):521–30.
27. Kim JY, et al. Autophagy induction can regulate skin pigmentation by causing melanosome degradation in keratinocytes and melanocytes. Pigment Cell Melanoma Res. 2020;33(3):403–15.
28. Murase D, et al. Autophagy has a significant role in determining skin color by regulating melanosome degradation in keratinocytes. J Invest Dermatol. 2013;133(10):2416–24.
29. Sheth VM, Pandya AG. Melasma: a comprehensive update: part I. J Am Acad Dermatol. 2011;65(4):689–97.
30. Evans AG, et al. Rejuvenating the periorbital area using platelet-rich plasma: a systematic review and meta-analysis. Arch Dermatol Res. 2021;313(9):711–27.
31. Mehryan P, et al. Assessment of efficacy of platelet-rich plasma (PRP) on infraorbital dark circles and crow's feet wrinkles. J Cosmet Dermatol. 2014;13(1):72–8.
32. Xie H, et al. Vitiligo: how do oxidative stress-induced autoantigens trigger autoimmunity? J Dermatol Sci. 2016;81(1):3–9.
33. Zhou L, et al. Increased circulating Th17 cells and elevated serum levels of TGF-beta and IL-21 are correlated with human non-segmental vitiligo development. Pigment Cell Melanoma Res. 2015;28(3):324–9.
34. Zaslavsky AB, et al. Platelet PD-L1 suppresses anti-cancer immune cell activity in PD-L1 negative tumors. Sci Rep. 2020;10(1):19296.
35. Salem SAM, et al. Effect of platelet-rich plasma on the outcome of mini-punch grafting procedure in localized stable vitiligo: clinical evaluation and relation to lesional basic fibroblast growth factor. Dermatol Ther. 2021;34(2):e14738.
36. Abdelghani R, Ahmed NA, Darwish HM. Combined treatment with fractional carbon dioxide laser, autologous platelet-rich plasma, and narrow band ultraviolet B for vitiligo in different body sites: a prospective, randomized comparative trial. J Cosmet Dermatol. 2018;17(3):365–72.
37. Garg S, Dosapaty N, Arora AK. Laser ablation of the recipient area with platelet-rich plasma-enriched epidermal suspension transplant in vitiligo surgery: a pilot study. Dermatol Surg. 2019;45(1):83–9.
38. Parambath N, et al. Use of platelet-rich plasma to suspend non-cultured epidermal cell suspension improves repigmentation after autologous transplantation in stable vitiligo: a double-blind randomized controlled trial. Int J Dermatol. 2019;58(4):472–6.
39. Gamea MM, et al. Comparative study between topical tranexamic acid alone versus its combination with autologous platelet rich plasma for treatment of melasma. J Dermatolog Treat. 2020;33:1–7.
40. Kim DH, et al. Can platelet-rich plasma be used for skin rejuvenation? Evaluation of effects of platelet-rich plasma on human dermal fibroblast. Ann Dermatol. 2011;23(4):424–31.
41. Merchan WH, et al. Platelet-rich plasma, a powerful tool in dermatology. J Tissue Eng Regen Med. 2019;13(5):892–901.
42. Chawla S. Split face comparative study of microneedling with PRP versus microneedling with vitamin C in treating atrophic post acne scars. J Cutan Aesthet Surg. 2014;7(4):209–12.
43. Na JI, et al. Rapid healing and reduced erythema after ablative fractional carbon dioxide laser resurfacing combined with the application of autologous platelet-rich plasma. Dermatol Surg. 2011;37(4):463–8.
44. Ulusal BG. Platelet-rich plasma and hyaluronic acid - an efficient biostimulation method for face rejuvenation. J Cosmet Dermatol. 2017;16(1):112–9.

Platelet-Rich Plasma and Bone Regeneration

9

Ting Yuan, Yiqing Zhou, Jian Zou, Xuetao Xie, Zhaoyuan Zhang, and Zhongmin Shi

In addition to the therapeutic effects of PRP on skin and soft tissues and skin appendages, it also has a wide range of clinical applications in the field of bone tissue repair and regeneration. Therefore, a large number of basic researches focus on this direction. At the same time, PRP is used in clinical diseases such as bone injury and osteoarthritis and so on. The treatment has once again proved the application prospect and value of PRP in the field of regeneration.

The initial theory behind the use of PRP for bone regeneration was that PRP contains a variety of growth factors that promote bone regeneration. As PRP research developed, the theory that it promotes bone regeneration was gradually refined to that PRP regulates inflammation, vascular regeneration, and bone matrix deposition, provides scaffolding for bone regeneration, affects the local microenvironment of bone formation, and so on. Compared to other biological therapies in the field of bone regeneration such as stem cells, xenogeneic growth factors, and recombinant growth factors, PRP has the inherent advantages of being safe, easy to use, and inexpensive, without the medical ethical issues of the stem cell or xenogeneic growth factors that may cause damage to the human. Due to these characteristics, PRP was used in clinical repair of bone defects, osteonecrosis, and fractures decades ago. In contrast to the many years of basic stem cell research but slow advancement in clinical applications, the use of PRP started from the beginning with both clinical and basic researches together. This chapter will focus on the clinical applications of PRP in different areas of bone regeneration and the corresponding basic research, including the history of PRP in bone regeneration, different application scenarios, the efficacy of PRP in combination with other therapeutic approaches, current problems, and future developments.

9.1 History of PRP Research and Application

PRP (platelet-rich plasma) is used for clinical repair of bone and soft tissue, thanks to the discovery of growth factors in platelets. In 1974, Ross [1] used activated blood supernatant in monkey arterial smooth muscle cell (SMC) culture and found that the supernatant promoted cell proliferation. If the platelet-removed blood-activated supernatant was used in cell culture, it was found to have no significant effect on promoting SMC proliferation. This result suggested, for the first time, that platelets may contain some cell growth-promoting factors that, after releasing by activation, promote cell proliferation. Based on Ross' study, in 1978, Witte [2] identified a factor stored in platelet alpha granules that significantly promoted the proliferation of human SMC and mouse 3T3 cells and named it PDGF (platelet-derived growth factor). Subsequently, platelet growth factors such as TGF-β (transforming growth factor-β), IGF-1 (insulin-like growth factor-1), FGF (fibroblast growth factor), and VEGF (vascular endothelial growth factor) have been shown to promote cell growth, collagen formation, vascular regeneration, and accelerated wound healing, among other effects [3].

PRP initially used in orthopedic clinics was to repair chronic wounds. In 1990, Knighton [4] found that treatment of chronic hard-to-heal wounds with PRP reduced the healing time of wounds by 50%. In 1993, Ganio [5] treated hard-to-heal wounds that had not healed for an average of 75 weeks with PRP, and after 10 weeks of PRP treatment, all wounds were healed. Due to the remarkable efficacy of PRP to repair wounds, PRP was then gradually applied to repair more tissue diseases.

The first report on the use of PRP for bone repair and regeneration was by Robert E. Marx, a dentist. In this

T. Yuan (✉) · J. Zou · X. Xie · Z. Zhang · Z. Shi
Department of Orthopaedics, Shanghai Jiao Tong University Affiliated Sixth People's Hospital, Shanghai, China

Y. Zhou
Department of Orthopedics, Shanghai Changzheng Hospital, Naval Medical University, Shanghai, China

B. Cheng, X. Fu (eds.), *Platelet-Rich Plasma in Tissue Repair and Regeneration*, https://doi.org/10.1007/978-981-99-3193-4_9

Table 9.1 Quantity of articles on PRP published searched by PubMed

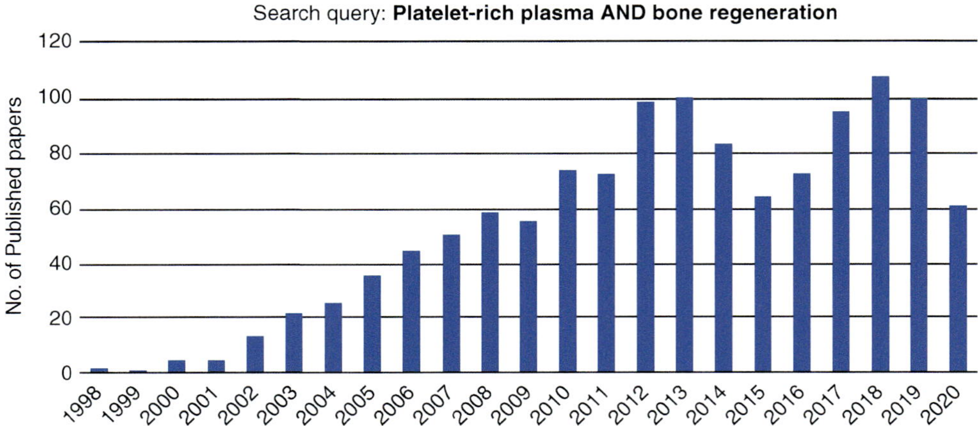

prospective clinical study by Marx [6], a total of 88 patients with mandibular tumors, with defects greater than 5 cm after tumor resection, underwent iliac bone graft reconstruction and were randomized to the PRP group versus the conventional treatment control group. The 6-month postoperative follow-up showed that the PRP group had 1.62–2.16 times more bone maturation and significantly faster bone regeneration than the control group (PRP group, 74.0% ± 11%; control group, 55.1% ± 8%; $p = 0.005$). This study describes in more detail the PRP-making method, clinical use procedure, and clinical efficacy of PRP and explores the mechanism of PRP in promoting bone regeneration. The publication of this article has given a great impetus to the clinical applications of PRP. By 2020, the study was cited more than 3000 times. Subsequently, studies on PRP in the field of bone regeneration have increased (Table 9.1).

9.2 Application of PRP in Bone Defect and Nonunion

Bone defects and nonunion caused by bone tumors, high-energy trauma, or bone infections have always been one of the challenges facing clinical orthopedic surgeons. Although with the development of orthopedic surgical techniques and the emergence of new biomaterials, the repair of bone defects and bone nonunion has improved to a great extent. It is still far from the standard of satisfactory clinical bone repair, and the shortcomings and complications of these treatments themselves limit their wide clinical application. For example, autologous bone graft can cause significant donor site morbidity, allogeneic bone graft has insufficient activity and poor bone formation, and Ilizarov technique and Masquelet technique have problems such as long treatment time and needle tract infection. The combination of PRP and these techniques can compensate for the shortcomings of these techniques and promote bone regeneration more significantly.

At the cellular level, PRP's ability to promote bone regeneration is that PRP can promote the proliferation and differentiation of osteoblasts. In 1995, Slater added PRP in bone marrow stromal cell culture in vitro and found that PRP not only accelerated cell proliferation but also promoted the differentiation of bone marrow stromal cells to osteoblasts. Compared to the control group, the cells in the PRP group had a significant ability to secrete ALP and increase calcification [7]. Subsequently, the number of studies using PRP for bone marrow stromal stem cells, bone precursor cells, osteoblasts, and other bone-related cells gradually increased, and PRP has also played a significant role in promoting the differentiation of different types of stem cells to osteoblasts in experimental studies.

Using PRP to repair bone defects and bone nonunions has also shown satisfactory results in many animal experiments. Changqing Zhang and Ting Yuan et al. [8] used PRP combined bioceramic bone material to repair radial defects in New Zealand white rabbits in 2004 (Fig. 9.1). PRP was combined with porous bioceramic to repair a 1 cm defect in the rabbit radius, with only bioceramic implantation as a control group. Radiographic and histological observations showed that the osteogenic quantity and quality of PRP group were significantly better than that of the control group. Fennis et al. [9] performed an experimental study on the repair of mandibular defects in sheep by combining PRP with the autologous bone. The mandibular defect area was fixed with titanium plate. In the control group, the same experimental method was used, but the same autologous cancellous bone without PRP was implanted. The histological and histomorphometric analyses showed that the PRP group had significantly more osteogenesis than the control group.

In 2008, Bielecki [10] reported a clinical study using percutaneous injection of PRP for the treatment of delayed union and nonunion. A total of 12 patients with delayed union and 20 patients with bone nonunion were enrolled, with 4 patients with bone nonunion having local infection. All patients with delayed union healed in a mean of

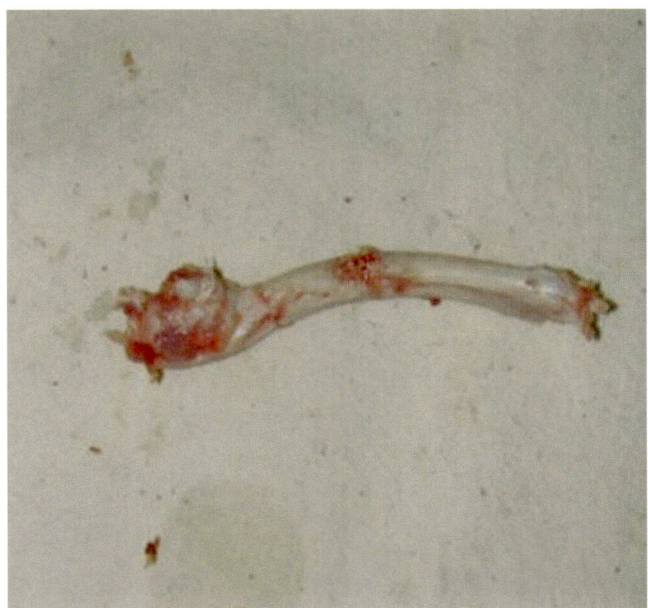

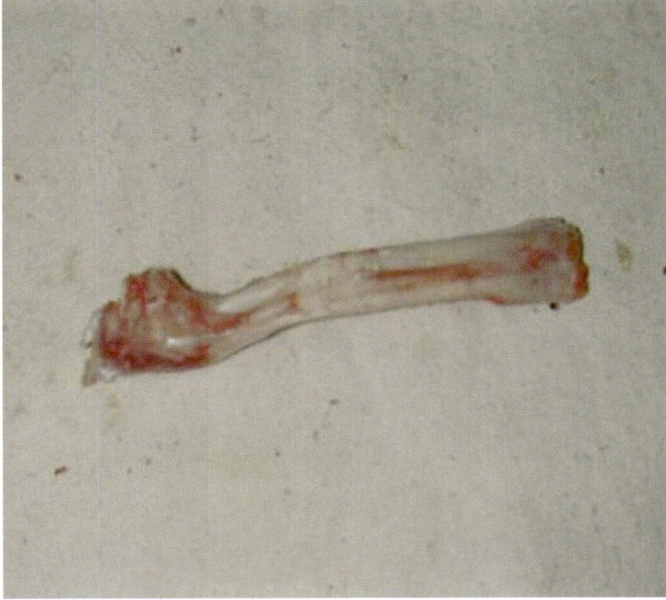

Fig. 9.1 New Zealand white rabbits with radial defects treated for 12 weeks (left is the control group, where the bone defect is not completely repaired and some implanted graft is still exposed; right is the PRP group, where the bone defect is completely repaired and new bone completely fills in and covers the bone defect area)

9.3 weeks after percutaneous injection of PRP. Thirteen patients with bone nonunion healed at 10.3 weeks after PRP treatment. Based on the duration of bone nonunion prior to treatment, the authors found that PRP treatment was ineffective if the duration of bone nonunion was longer than 11 months. If the duration of bone nonunion was less than 11 months, PRP treatment by percutaneous injection resulted in complete healing. The authors concluded that PRP percutaneous injection is a minimally invasive operation compared to traditional incisional debridement and bone grafting surgery, which does not disrupt the local blood supply, and that PRP contains a large amount of growth factors to stimulate bone cell regeneration, promote extracellular matrix synthesis, and enhance vascular regeneration. For patients with bone nonunion less than 11 months, percutaneous PRP injection can replace traditional surgery. Early percutaneous PRP injections were performed under fluoroscopy, and the surgeon was exposed to radiation during the percutaneous injection (Figs. 9.2 and 9.3). With the development of musculoskeletal ultrasound in recent years, percutaneous injection of PRP under the guidance of musculoskeletal ultrasound for the treatment of bone nonunion has gradually become a mainstream method. Ultrasound does not produce radiation exposure to the physician, and the ultrasound machine is small and convenient, allows observation of the bone nonunion site at multiple levels, and also allows determination of the local blood supply. Ultrasound-guided PRP percutaneous injection has many advantages. This procedure does not require the operating room and can be done in a common outpatient room (Figs. 9.4 and 9.5).

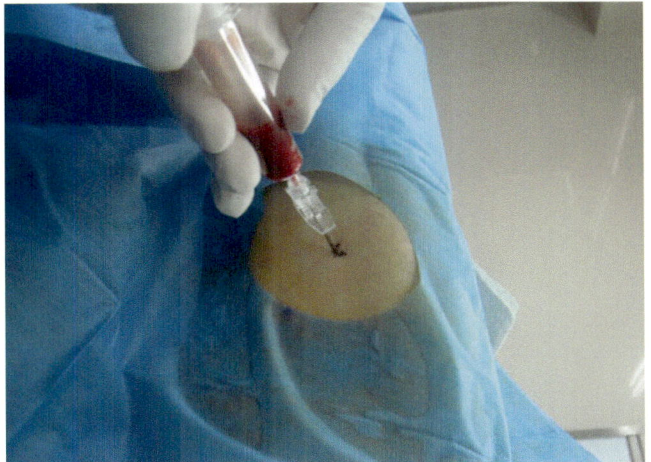

Fig. 9.2 Percutaneous PRP injection

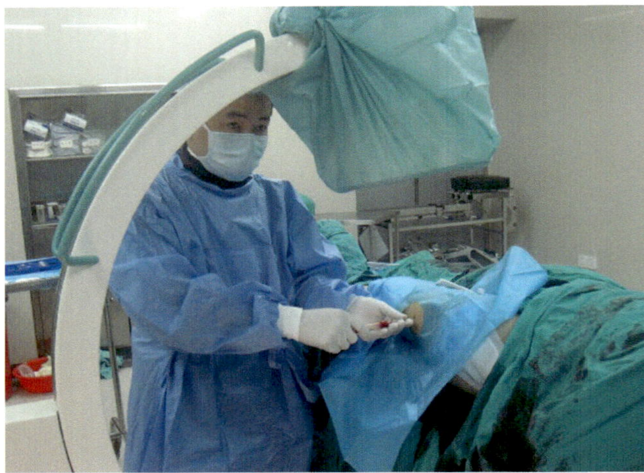

Fig. 9.3 Percutaneous PRP injection guided by c-arm X-ray machine in operation room

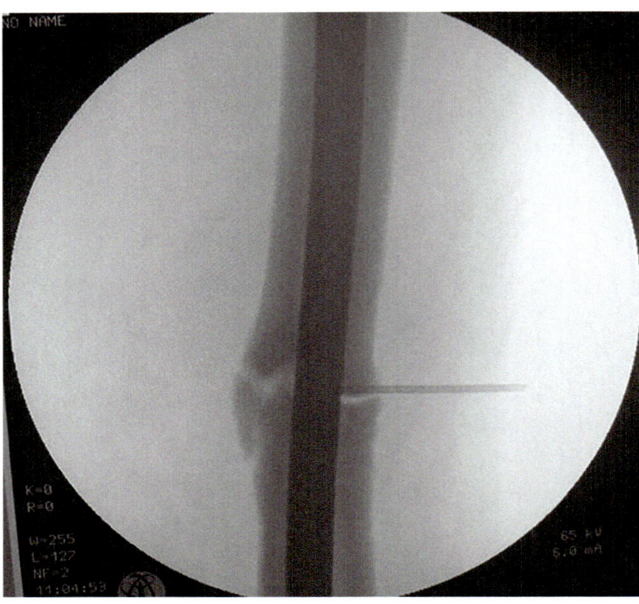

Fig. 9.4 Syringe needle was percutaneously inserted in fracture guided by c-arm X-ray machine

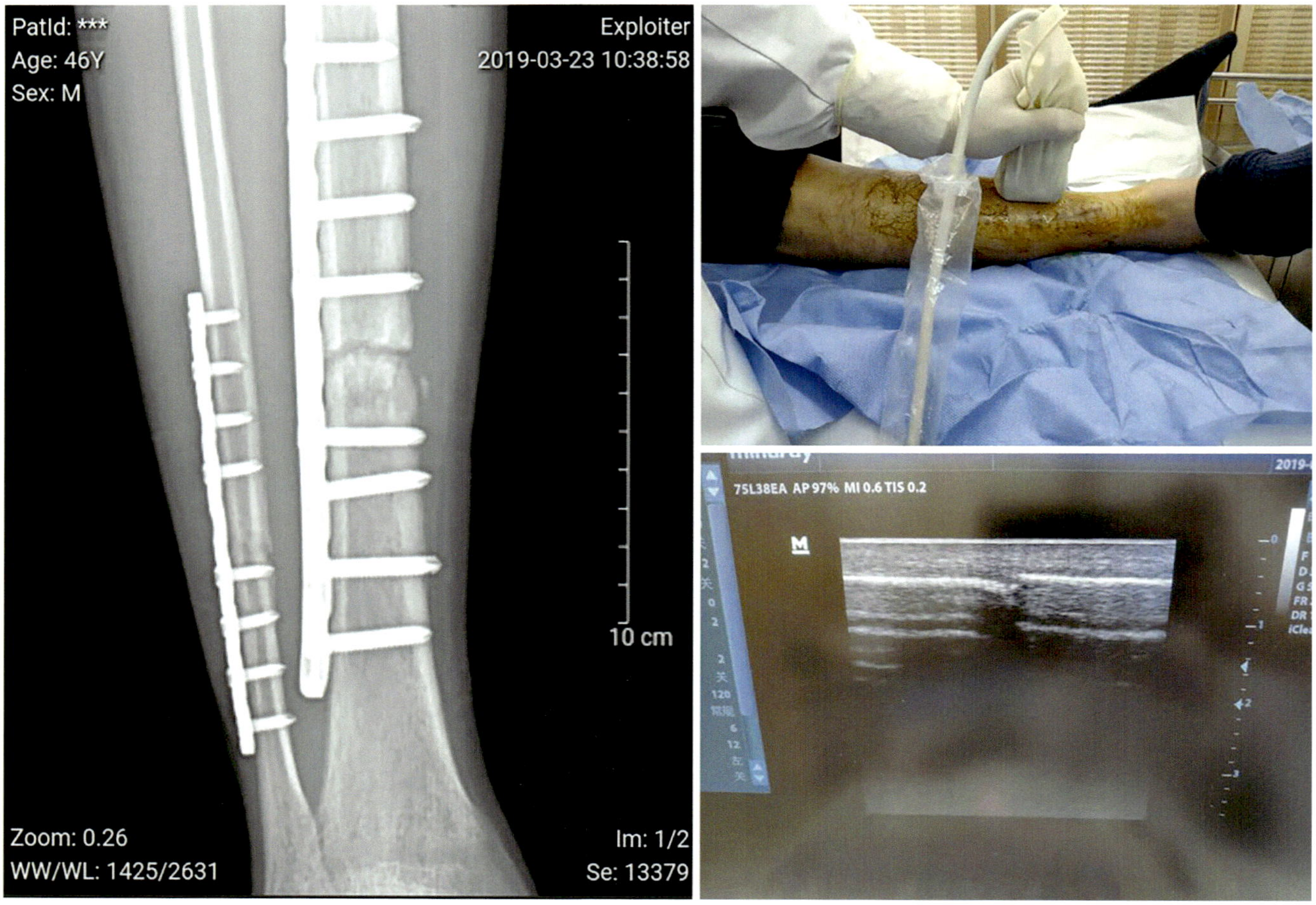

Fig. 9.5 Patients with nonunion received percutaneous PRP injection guided by musculoskeletal ultrasonography

9.3 Application of PRP in Bone Infection

PRP contains high concentrations of leukocytes, such as neutrophils, monocytes, and lymphocytes. These leukocytes play an important role in inflammation. In vitro studies have shown that PRP can inhibit the growth of *Staphylococcus aureus* and *Escherichia coli*. In particular, the inhibitory effect of PRP on methicillin-sensitive *Staphylococcus aureus* (MSSA) was comparable to that of gentamicin and benzocillin [11]. This antimicrobial effect correlates with the leukocytes contained in PRP [12]. PRP also contains many kinds of antibacterial proteins that inhibit the growth of bacteria and fungi [13].

In addition to the specific anti-infective effects of leukocytes in PRP, platelets themselves, the main component of PRP, have strong anti-infective effects. Platelets are the first cells in the body to detect and react to endothelial cell damage and pathogen invasion; therefore, platelets are at the forefront of the body's reaction against infection and also play an important role in regulating the immune system response [14]. The alpha granules of platelets are rich in antimicrobial peptides, and lysosomes contain a variety of proteins with bactericidal activity [15].

Platelets can suppress infections directly or indirectly in vivo by endocytosis of pathogens, release of antimicrobial proteins and chemokines, activation and involvement of leukocytes in bactericidal activity, activation of the complement system and antigen-presentation function (Figs. 9.6 and 9.7).

Jia [16] from Prof. Changqing Zhang's team in 2010 used PRP for the treatment of rabbit tibial osteomyelitis, and the animal model of osteomyelitis was constructed by injecting *Staphylococcus aureus* into the tibial marrow medullary. It was found that PRP also showed better anti-infective ability in animals. Subsequently, Li [17], also a member of Changqing Zhang's team, combined PRP with vancomycin for the treatment of MRSA-induced tibial osteomyelitis in New Zealand rabbits and found that the anti-infective effect of PRP in combination with vancomycin was superior to that of the PRP alone or vancomycin alone, suggesting that PRP not only has a good anti-infective effect on its own but also has a reinforcing effect in combination with antibiotics.

Although there are no high-quality clinical studies of PRP for osteomyelitis, the case reports published to date have shown that PRP is also clinically effective in the treatment of osteomyelitis. In the following case, infection occurred after internal fixation of the calcaneus fracture, and the wound has been oozing pus heavily since the surgery (Figs. 9.8 and 9.9), requiring daily dressing changes to keep from wetting the patients' socks and shoes. Because of this disease, the patient's quality of life was very poor. The patient underwent four debridement surgeries during the 2 years after the initial surgery, but the wound never healed. Changqing Zhang and Ting Yuan's team performed two PRP treatments on the patient (Fig. 9.10). Two weeks after the first treatment, the patient's wound was significantly reduced to the size of a green bean (Fig. 9.11), and after the second PRP treatment,

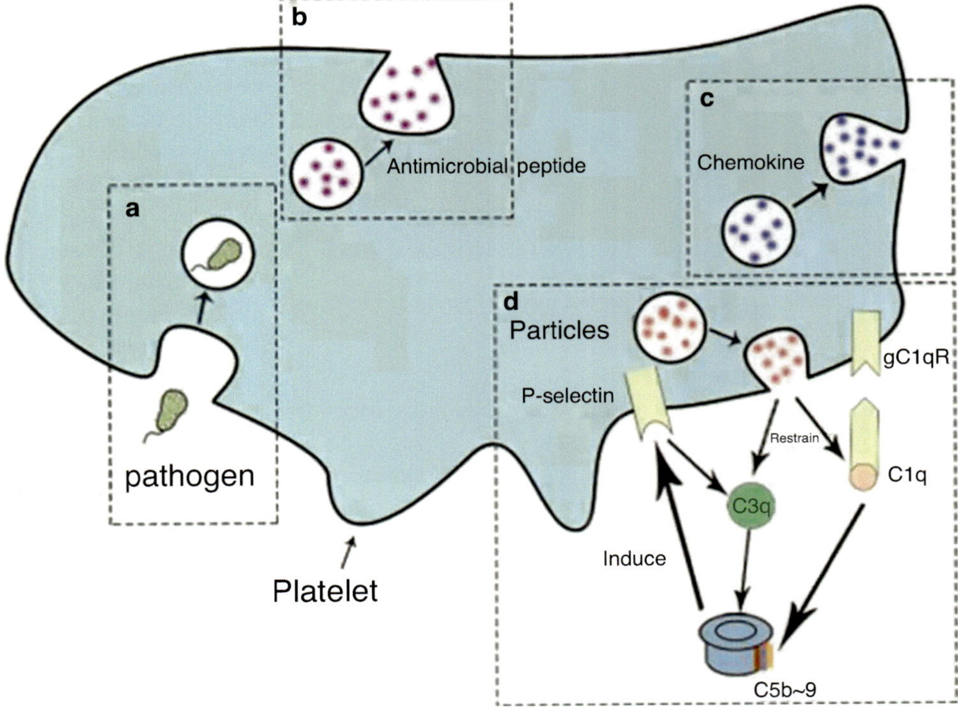

Fig. 9.6 Anti-infection mechanism schemes of platelets: (**a**) internalizing pathogens; (**b**) releasing antibacterial peptide; (**c**) secreting chemokines; and (**d**) activating and regulating complement system

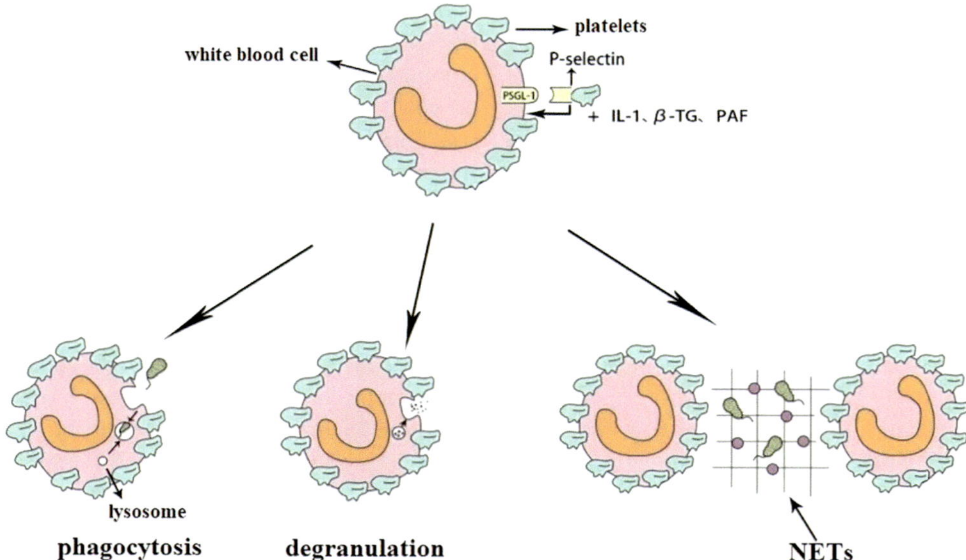

Fig. 9.7 Anti-infection mechanism schemes of platelets. Platelets combine with and adhere to leukocytes via combination of p-selectin expressed on platelets and p-selectin glycoprotein ligand-1 (PSGL-1) expressed on leukocytes, form garland-like structure, and release interleukin 1 (IL-1), β-thromboglobulin (β-TG), and platelet-activating factor (PAF), which finally activate leukocytes. When activated, leukocytes phagocytose pathogens, produce degranulation effects (release of superoxide and lysosomal enzymes to remove invading pathogenic microorganisms), and form NETs (neutrophil extracellular traps)

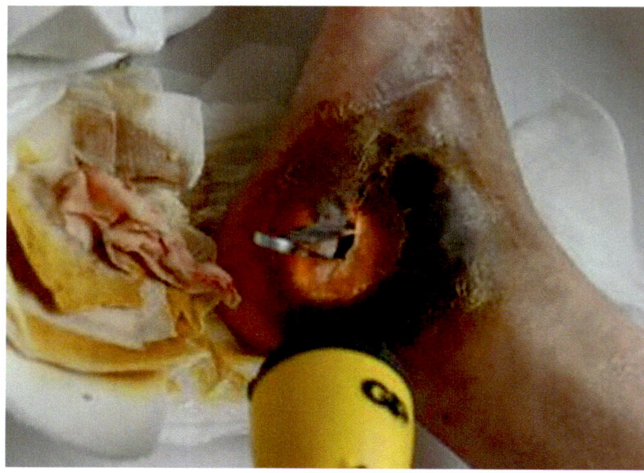

Fig. 9.8 Calcaneus osteomyelitis, a large amount of pus oozed from the wound everyday

the wound was completely healed and has been recurrence-free for 2 years of follow-up (Fig. 9.12).

Guo Yanjie et al. [18] treated 47 clinically infected chronic wounds with PRP, including 10 cases of tibial osteomyelitis and 1 case of femoral osteomyelitis, with a total of 38 cases of positive trauma bacterial cultures, and the majority of cases showed significant improvement without exacerbation of infection after PRP treatment. The rate of positive bacterial culture decreased from 80.9% to 31.9% before surgery.

The rationale for PRP treatment of osteomyelitis may lie in the following:

1. Chronic osteomyelitis due to rapid degradation and low concentration of growth factors: PRP provides a large amount of high concentration of growth factors to make up for the lack of local growth factors and stimulate tissue regeneration.
2. The high concentration of leukocytes in PRP can inhibit or even phagocytose and kill harmful bacteria, remove necrotic tissues, reduce the inflammatory response, and decrease purulent exudate.
3. Osteomyelitis has serious destruction of blood transport and slow vascular regeneration and poor blood supply due to high pressure in the early pulp cavity and long-term inflammatory fluid infiltration. PRP contains high concentrations of PDGF, VEGF, and EGF, which have a synergistic effect of strongly stimulating vascular regeneration. In a study of treating maxillofacial bone defects with PRP composite iliac bone, Marx found that new blood vessels were seen to grow into the wound from the surrounding tissue on the third day after PRP application.
4. PRP significantly promotes soft tissue repair, and good soft tissue conditions are an important basis for osteomyelitis healing.
5. PRP in liquid form forms a gel after injection into the sinus tract and can be used to fill and cover the wound cavity [19].

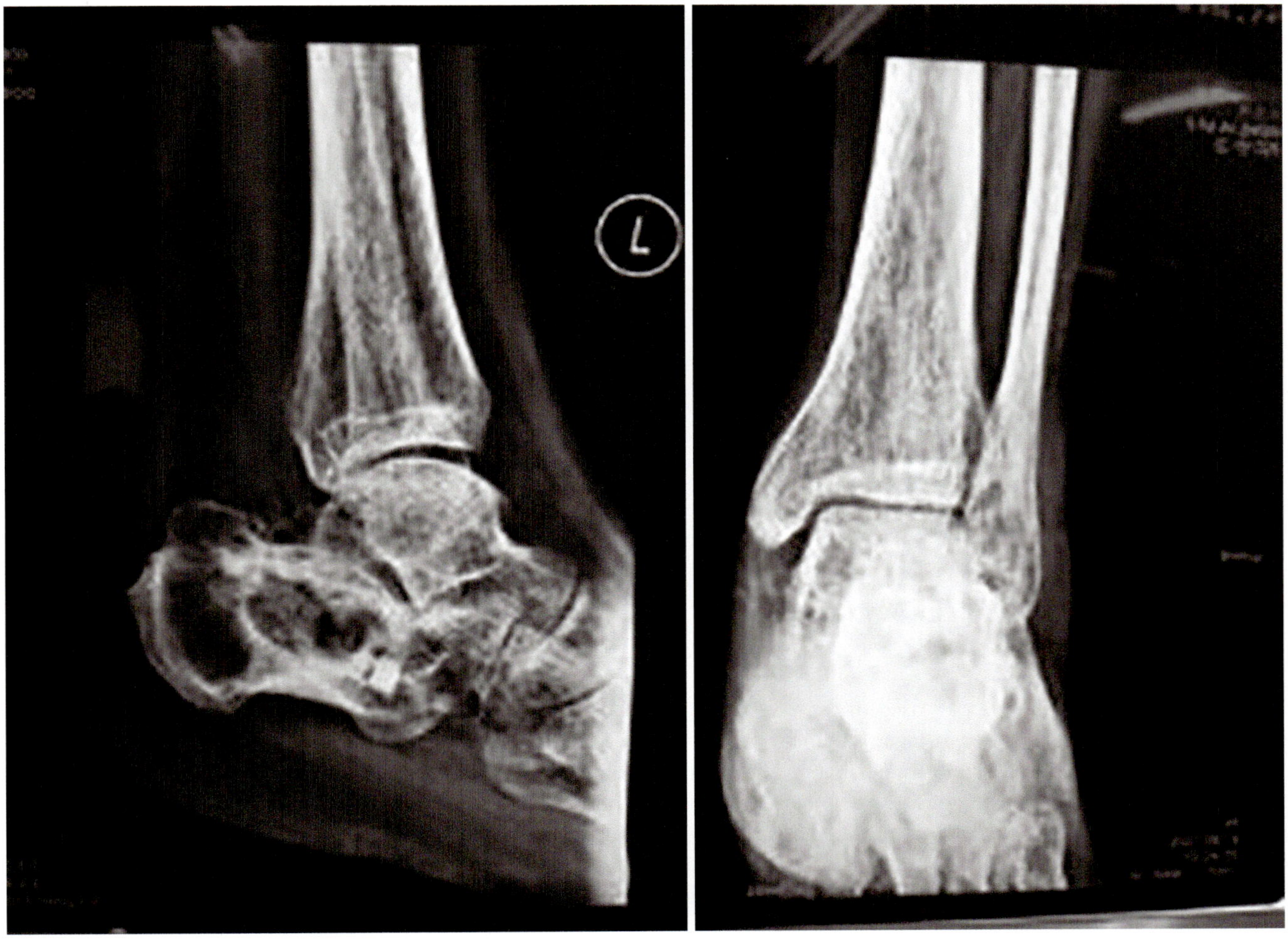

Fig. 9.9 Low density lesions of calcaneus were shown in X-ray, and remaining bone graft implanted previously could be seen

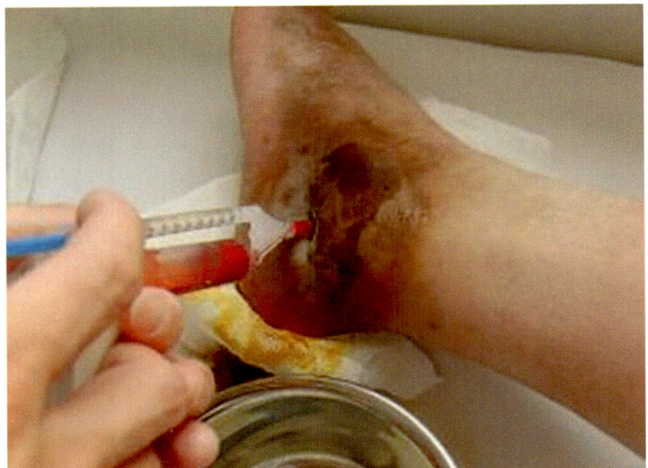

Fig. 9.10 PRP was injected to the wound

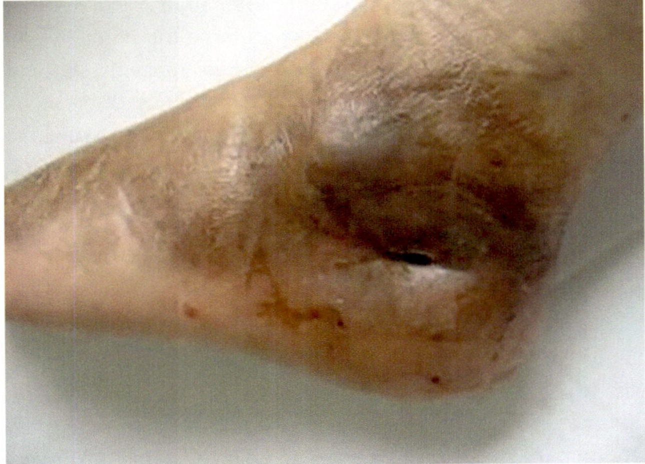

Fig. 9.11 Two weeks after the first PRP injection treatment, the patient's wound shrunk to the size of a green bean with no significant exudate

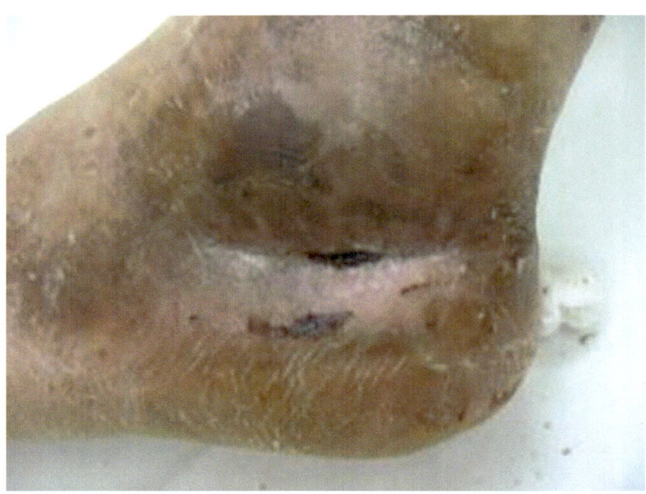

Fig. 9.12 The wound was healed 4 weeks after the second treatment, without recurrence during 2-year follow-up period

9.4 Application of PRP in Tendon-Bone Healing

The tendon-bone junction is composed of four types of tissue: tendon, uncalcified fibrocartilage, calcified fibrocartilage, and bone tissue. The tendon-bone junction is mainly responsible for the transmission of force between the tendon and bone. This special tissue can resist strong stresses, enhance the strength of the tendon-bone junction, and reduce the probability of the tendon and bone separating and being injured due to excessive tension. At the same time, due to the complex structure of the tissue, it is very difficult to reconstruct the tendon-bone connection once it is damaged. Generally speaking, the tendon-bone junction cannot naturally return to its normal structure after injury. In addition, clinicians have tried and failed to promote the regeneration and repair of the tendon-bone junction through surgical procedures and the use of various materials or drugs. It is easy to imagine the challenge of fixing a hard tissue like bone to soft tissue like tendon in order to reconstruct and repair the tendon-bone junction area.

PRP is enriched with high concentrations of platelets, which upon activation can release a large number of factors, including PDGF, TGF-β, VEGF, and HGF, which are beneficial for tissue repair. It has also been studied that PRP alone can promote the proliferation of tendon cells and osteoblasts, which may also facilitate the healing of the tendon-bone interface. However, tendon-bone healing is different from tendon tissue healing and repair, and the key to the healing of the tendon-bone interface is the regeneration of the migration zone, especially the regeneration of fibrocartilage, which is the key to the mechanical stability of the tendon-bone junction and is the focus of tendon-bone healing observation. And it is important for the prevention of re-injury to the tendon-bone junction. Thus, the ability to promote the regeneration of fibrocartilage at the tendon bone interface is the key to whether PRP can truly promote tendon bone healing.

In terms of in vitro studies, TSC and MSC may theoretically exist at the tendon bone interface, but there is no evidence from current studies that PRP can effectively promote TSC as well as BMSC into cartilage differentiation and promote fibrocartilage regeneration. In addition, for in vivo studies, Zhou et al. [20] established a tendon bone injury healing model in rat ankle and found that the PRP group significantly accelerated the healing of the gap at the tendon bone interface by adding PRP compared with the control group. However, as observed by a 3-month pathological follow-up, the use of PRP mainly promoted the healing rate of scar junctions at the interface between bone and tendon tissue junctions and did not promote the regeneration of fibrocartilage and migrating bands at the tendon bone interface. Thus, the final biomechanics showed that the use of PRP did not significantly increase the mechanical properties of the tendon bone interface such as resistance to pulling. The efficacy of PRP alone in repairing the tendon bone injury interface is not positive enough, but as a cofactor, PRP has the dual function of being a carrier of intervening factors and releasing cytokines to assist in repair and can still play an important role in tendon bone healing.

PRP has been used clinically to treat lesions caused by combined tendon-bone injuries such as plantar fasciitis, Achilles tendinopathy, tennis elbow, and tarsal sinus syndrome and has shown good results in most cases. Shi Zhongmin's team at the Department of Orthopaedics, Sixth People's Hospital of Shanghai Jiao Tong University, treated 16 patients with insertion site (bone-tendon interface) Achilles tendinopathy and 12 patients with non-interface Achilles tendinopathy with PRP. The patients were treated with PRP injections. All patients had received regular treatment before PRP injection, including gastrocnemius stretching, oral nonsteroidal anti-inflammatory drugs, rest, and hindfoot insoles, but no pain relief. Magnetic resonance imaging (MRI) also showed edema at both the Achilles tendon-calcaneus interface and the non-interface site. The patients received PRP injections at the point of pain once a month for three times; during the injection period, the patients continued to perform regular stretching of the gastrocnemius muscle for 20 min daily. Six patients with Achilles tendinopathy interface site and three patients with non-interface Achilles tendinopathy had their symptoms relieved within 6 months, and the pain VAS score decreased from 6.2 to 0.3. Three and two patients had their symptoms relieved within 1 year of PRP injection, respectively. Therefore, 56.25% (9/16) of patients with Achilles tendinopathy and 41.67% (5/12) of patients with non-interface Achilles tendinopathy had symptom relief within 1 year. Overall, PRP injections were effective in treating Achilles

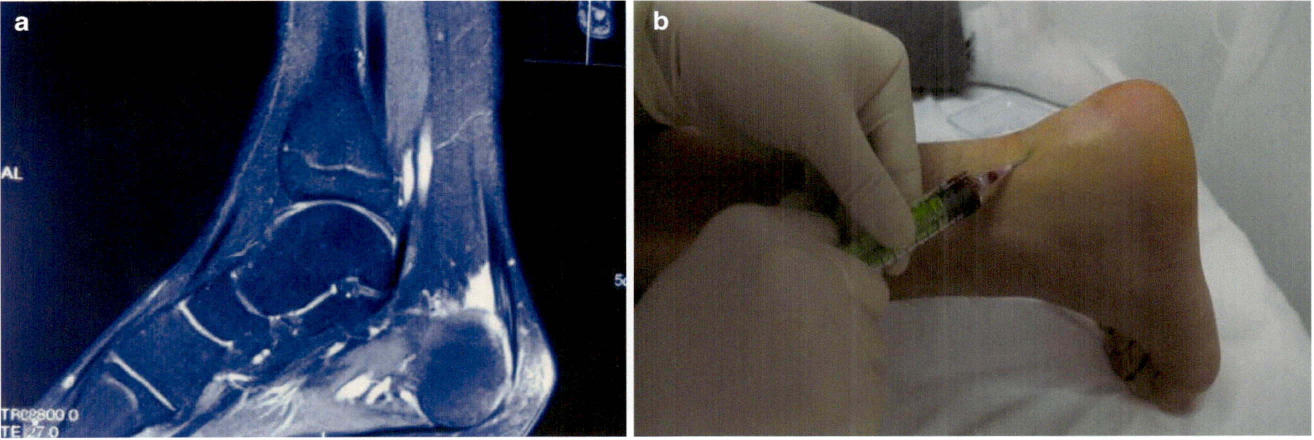

Fig. 9.13 Treatment of PRP for Achilles tendon's enthesiopathy. (**a**) MRI indicated edema appeared at the insertion of the Achilles tendon and the patient felt pain. (**b**) PRP was injected into the insertion of the Achilles tendon

tendinopathy but does not benefit non-interface Achilles tendinopathy. All patients with symptom relief have not relapsed to date (Fig. 9.13).

Shi's team treated a total of 12 patients with diagnosis of tarsal sinus syndrome who had undergone one or more (≤3) treatments with little or no relief. After informing the patients of their condition and injection instructions, intra-tarsal sinus PRP injections were performed. Four of the 12 patients had complete remission of symptoms at 4 and 6 months after the injection, and no recurrence of symptoms occurred in 1 year of observation; five patients had remission of symptoms, and the VAS score decreased from 6.6 to 2.4 before surgery; three patients still had no remission of symptoms.

9.5 Research of PRP-Derived Exosomes on Bone Generation

The vast majority of extracellular vesicles in PRP are secreted by platelets. The extracellular vesicles secreted by platelets include two main types of extracellular bodies ectosomes and exosomes (PRP-Exos). Extracellular vesicles are 100 nm–1 μm in diameter and are formed by means of platelet cytoplasmic membrane outgrowth and are mainly involved in the coagulation process. Exosomes are stored in the multivesicular bodies and alpha granules of platelets and are released outside the platelet by extracellular secretion after activation to participate in various physiopathological processes, including tissue repair. Since PRP-derived exosomes do not bind to coagulation factor X and prothrombinogen as extracellular bodies do, it is suggested that PRP-derived exosomes may not be involved in the coagulation process.

Extracellular vesicles originating from different cells possess specific proteins reflecting their cellular origin. For example, platelet-derived exosomes have vascular hemophilia factor and fusion protein CD41a on their plasma membrane and contain platelet-specific mRNAs and miRNAs. Extracellular bodies are synthesized by means of platelet plasma membrane outgrowth, and exosomes are formed by invagination of the outer membrane of multivesicular bodies in platelets. When multivesicular bodies fuse with the platelet plasma membrane, exosomes are released outside the platelet by endocytosis.

There are very few reports on PRP-Exos and tissue repair. In an experiment by Torreggiani [21] to repair bone tissue with PRP-Exos, PRP-Exos was co-cultured with BMSC in vitro for 20 h. It was found that PRP-Exos labeled with PKH26 was detectable in (98 ± 1.8)% of BMSC and PRP-Exos significantly promoted the proliferation of BMSC (1.2 times faster than the control group), and the higher the concentration of PRP-Exos, the more obvious the promotion of proliferation. Also, PRP-Exos significantly promoted the migration and differentiation of BMSC, and the mineralization of calcium deposition after osteoinduction was more pronounced in the PRP-Exos group compared with the control group. It is suggested that when PRP is used for bone tissue repair, a large amount of PRP-Exos is released locally, and these PRP-Exos can interact with repair cells in the local environment such as stem cells and bone precursor cells to promote the migration of repair cells to the bone injury and promote the proliferation and differentiation of repair cells to osteoblasts, thus achieving the effect of promoting the repair of bone tissue. The promotion of BMSC-induced osteogenesis by PRP-Exos differentiation was dose-dependent at low doses. However, when PRP-Exos was administered to BMSC bone at a high concentration of 50 μg, its osteo-differentiation effect was found to be reduced. This may be due to the fact that the effect of PRP-Exos lies more in promoting cell proliferation, which is in accordance with the mechanism of human bone tissue repair. In bone defects, firstly, bone precursor cells proliferate to fill the bone defect and form a bone bridge; later on, bone precursor cells differentiate toward mature osteocytes, which are shaped by mechanics and gradually form mature bone structures. The concentrations of growth factors such as bFGF, VEGF, PDGF-BB, and TGF-β1 in PRP-Exos and PRP were measured by ELISA, and it was found that the same volume of PRP-Exos showed clearly higher concentrations of growth factors compared to PRP group. The concentrations of bFGF, PDGF-BB, and TGF-β1 were 3.3, 2.7, and 35.5 times higher than those of PRP, respectively. It indicates that most of the growth factors, which are the most important active components in PRP, are stored in PRP-Exos, especially TGF-β1.

In a recent experiment by Changqing Zhang's team [22, 23] to repair femoral head necrosis with PRP-Exos, it was found that PRP-Exos promotes cell proliferation and angiogenesis through the Akt/Erk signaling pathway and inhibits glucocorticoid-induced apoptosis. For osteoblasts, PRP-Exos enhanced the expression level of osteogenic proteins through the Wnt/β-linked protein signaling pathway and promoted bone precursor cell differentiation and bone regeneration.

There are many mechanisms that have not been elucidated so far in the study of PRP-EVs. According to the current studies of PRP-EVs, growth factors are mainly stored in exosomes in platelets, and after platelet activation, the outer membrane of exosomes can protect growth factors from destruction by lytic enzymes in the external environment. Therefore, exosomes are more stable extracellularly and have enough time to bind to the target cell receptor, thus changing its biological function; exosomes are less immunogenic, which facilitates the use of allogeneic exosomes, that is, exosomes extracted from platelet fluid from blood banks, which is conducive to large-scale production and standardization; a very small amount of exosomes can achieve the repair effect of PRP, which is convenient for clinical use and portability. In addition, PRP-EVs contain genetically informative DNA and RNA, which have the potential to cause genetic mutations in target cells. Exosomes play a very important role in tumor formation and metastasis, and it remains to be verified whether PRP-Exos can cause or promote cancer formation when applied in a non-tumor setting.

Although animal studies and some clinical trials have initially demonstrated the safety of exosomes, further experiments are needed to demonstrate their multifaceted and long-term safety.

References

1. Ross R, Glomset J, Kariya B, Harker L. A platelet-dependent serum factor that stimulates the proliferation of arterial smooth muscle cells in vitro. Proc Natl Acad Sci. 1974;71(4):1207–10.
2. Witte LD, Kaplan KL, Nossel HL, Lages BA, Weiss HJ, Goodman DS. Studies of the release from human platelets of the growth factor for cultured human arterial smooth muscle cells. Circ Res. 1978;42(3):402–9.
3. Yuan T, Guo SC, Han P, Zhang CQ, Zeng BF. Applications of leukocyte- and platelet-rich plasma (L-PRP) in trauma surgery. Curr Pharm Biotechnol. 2012;13(7):1173–84.
4. Knighton DR, Ciresi K, Fiegel VD, Schumerth S, Butler E, Cerra F. Stimulation of repair in chronic, nonhealing, cutaneous ulcers using platelet-derived wound healing formula. Surg Gynecol Obstet. 1990;170(1):56–60.
5. Ganio C, Tenewitz F, Wilson R, Moyles B. The treatment of chronic nonhealing wounds using autologous platelet-derived growth factors. J Foot Ankle Surg. 1993;32(3):263–8.
6. Marx RE, Carlson ER, Eichstaedt RM, Schimmele SR, Strauss JE, Georgeff KR. Platelet-rich plasma: growth factor enhancement for bone grafts. Oral Surg Oral Med Oral Pathol Oral Radiol Endod. 1998;85(6):638–46.
7. Slater M, Patava J, Kingham K, Mason RS. Involvement of platelets in stimulating osteogenic activity. J Orthop Res. 1995;13(5):655–63.
8. Zhang CQ, Yuan T, Zeng BF. Experimental study of the effect of platelet-rich plasma on osteogenesis in rabbit. Chin Med J. 2004;117(12):1853–5.
9. Fennis J, Stoelinga P, Jansen J. Mandibular reconstruction: a histological and histomorphometric study on the use of autogenous scaffolds, particulate cortico-cancellous bone grafts and platelet rich plasma in goats. Int J Oral Maxillofac Surg. 2004;33(1):48–55.
10. Bielecki T, Gazdzik TS, Szczepanski T. Benefit of percutaneous injection of autologous platelet-leukocyte-rich gel in patients with delayed union and nonunion. Eur Surg Res. 2008;40(3):289–96.
11. Bielecki TM, Gazdzik TS, Arendt J, Szczepanski T, Krol W, Wielkoszynski T. Antibacterial effect of autologous platelet gel enriched with growth factors and other active substances: an in vitro study. J Bone Joint Surg Br. 2007;89(3):417–20.
12. Cieslik-Bielecka A, Gazdzik TS, Bielecki TM, Cieslik T. Why the platelet-rich gel has antimicrobial activity? Oral Surg Oral Med Oral Pathol Oral Radiol Endod. 2007;103(3):303–5. author reply 305-306
13. 袁霆, 张长青, 余楠生: 富血小板血浆在骨关节外科临床应用专家共识(2018年版). 中华关节外科杂志(电子版) 2018;12(5):596–600.
14. 张昭远, 杨帆, 卢年芳, 袁霆, 张长青: 血小板抗感染的机制研究进展. 中华关节外科杂志 (电子版) 2019;13(4):443–7.
15. Deppermann C, Kubes P. Platelets and infection. Semin Immunol. 2016;28(6):536–45.
16. Jia WT, Zhang CQ, Wang JQ, Feng Y, Ai ZS. The prophylactic effects of platelet-leucocyte gel in osteomyelitis: an experimental study in a rabbit model. J Bone Joint Surg Br. 2010;92(2):304–10.
17. Li GY, Yin JM, Ding H, Jia WT, Zhang CQ. Efficacy of leukocyte- and platelet-rich plasma gel (L-PRP gel) in treating osteomyelitis in a rabbit model. J Orthop Res. 2013;31(6):949–56.
18. Guo Y, Qiu J, Zhang C. [Follow-up study on platelet-rich plasma in repairing chronic wound nonunion of lower limbs in 47 cases]. Zhongguo Xiu Fu Chong Jian Wai Ke Za Zhi. 2008;22(11):1301–5.
19. Yuan T, Zhang C, Zeng B. Treatment of chronic femoral osteomyelitis with platelet-rich plasma (PRP): a case report. Transfus Apher Sci. 2008;38(2):167–73.
20. Zhou Y, Zhang J, Yang J, Narava M, Zhao G, Yuan T, Wu H, Zheng N, Hogan MV, Wang JH. Kartogenin with PRP promotes the formation of fibrocartilage zone in the tendon-bone interface. J Tissue Eng Regen Med. 2017;11(12):3445–56.
21. Torreggiani E, Perut F, Roncuzzi L, Zini N, Baglio SR, Baldini N. Exosomes: novel effectors of human platelet lysate activity. Eur Cell Mater. 2014;28:137–51; discussion 151.
22. Tao SC, Yuan T, Rui BY, Zhu ZZ, Guo SC, Zhang CQ. Exosomes derived from human platelet-rich plasma prevent apoptosis induced

by glucocorticoid-associated endoplasmic reticulum stress in rat osteonecrosis of the femoral head via the Akt/Bad/Bcl-2 signal pathway. Theranostics. 2017;7(3):733–50.

23. Guo SC, Tao SC, Yin WJ, Qi X, Yuan T, Zhang CQ. Exosomes derived from platelet-rich plasma promote the re-epithelialization of chronic cutaneous wounds via activation of YAP in a diabetic rat model. Theranostics. 2017;7(1):81–96.

10 Platelet-Rich Plasma and Its Derivatives and Oral and Maxillofacial Surgery

Zhifa Wang

This chapter will focus on the clinical research and typical cases of PRP and its derivatives and oral and maxillofacial surgery and further elaborate on the research and progress of PRP and its derivatives in clinical related fields.

10.1 Introduction

The repair and reconstruction of bone and soft tissue defects resulted from tumor resection; congenital and acquired deformities remain a critical issue in clinic. In addition, due to the characteristics of easy exposure and difficult protection, the oral and maxillofacial area is prone to be damaged, such as in traffic accident injuries, leading to facial fractures and soft tissue defects and deformities. There are many kinds of oral diseases, including but not limited to pulpitis, apical periodontitis, periodontitis, gingival recession, insufficient height and width of jaws, benign and malignant tumors and trauma, etc. These abovementioned diseases will not only affect the chewing function, swallowing function, and speech function of the patient but also increase the gastrointestinal burden of the patient. Moreover, some of these oral diseases can also affect the appearance of the patient, causing the patient to have severe inferiority mentality and social dysfunctions. A lot of surgery treatments were invented or introduced into oral surgery to deal with the varied diseases, such as connective tissue graft (CTG), guided bone regeneration (GBR), sinus floor elevation, alveolar ridge preservation, and so on. Encouragingly, tissue engineering and regenerative medicine, as a hopeful strategy for reconstruction of defected tissues and organs, have been widely used in the field of basic medical research and clinical applications of stomatology and also achieved some satisfactory results. It is understood that a good blood supply is quite essential for the self-repairing of defective tissues and self-healing of wounds. There are three important factors: appropriate scaffold materials, sufficient stem cells, and growth factors in tissue engineering [1]. Several kinds of stem cells are able to use in lab research because there are sufficient quality and quantity of stem cells, such as bone marrow mesenchymal stem cells (BMSCs), adipose-derived stem cells (ADSCs), human dental pulp stem cells (hDPSCs), human periodontal ligament stem cells (hPDLSCs), etc. [2, 3]. However, there are not so many kinds of stem cells that can be used in clinical practice due to various reasons, such as the restrictions of policies and regulations, the patient's own health status, age and other unpredictable factors. Thus, growth factors and proper scaffold materials are well investigated to restore defective tissues in oral and maxillofacial regions. For instance, several bone substitutes (such as Bio-Oss®, Geistlich Pharma North America, Inc., Princeton, NJ, USA) have been successfully introduced in guided tissue regeneration (GTR) procedures for sinus floor elevation. And for the treatment of bone intrabony defects in patients with severe periodontitis, the use of platelet-rich fibrin (PRF) membrane combined with GTR would present a better repair result than GTR used alone by analyzing probe depth (PD) and the height of newly formed bone detected by cone beam computed tomography (CBCT) and panoramic radiography scanning, which could be attributed to plentiful growth factors (GFs) in PRF. Besides, bone morphogenetic proteins (including BMP-2 and BMP-7) and growth differentiation factor-5 (GDF-5) have also been proved to accelerate local bone augmentation during tooth extraction socket preservation [4]. All of these indicate that growth factors, especially autologous growth factors, play an important role in the repair of tissue defects and have a wide range of clinical applications. Among them, platelet aggregates are the most widely used and the most in-depth researched.

Z. Wang (✉)
Department of Stomatology, General Hospital of Southern Theater of PLA, Guangzhou, Guangdong, China

B. Cheng, X. Fu (eds.), *Platelet-Rich Plasma in Tissue Repair and Regeneration*, https://doi.org/10.1007/978-981-99-3193-4_10

10.2 The Classification and Characterization of Platelet Aggregates

Fibrin glues, as one of the autologous blood-derived products, are first introduced into stimulating wound healing about 50 years ago. Then platelet concentrates were used to ameliorate wound healing. Platelets contain plenty of essential growth factors, such as VEGF, TGFβ-1, and PDGF-AB, which are verified to be able to improve cell proliferation and differentiation, angiogenesis, and matrix remodeling [5]. PRP is the first generation of platelet concentrates that are prepared by two centrifugation steps. A first centrifugation step is aimed to divide the collected blood into three layers, "buffy coat" layer (PRP) in the middle and platelet-poor plasma (PPP, also called acellular plasma) in the supernatant. Platelets are concentrated in the middle layer. The second centrifugation step is designed to collect the "buffy coat" layer and to abandon the acellular plasma and the RBC layers. Lastly, the collected PRP could be administrated into the defect sites via injection with a syringe or be combined with other bone substitutes to be transplanted into the bone defect regions.

Leucocyte-platelet-rich fibrin (L-PRF, also known as Choukroun's PRF) is the second generation of platelet-rich concentrates because it only requires one centrifugation step (3000–3200 rpm, about 10–12 min centrifugation varied according to different preparation protocols) during its preparation process without any additional biomedical agents such as anticoagulant, thrombin, and calcium chloride [6]. Like PRP, L-PRF also contains a lot of autologous GFs including VEGF, TGFβ-1, and endothelial cell growth factor (ECGF), which could release slowly and continuously for more than 2 weeks, thus providing an alternative solution for GF administration. The functions of these GFs are as follows: PDGF could promote the recruitment and the activation of inflammatory cells such as macrophages, endothelial cells, and neutrophils and stimulate matrix formation and remodeling. TGF-β has mostly appeared in angiogenesis and re-epithelialization processes during wound healing; it also could inhibit the proliferation of mesenchymal stem cells, macrophages, and lymphocytes and increase matrix formation and remodeling. VEGF plays a key role in the wound healing process because it could be able to promote angiogenesis and increase vessel permeability. FGF also could increase angiogenesis and has mitogenic effect on mesenchymal stem cells, chondroblasts, endothelial cells, osteoblasts, and fibroblasts. Except for growth factors in L-PRF, leucocytes and fibrin matrix are the other two important parameters for tissue engineering and repair. Leucocytes not only be proved to be able to regulate immune and present anti-infectious action; they also could produce a great deal number of VEGFs, which is extremely essential for the promotion and development of angiogenesis. Moreover, L-PRP also be verified to be able to motivate anabolism and remodeling potential of tendons and be triumphantly applied in the repair of tendonitis and long bone delayed healing with an injectable form. However, the individual effects of leucocytes and platelets in the L-PRP and L-PRF have not yet been clearly elucidated, though the synergistic effects could be hypothesized. Therefore, further studies need to be performed to address this issue of platelet concentrate function to distinctly analyze the respective effects of the concentrate components, thus helping to process concentrates with targeted and specific effects. Although the biological effects of platelet concentrates were proclaimed to be contributed to the platelet-derived growth factors in many researches, the cytokines within their fibrin matrix and the microenvironment established by fibrin matrix structures, which help to release growth factors, should be focused and investigated. Thus, PRFs are often considered as improved biomaterials. L-PRF can be taken as a biological healing matrix via regulating and improving cell proliferation and migration and cytokine release and expanding the potential application range of PRF greatly [7].

Besides, this technique for L-PRF preparation is simpler and easier and also cost-less when compared with PRP preparation. Because no anticoagulants were used in this process, platelet activation and fibrin polymerization are initiated immediately. Thus, three layers are displated after centrifugation: the RBC layer at the bottom, a PRF clot in the middle, and acellular plasma at the top (Fig. 10.1). A stable fibrin matrix with a three-dimensional structure was formed in the obtained PRF clot, in which the harvested platelets and leucocytes are concentrated. After being pressed with two gauzes or commercial tailor-made tools, the PRF clot transforms a membrane (Fig. 10.1c), which expands the application scope of PRF, and has been successfully introduced in oral and maxillofacial surgery [8].

One of the advantages of L-PRF is that it will not be dissolved quickly after being implanted into defect sites in vivo, which could be attributed to the strong fibrin matrix remodeling slowly in a parallel way to the natural blood clots. The H&E staining presented that PRF was composed of a mass of red-stained fiber bundles containing a great deal of blue-stained leukocytes (Fig. 10.2a). Scanning electron microscope (SEM) views demonstrated that fibrin fibers were arranged regularly in the L-PRF (Fig. 10.2b). Transmission electron microscope (TEM) views showed a mass of fibrin bundles in PRF (Fig. 10.2c). In addition, SEM examination also showed that BMSCs (black arrow, Fig. 10.2d) could adhere to the surface of L-PRF and presented a good status of survival (Fig. 10.2d).

Besides, leucocytes, platelets, and plenty of growth factors from leucocytes and activated platelets are also collected and preserved in L-PRF. This preparation method of L-PRF

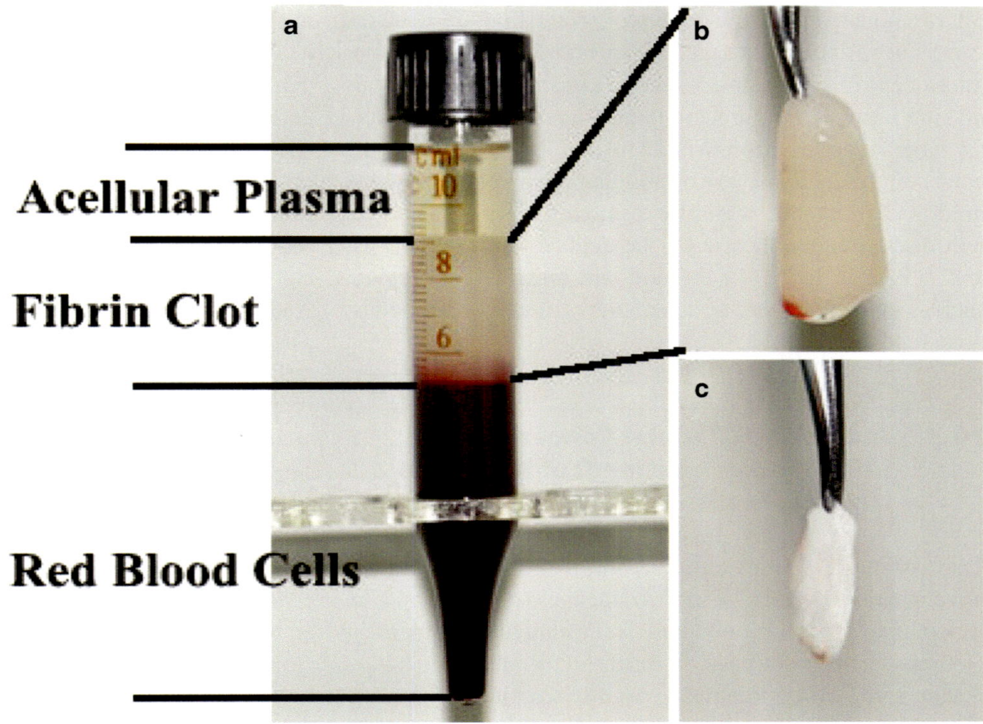

Fig. 10.1 The preparation process of L-PRF. (**a**) The samples of blood were separated into three layers after centrifugation. Acellular plasma was located on the top layer with pale yellow liquid, the red blood cell layer was collected at the bottom layer, and the fibrin clot was located in the middle. (**b**) A PRF clot was obtained easily. (**c**) A pale yellow fibrin membrane was regarded as the PRF membrane and was harvested by removing the fluids

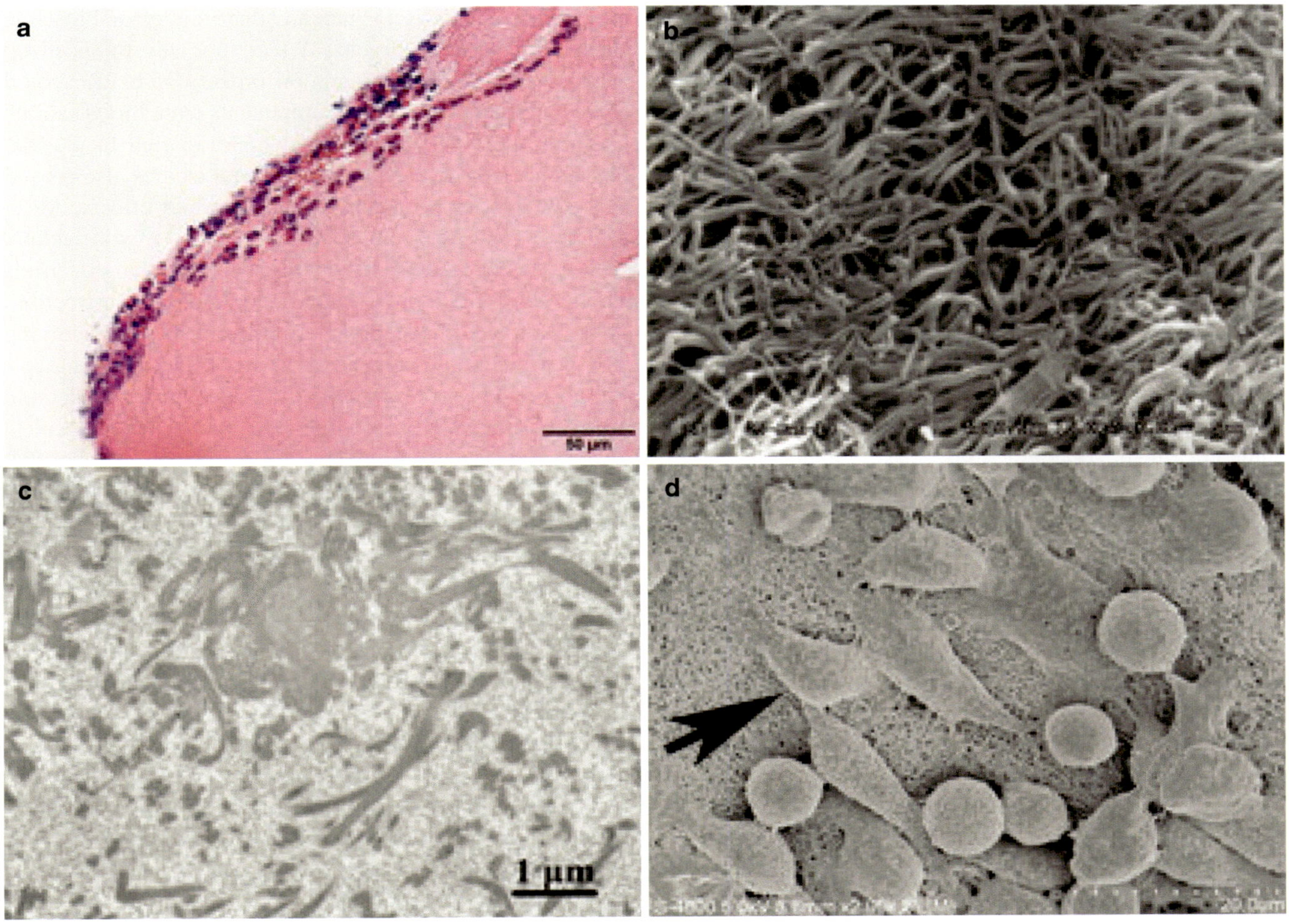

Fig. 10.2 The characterization of L-PRF. (**a**) H&E staining presented that PRF was composed of a mass of red-stained fiber bundles containing a great deal of blue-stained leukocytes. (**b**) SEM views demonstrated that fibrin fibers were arranged regularly in the L-PRF. (**c**) TEM views showed a mass of fibrin bundles in PRF. (**d**) SEM examination also showed that BMSCs (black arrow) grew well on the surface of L-PRF

offers a high quantity and quality of production of PRF clots simultaneously using a specific centrifuge tube with a laboratory centrifuge or some modified clinical centrifuge, thus making it possible to process large amounts of L-PRF clots for large surgeries. Moreover, thanks to its low cost and the great convenience and ease of this method, it could be widely used in daily practices and serve more patients. Below, we will discuss and elaborate on the applications of PC (PRP and L-PRF included) in the oral and maxillofacial region, such as in the treatment of dental pulp disease, orthodontics, bone regeneration, etc.

10.3 Autologous Platelet Concentrates (APCs) in the Treatment of Immature Necrotic Teeth

The treatment of immature necrotic teeth remains a great issue in clinic. Because of the low thickness of dentin and the lack of apex closure in immature teeth, endodontic treatment of these teeth is not easy to finish and is also difficult to obtain satisfactory treatment results. Calcium hydroxide ($Ca(OH)_2$) and mineral trioxide aggregate (MTA) are mostly used in the treatment of these teeth, such as apexification. Although $Ca(OH)_2$ could induce the appearance of an apical barrier, this method claims patient visits several times and a total treatment time of 10 months. Moreover, there is a possibility of cervical root fracture when exposed to $Ca(OH)_2$ in a long time, and the apical closure is changeable and unpredictable. MTA seems to be more biocompatible than $Ca(OH)_2$ because it offers an effective artificial apical barrier and does not weaken the root canal dentin and may stimulate more apexification completion in a single session. However, MTA is not easy to operate during the treatment, and it would release, to some extent, toxic elements, which might lead to tooth discoloration. In addition, only a small amount of root regenerated with regard to the length and width of the dentin walls when $Ca(OH)_2$ or MTA was used in the remedy of immature teeth. Encouragingly, tissue engineering and regenerative endodontics were considered as promising alternatives for the treatment of immature necrotic teeth. As our aforementioned explanations in tissue engineering, three key elements are also required to obtain the successful revascularization of a tooth: first, proper stem cells that are needed in the periapical tissues and in the apical papilla of a necrotic immature tooth; second, appropriate growth factors that could improve the migration, proliferation, and differentiation of stem cells; and third, suitable scaffold materials that possess a specific three-dimensional structure which offers support for the migration and proliferation of stem cells.

Autologous platelet concentrates (APCs) could be administrated into the targeted sites, thus inducing collagen production, stimulating migration of stem cells, accelerating the vascularization, and finally facilitating the wound healing process. Therefore, APCs may be able to use in the treatment of immature necrotic teeth by improving the defected pulp revascularization and increasing the width and length of root dentin [9]. PRP and PRF are the most famous platelet concentrates that could be delivered into the root canal systems and be helpful for the regeneration of root dentin. PRP is a high amount of platelet concentration and requires anticoagulants during the preparation process. And PRF maintains the most leucocytes and platelets within a dense fibrin matrix without anticoagulants needed. Several researches were conducted to assess the utility of APCs for pulp regeneration and radicular development. PRP and PRF were used in the experimental groups. And the platelet concentrate was used alone, combined with collagen sponge or in junction with blood and collagen sponge, which were delivered into the root canal. Then MTA was placed into the root canal over the APCs. Although the statistical significance was not observed, the APC treatment group showed an improved result in terms of periapical healing and apical closure [10]. Thus, APCs still presented a promising potential effectiveness in stimulating root development and reconstruction of the pulp-dentin complex in immature necrotic teeth, which needed further investigations. The fundamental principle of APCs is to increase the number of bioactive cues from blood in targeted defect sites and to speed up healing process. The preparation process of L-PRF could harvest numerous bioactive components from blood sample (approximately 10 ml) among which are rich in plasma, fibrin, platelets, and leucocytes. Several studies also proved that APCs have the potential antimicrobial effects. APCs contain a great deal number of autologous growth factors, such as VEGF and FGF, which may initiate angiogenesis ameliorating tissue revascularization and reconstruction. Thus, APCs hold the potent improvement ability of the pulp-dentin complex regeneration process by inducing apical closure and root dentin wall thickening in a quite safe manner for patient blood-derived bioactive molecules. Moreover, when compared to PRP and blood clot, PRF holds a huge potential of increasing the growth characteristics in necrotic immature permanent teeth. However, due to the lack of histological results, for histological observation needs, the experimental tooth was extracted, which is forbidden by ethical concerns and legal provisions; it is impossible to evaluate the thickness and length of the neo-formed root tissue. But the histological outcomes in animal studies demonstrated that the neo-formed tissue is largely bone-like and cementum-like rather than pulp-like tissues. Conversely, few loose connective tissues resemble immature pulp containing mesenchymal cells, and fibroblasts were observed in the root canal space of an immature tooth diagnosed with irreversible pulpitis without apical periodontitis after revascularization for 4 weeks.

Although there is insufficient evidence to verify the possible effectiveness of autologous PCs in stimulating root development of immature teeth, they still hold the promising application potential in regenerative endodontics due to their biological safety with simple and cost-efficient preparation procedures and the potential effectiveness.

10.4 Leucocyte-Platelet-Rich Fibrin (L-PRF) in the Treatment of Periodontal Diseases

Autologous platelet concentrates, as a human blood-derived extracts, have been considered as a promising regenerative material, applied alone or in combination with other bone substitutes in the last decades [3]. Although PRP and platelet derived growth factors (PDGF) were first introduced to oral surgery, PRF was more popular to accelerate wound healing now, for the use of it is simpler, avoiding any kinds of anticoagulants and collecting the most leucocytes and platelets from blood samples. Except for facilitating the migration, proliferation, and differentiation of progenitor and stem cells in the targeted local microenvironment, PRF also was regarded as an anti-inflammation niche with immune regulation capacity and held the ability of releasing growth factors continuously and slowly for 7–14 days. Moreover, due to being rich in dense fibrin matrix, L-PRF also can be further changed into a membrane by gently pressing with two gauzes or specific instruments, approximately 1 mm in thickness, by which the application range of L-PRF membrane was greatly enlarged. With the exception of the mechanical and biological characteristics, L-PRF also has been proved to present the antimicrobial effects.

The periodontal tissue contains three parts: periodontal ligaments, alveolar bone, and gingival tissues (also be named as dental gum). Periodontal ligaments are a kind of dense fibrous tissue, which one end is connected to the cementum of teeth and the other end is embedded in the alveolar bone. In other words, periodontal ligaments are essential for the teeth suspended in the alveolar socket. And these ligaments have a certain degree of elasticity, which helps to cushion the chewing force. The alveolar bone surrounds the root of the tooth to form an alveolar socket. Thus the root is erected so that the teeth and the alveolar bone are tightly connected together, which is convenient for chewing. Gingivae wrapped around the cervical part of the tooth with the edge. The gingivae between the two adjacent teeth is wedge-shaped, also be named as the gingival papilla. As we all know, healthy gums are pink and tough elastic so that they can withstand the pressure of chewing and the friction force of food. In addition, the blood vessels and nerves in the dental pulp are also directly connected with the blood vessels and nerves of the alveolar bone via the apical foramen. Therefore, the teeth and periodontal tissue are closely related. In terms of the classification of periodontal diseases, it could be classified into inflammation, degeneration, atrophy, trauma, hyperplasia, etc. according to the pathological type. A brief introduction to the applications of L-PRF in the treatment of periodontal disease is as follows.

Gingival recession, commonly leading to the exposure of the root surface, would result in some complications including dentin hypersensitivity, the issue of esthetics, and a higher risk of dental caries if not treated well. Several treatment approaches are suitable to use in the clinic: (1) connective tissue grafts (CTG), (2) subepithelial connective tissue grafts (SCTG), and (3) coronally advanced flap (CAF) technique [11]. However, the indications of these abovementioned approaches are quite strict, and the results are unpredictable in a long-time follow-up. Several studies were performed to assess the effectiveness of PRF in the treatment of gingival recession. Encouragingly, the addition of PRF to CAF ameliorated both the posttreatment stability of CAF and the clinical outcomes, including obtained more recession depth (RD) reduction, keratinized tissue width (KTW) increase, and average clinical attachment level (CAL) gain than CAF group, which is considered as control group. Moreover, gingival margin stability (GMS) after treatment in the experimental group was also better after 6 months of operation than that in the control groups. Herein, due to PRF being applied in the operations, more fast healing and fewer complications, such as pain, swelling, and discomfort, were presented in the test group [12]. Therefore, the combination of PRF and CAF could be regarded as a less invasive and safer method to conventional grafting approaches.

A large proportion of molars in the patients with periodontitis suffers from furcation involvement, thus leading to higher risks of periodontal tissue breakdown and weaker prognosis than single-rooted teeth. Current mostly approved treatment approach for periodontal furcation defects (PFDs) is the guided tissue regeneration (GTR) based on the bone substitutes and regenerative materials, such as Bio-Oss grafts and absorbable collagen membrane [13]. Interestingly, the addition of PRF to GTR has been proved to present better therapeutic results [13, 14]. For example, open flap debridement and the combination of PRF and open flap debridement were performed and compared to analyze the effectiveness of PRF in PFD treatment. The results of this study demonstrated that PRF could significantly ameliorate clinical and radiographic outcomes of open flap debridement. In detail, more CAL gain, higher PD reduction, and greater vertical defect fill verified by radiographical examination were shown in the experimental group versus control groups.

Due to the inflammation and the deficient intrinsic regenerative ability, intra-bony defects (IBDs) in severe periodontitis remain a challenge in the clinic. Conservative open flap

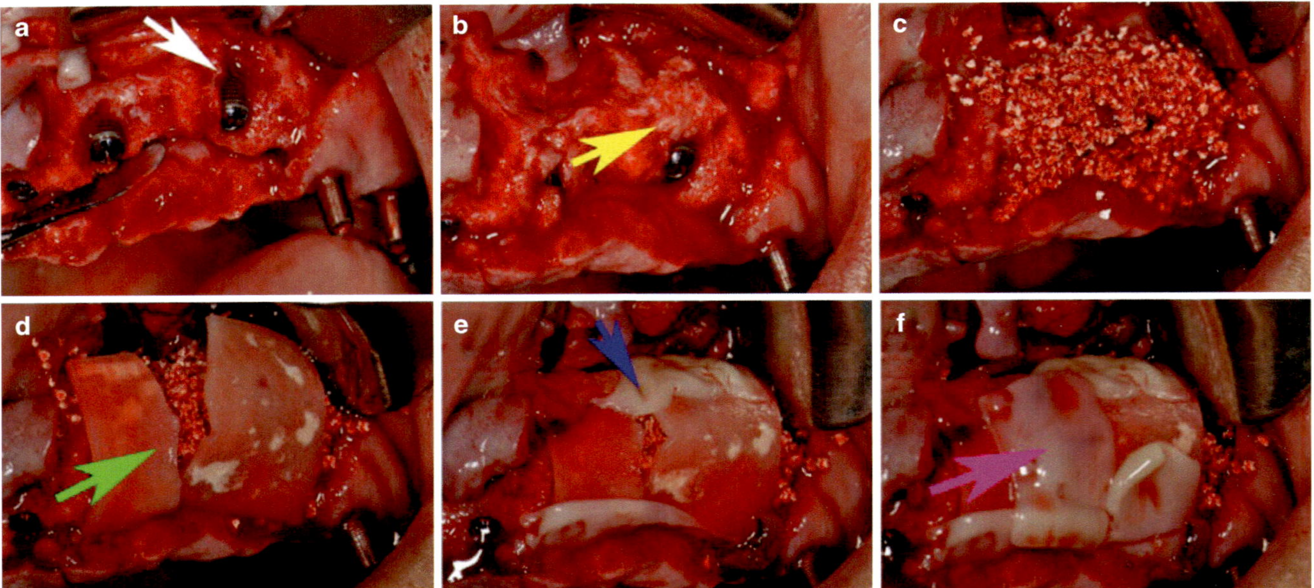

Fig. 10.3 PRF used in the dental implanting surgery that suffered with bone defects in the buccal region of dental implant. (**a**) The obvious bone defects (white arrow) in the buccal region of dental implant. (**b**) PRF membrane (yellow arrow) fragments were implanted into the bone defect sites around the implants. (**c**) Bone substitutes were then placed on the surface of PRF. (**d**) Collagen membranes (green arrow) were covered on the bone grafting based on the principle of GBR. (**e**) PRF membrane (blue arrow) were placed on the surface of collagen membrane. (**f**) Double PRF membrane (pink arrow) was used to cover the collagen membrane. (The case was provided by Dr. Duan Jianmin, from the Department of Stomatology, General Hospital of Southern Theater of PLA, Guangzhou, China)

debridement technique could increase an average 2 mm of CAL gain, in which approximately 1.5 mm may be resulted from the newly formed bone tissue. In our previous study, we found that PRF could stimulate the growth, proliferation, and differentiation of BMSCs in a dose-dependent manner and thereby improve the osteogenic potential of BMSCs significantly in vitro and in vivo. Thus, PRF seems a promising alternative for the treatment of periodontal tissues [4, 12]. PRF combined with Bio-Oss bone grafts or open flap surgery or inorganic bovine bone mineral (ABBM) or demineralized freeze-dried bone allograft (DFDBA) or collagen membrane was conducted as test group, while Bio-Oss bone grafts or open flap surgery or ABBM or DFDBA or collagen membrane without PRF was considered as control group. Thanks to the pain-abating and improved wound healing characteristics, the application of PRF holds a higher acceptance of patients. Thus, the addition of PRF membrane to the GBR has been widely used in the treatment of bone defects in patients with periodontitis and/or patients who need dental implanting surgery (Fig. 10.3). The addition of PRF to bone grafts, such as Bio-Oss and ABBM, significantly improved the clinical results, including higher PD reduction, CAL gain, and newly formed bone tissue as compared to grafts used alone.

10.5 Leucocyte-Platelet-Rich Fibrin (L-PRF) in the Treatment of Bone Regeneration in Oral and Maxillofacial Region

10.5.1 Alveolar Ridge Preservation

A remarkable bone resorption of the alveolar ridge including vertical and horizontal appears after tooth extraction because of the relationship of tooth and bundle bone. Especially in terms of implanting, these issues of bone resorption in the alveolar ridge caused by tooth extraction have to be taken into consideration seriously for obtaining satisfactory primary stability of dental implants and acceptable aesthetic outcomes. Thus, in order to achieve better aesthetic results in maxillary anterior region, the majority of the immediate implant surgeries and immediate restorations performed in aesthetic areas required instant bone augmentation by guided bone regeneration (GBR) due to the bone deficiency in the buccal zones [15]. Moreover, the addition of growth factors has also been proved to be able to increase the bone regeneration in GBR. VEGF and BMP-2 and BMP-7 were introduced into the bone augmentation in the preservation procedures of alveolar ridge. Platelet concentrates have been used in wound healing for decades. In need of special is that L-PRF, as the second generation of platelet concentrates, is more acceptable and widely used in the GBR for it contains plenty of leucocytes and platelets which were embedded in the dense fibrin network and it can also be regarded as scaffold for several types of cells. In our previous study, we found that the proliferative potential of BMSCs was significantly increased when BMSCs were exposed and cultured in the medium containing PRF (Fig. 10.4a). Moreover, the proliferative ability of BMSCs also remarkably increased with increasing PRF concentration in the culture medium (Fig. 10.4b). In a word, L-PRF could remarkably activate BMSC proliferation in a dose-dependent manner [8].

When it comes to the effect of L-PRF on osteogenic differentiation potential of BMSCs, we also found that the alkaline phosphatase (ALP) activity of BMSCs cultured in the osteogenic medium added with L-PRF was significantly higher than those cultured in osteogenic medium without L-PRF. Furthermore, the mRNA expression levels of osteogenic biomarkers, including BMP-2, osteopontin (OPN), and osteocalcin (OCN), were remarkably increased in the L-PRF group when compared to the control group, which indicated that L-PRF was able to significantly stimulate the osteogenic differentiation capacity of BMSCs in vitro. Next, we injected the osteogenic BMSC sheets combined with L-PRF subcutaneously in SCID and evaluated the formation of new bone by micro-CT and H&E staining, and we found that the new bone tissue in the L-PRF group was significantly greater than that in the control group without L-PRF (Fig. 10.5), which demonstrated that L-PRF can increase the osteogenic capacity of BMSC sheets in vivo [8, 9]. The possible reasons for these enhanced effects may be that L-PRF has lots of crucial growth factors. Second, the potential of sustained slow releasing of growth factors and protection of endogenous fibrogenic factors provided by L-PRF plays an important role in wound healing. Third, because it consisted dense fibrous network, structural glycoproteins, and cytokines, L-PRF could be considered as a biomaterial that is beneficial for cell migration, proliferation, and differentiation, thus stimulating defected tissue repair and regeneration.

Furthermore, we further investigated that the osteogenic BMSC sheets and L-PRF fragments improve bone regeneration in rabbits (Fig. 10.6), thus offering a promising approach for increasing skeletal repair; thus indicating L-PRF could be used in bone regeneration and repair [16].

Therefore, L-PRF was proved to be able to ameliorate the preservation of the alveolar ridge and led to less bone resorption in buccal areas when compared to the natural healing without PRF implanted. Besides, the addition of L-PRF also resulted in less post-extraction pain and better soft tissue healing. However, the controversial issue is that L-PRF did not increase bone heal-

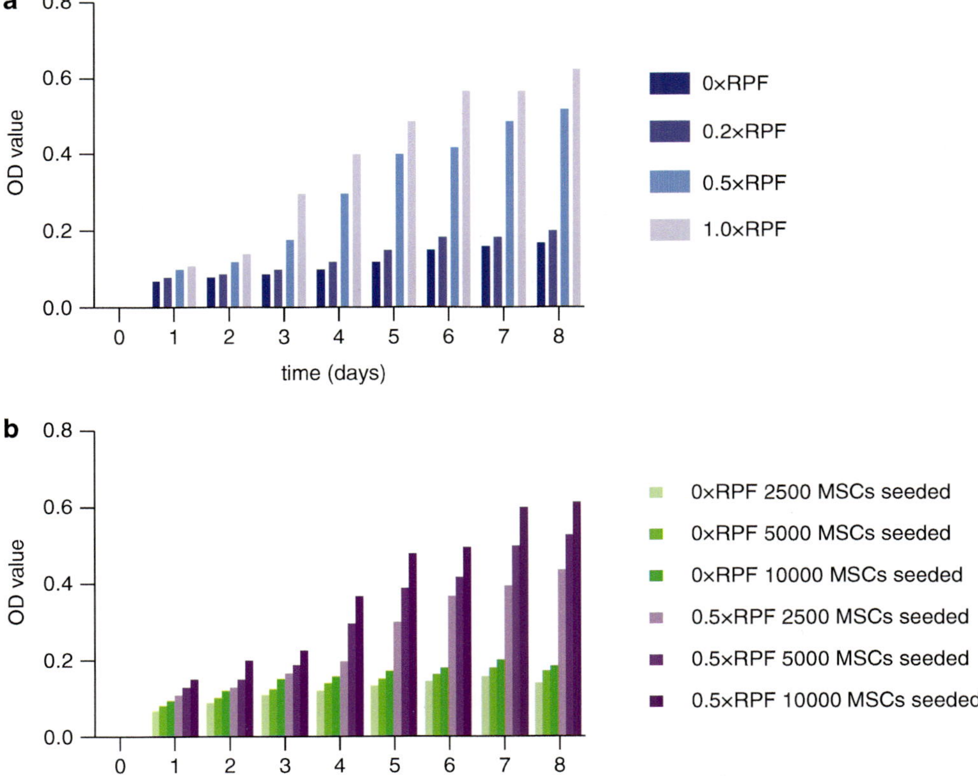

Fig. 10.4 The effects of L-PRF on BMSC proliferation. (**a**) The proliferation of BMSCs was remarkably improved when the concentration of L-PRF was increased. (**b**) Few L-PRF (0.5× PRF) also improved proliferative potential of BMSCs

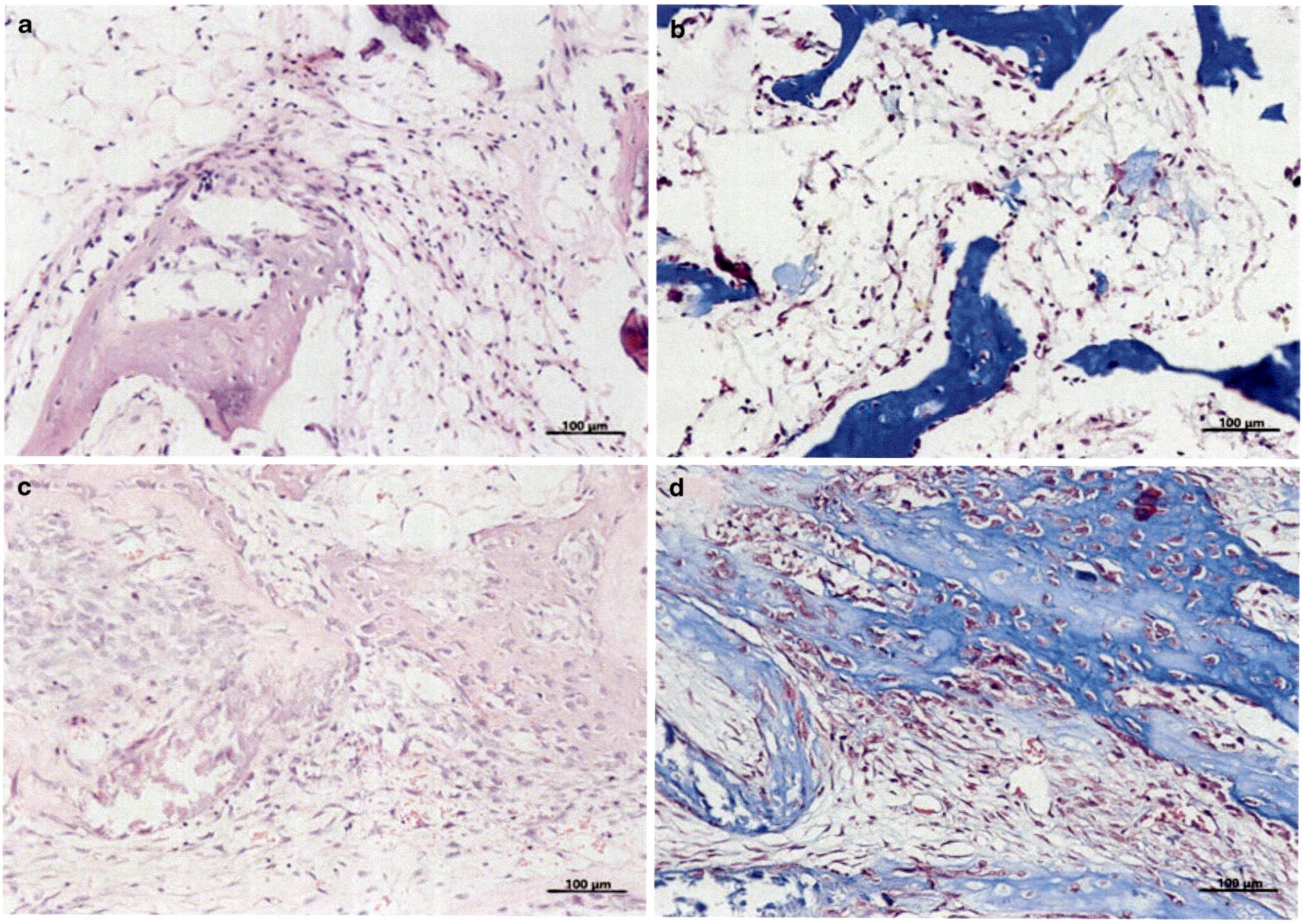

Fig. 10.5 Osteogenic BMSC sheets combined with L-PRF membrane were implanted into nude mice. (**a**, **c**) H&E staining showed more osteogenesis in the L-PRF group (**c**) than the control group (**a**). (**b**, **d**) Masson's trichrome staining presented a mass of cartilage-like tissue were observed in the L-PRF group. High-magnification, 200×

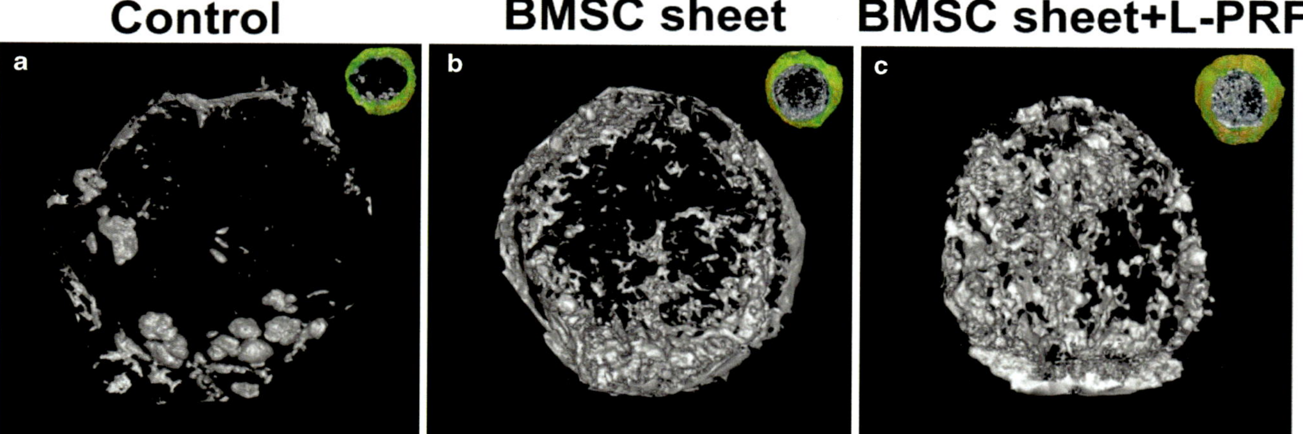

Fig. 10.6 BMSC sheets with or without L-PRF membrane were transplanted into critical-size calvarial defects in rabbits. (**a–c**) Micro-CT views proved that regenerated bone or bone-like tissues could repair the calvarial bone defects, but the combination of BMSC sheets and PRF group possessed a larger area of the bone (**c**)

ing in PRF-implanted sites. On the other hand, autogenous iliac crest bone graft with or without L-PRF was also used in the reconstruction of congenital alveolar defects (cleft lip and palate); some studies reported that there was a higher amount of newly formed bone in the L-PRF group, while the other studies suggested that the addition of L-PRF to autogenous bone failed to present a significant increase in the height, thickness, and density of alveolar bone graft [17–19]. Therefore, more clinical studies need to be performed to illustrate the effectiveness of PRF in the treatment of preservation of alveolar ridge and reconstruction of alveolar cleft.

10.5.2 Sinus Augmentation

Sinus augmentation is mainly used to deal with these issues of insufficient bone and soft tissues that are accompanied by atrophic maxilla. Several surgical techniques, including lateral window approach and trans-alveolar technique, were developed to increase the height and density of the maxillary bone in posterior alveolar bone [20]. The sinus membrane can be finished with or without the addition of bone grafting substitutes. If the residual vertical alveolar bone height is sufficient, there is no need to implant grafting substitutes for the satisfactory primary stability of the immediately placed implants that has been achieved and a blood clot formation around the part of the implant in the sinus cavity, which may be attributed to the augmented Schneiderian membrane which is maintained intact. On the other hand, several kinds of different bone grafting substitutes are introduced into sinus floor augmentation, such as autologous bone graft and growth factors. Although autologous bone grafting is the most suitable for bone regeneration, the inevitable morbidity and undesirable bone absorption remain great issues that need to be addressed. Indeed, a lot of studies about the use of platelet concentrates and growth factors in oral surgery have been well investigated, and some of them actually achieved to some extent some satisfactory results [21]. However, in terms of newly formed bone height and percentage of soft tissue zones, there is no significant additional effects of PRF in sinus floor augmentation. In detail, the percentage of residual bone substitutes in the PRF group was remarkably lower than that in the control (without PRF) group. But interestingly, no statistical significance was observed; the percentage of newly formed bone in the PRF group was slightly higher than that in the control (without PRF) group. This advantage may be attributed to the osteoinductive characteristics of bone grafting substitutes and the improved revascularization process of PRF, which synergistically ameliorated the healing process of the bone tissue as well. In summary, the use of PRF in sinus augmentation failed to provide significant beneficial effects, although they may ameliorate the bone formation and healing period [17, 18].

10.5.3 Implant Therapy

Due to its potential of speeding up revascularization and wound healing, PRF was also used in dental implants for accelerating the osseointegration process. Herein, implant stability quotients (ISQ values) were measured by resonance frequency analysis and were used to evaluate the implant stability when the implant was coated with L-PRF [15]. The application of L-PRF for implant leads to remarkably higher ISQ values, which would increase continuously overtime during the prearranged observation period. When the implants coated with L-PRF were implanted, about 50% less initial bone loss was presented in the L-PRF-coated implants. Besides, L-PRFs also have been verified to be used in the treatment of periimplantitis bone loss. In the L-PRF group, more PD reduction and CAL gain were shown. Detailedly, the PD reduction in the L-PRF sites (2.4 ± 1.1 mm) was significantly higher than that in the non-L-PRF sites (1.65 ± 1.0 mm) at three months after operation. The CAL gain in the L-PRF sites (2.9 ± 1.0 mm) was also significantly higher than that in the non-L-PRF sites (1.4 ± 1.0 mm). Moreover, a better bone-to-implant contact was also obtained in an animal study when the L-PRF was used in the treatment of periimplantitis defects. Moreover, the addition of PRF to bone grafting substitutes also presented favorable results in terms of bone gain and implant survival (Fig. 10.7). In conclusion, due to its ease and simple of preparation, low cost, and satisfactory biological properties, L-PRF could be regarded as an acceptable alternative for the bone regeneration in implant surgery [12, 15, 16]. However, the standard preparation and application protocol are needed to achieve more reproducible results, and furthermore researches with long-term follow-up are also required to perform for evaluating the potential effect of L-PRF on bone regeneration and osseointegration in dental implant surgery.

Furthermore, in order to reduce the postoperative complications, such as swelling and pain and promote bone regeneration, L-PRF was also used for the treatment of cyst cavity filling after curettage of jaw cyst (Fig. 10.8).

10.5.4 Orthodontics

Due to a high proportion of patients needing both orthodontic treatment and bone regeneration, the approach of tissue engineering and regenerative medicine has also been introduced into orthodontics. Many patients may require this approach for different reasons. For example, children who suffered from cleft lip and/or palate need the repair of alveolar cleft; older patients suffered with alveolar bone defect resulted from tooth loos need both the treatment of orthodontic and bone repair [22]. The fundamental principle of tooth movement in orthodontic is the proper mechanical force

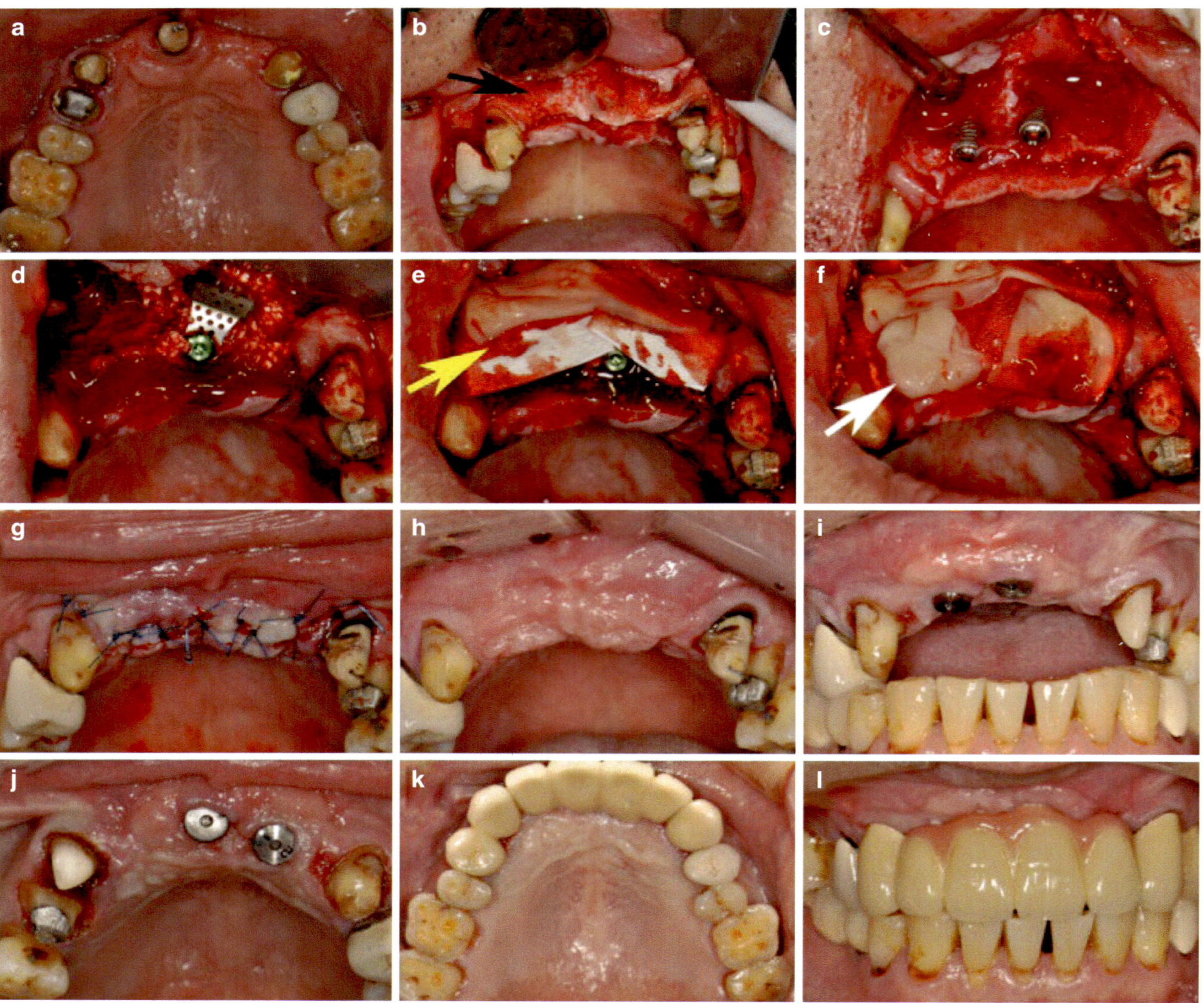

Fig. 10.7 PRF was applied in the dental implant surgery. (**a**) Patient with insufficient bone width for the placement of dental implants in the maxillary anterior area. (**b**) A mucoperiosteal tissue flap was elevated with vertical releases to the canines and the obvious insufficient bone width and sunken bone in the buccal area (black arrow). (**c**) After the implants were placed, the buccal side of the implants was exposed. (**d**) The titanium mesh was used to fix the implanted bone substitutes and provide a stable microenvironment for osteogenesis. (**e**) An absorbable collagen membrane (yellow arrow) was placed over the titanium mesh and bone substitutes. (**f**) Then PRF membranes (white arrow) were used to cover the collagen membrane for offering growth factors. (**g**) The recipient site was closed in a tension-free manner with nonabsorbable sutures. (**h**) Tissue condition and alveolar ridge width after 6 months of operation. (**i**) The buccal view at 2 weeks of the healing abutment was placed. (**j**) The occlusal view at 2 weeks of the healing abutment was placed. (**k**) The occlusal view after the permanent porcelain-fused metal prosthesis was placed. (**l**) The buccal view after the permanent porcelain-fused metal prosthesis was placed. (The case was provided by Dr. Duan Jianmin, from the Department of Stomatology, General Hospital of Southern Theater of PLA, Guangzhou, China)

applied on the teeth that allows for the remodeling of the alveolar bone and the periodontal ligament. For orthodontic patients with thin alveolar bone, the technique of periodontally accelerated osteogenic orthodontics (PAOO) was used to accelerate the tooth movement and shorten the therapeutic time [23, 24]. The general process is to open the gums under local anesthesia and cut the outer (or inner) bone cortex of the root of the orthodontic tooth sites that need to perform bone grafting. The cut depth is commonly only a single layer of cortical bone, and then the surface of the cut bone is covered with artificial bone substitutes for increasing bone mass, and then collagen membrane and L-PRF membrane are used to cover bone grafting, which can be regarded as a procedure of GBR in orthodontic treatment. However, the potential effect of L-PRF on this process remains controversial, though there was an obvious trend that the tooth movement was accelerated when L-PRF was applied [25]. Therefore, further study with a longer follow-up and larger sample size need to

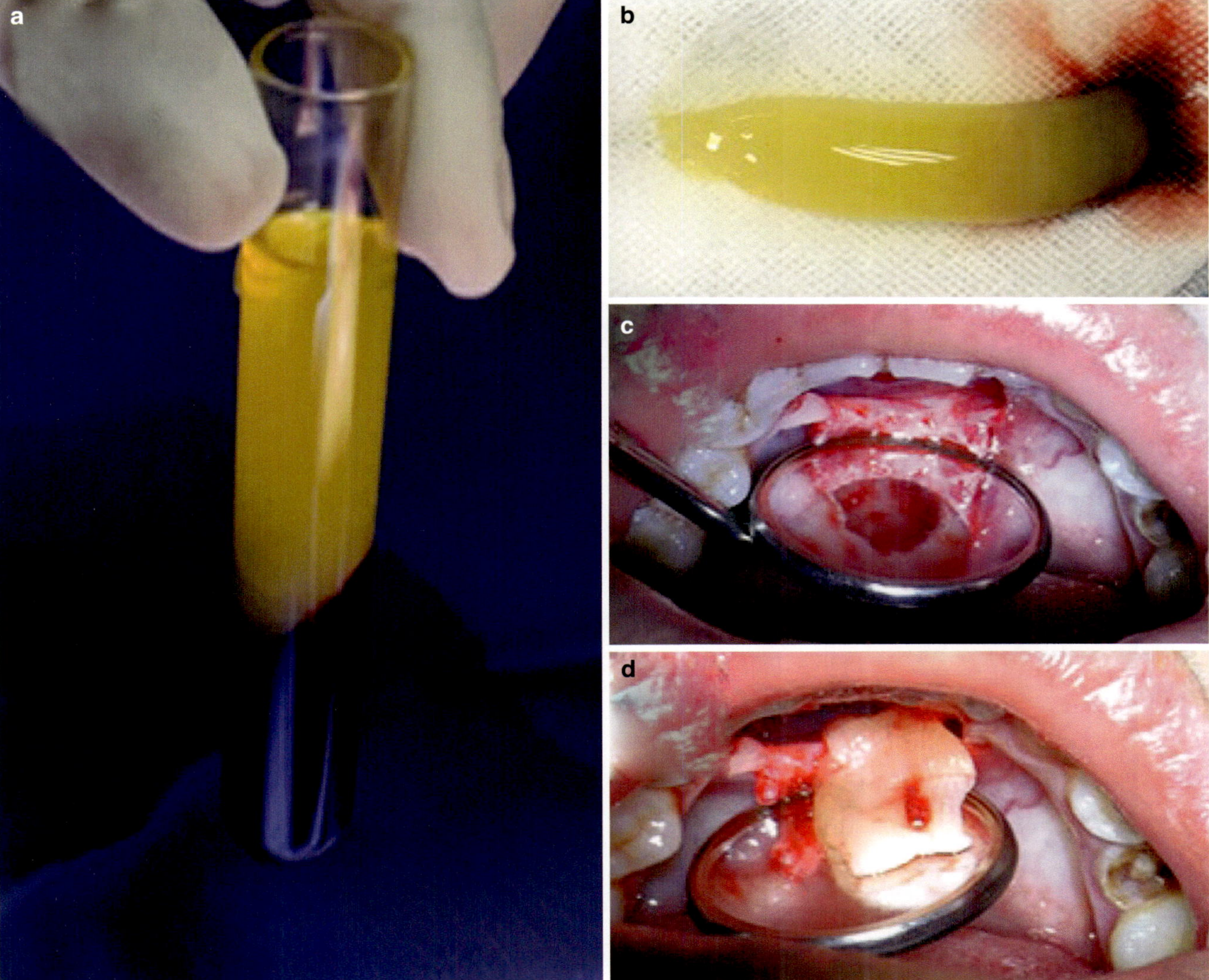

Fig. 10.8 L-PRF in the treatment of jaw cyst. (**a**) The 10 ml of autologous blood sample was centrifugated for 10 min at 3000 rpm, and three layers were formed. (**b**) The prepared L-PRF was harvested and placed on the gauze for further gentle pressing to obtain L-PRF membrane. (**c**) The cyst cavity is obvious and huge after curettage of maxillary cyst. (**d**) The prepared L-PRF membrane was ready to be implanted into the cyst cavity

be performed to assess the application and effectiveness of L-PRF in the orthodontic treatment.

10.6 Leucocyte-Platelet-Rich Fibrin (L-PRF) in the Treatment of Soft Tissue Repair

Soft tissue defects resulting from congenital malformations, tumor resection, and trauma would affect patients functionally and cosmetically. Contour defect remains a great challenge for restoration treatment in the clinic, thus making adipose tissue regeneration a strong clinical need. Autologous adipose tissue grafting is considered as a good alternative for the treatment of soft tissue defects for it avoids the unpredictable complications associated with foreign materials. However, the low survival rate of adipose grafts and the unpredictability are the main issues for adipose transplantation. Adipose-derived stem cells (ADSCs), as an ideal choice for improving the survival rate of transplanted fat tissue, could maintain large parts of the transplanted fat for over half a year and improve the fat remodeling, but the survival rate of fat transplants could be further enhanced. And encouragingly, the L-PRF-mixed fat performed better than PRP-mixed fat in facial lipotamponade surgery, which may be resulted from L-PRF releasing multiple growth factors at a steady rate for up to 4 weeks and serving as a biomaterial

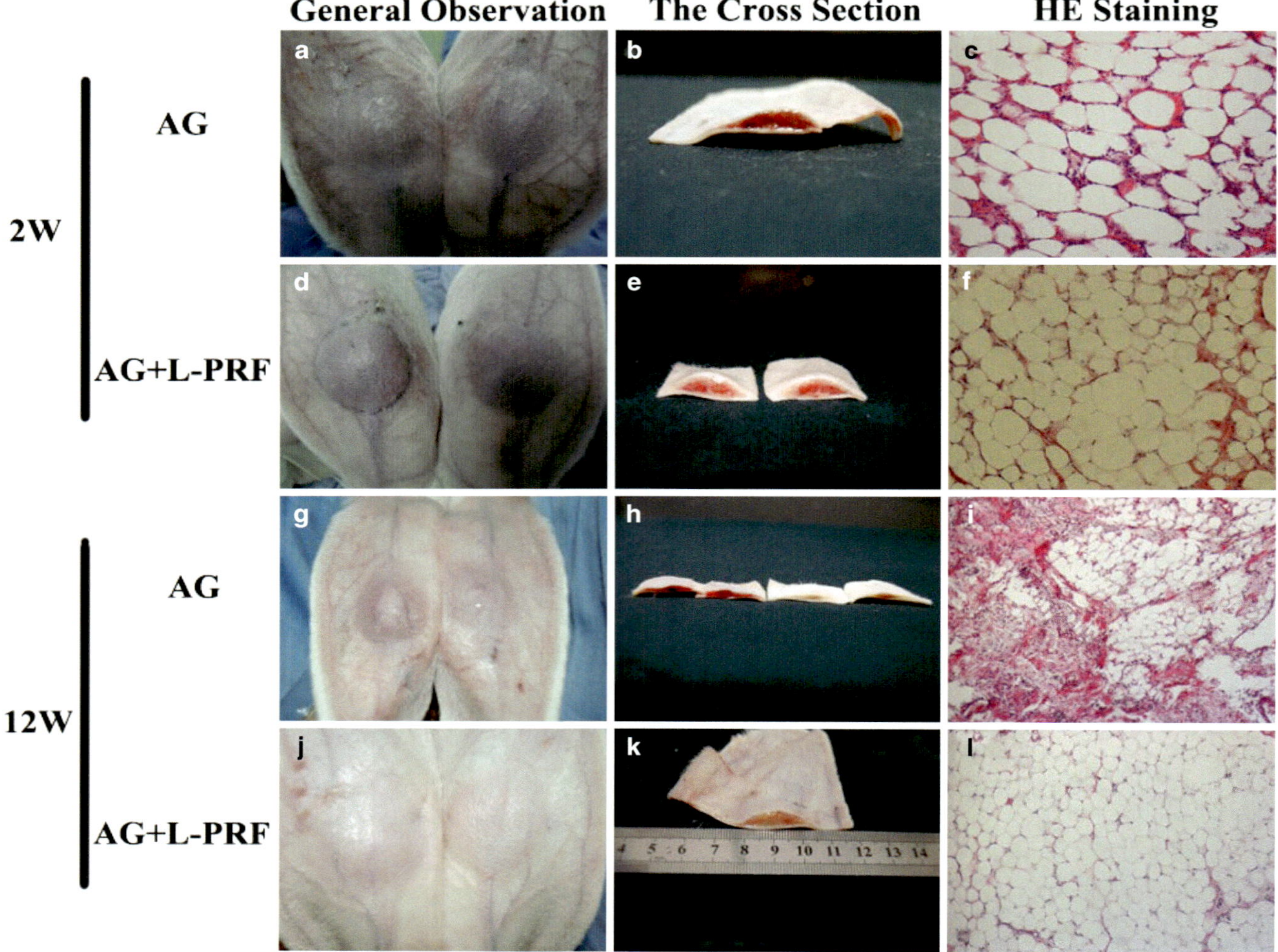

Fig. 10.9 L-PRF improve the efficacy of transplanted fat tissue. (**a**, **d**, **g**, **j**) A general view of remaining fat volume at 2 weeks and 12 weeks after transplantation. (**b**, **e**, **h**, **k**) The cross section of middle point of transplanted fat tissue. (**c**, **f**, **i**, **l**) H&E staining: the only AG group had the lower tissue remodeling, higher degree of fiber liquefaction necrosis, and lower angiogenesis when compared to the AG + L-PRF group. *AG* adipose granules. (These pictures were provided by Dr. Li Long, from the Department of Stomatology, ShenZhen Qianhai Shekou Free Trade Zone Hospital, Shenzhen, China)

scaffold that is beneficial for cell proliferation and differentiation [26, 27]. In summary, the potential of ADSCs to differentiate into different types of cells could be enhanced by L-PRF in a dose-dependent manner. The fat composite containing both L-PRF and ADSCs presented a higher fat survival rate and stronger angiogenesis compared to control group (Fig. 10.9), indicating that L-PRF-mixed ADSCs and fat tissues could be a promising composite biomaterial for the treatment of soft tissue defects. Furthermore, L-PRF, which serves as both a source of growth factors and a bioscaffold, has also been used in many applications as choice of biomaterial.

10.7 Leucocyte-Platelet-Rich Fibrin (L-PRF) in the Treatment of Irradiation-Induced Salivary Gland Damage

The decrease in the amount of saliva certainly leads to many accompanying complications, including dry mouth, oral mucous inflammation, and secondary rampant caries, which would remarkably depress the quality of life of patients. It was reported that about 500,000 novel cases of head and neck cancers diagnosed every year and approximately 40% of the cancer patients who receive radiotherapy suffered from salivary hypofunction or xerostomia. Salivary substitutes or sial-

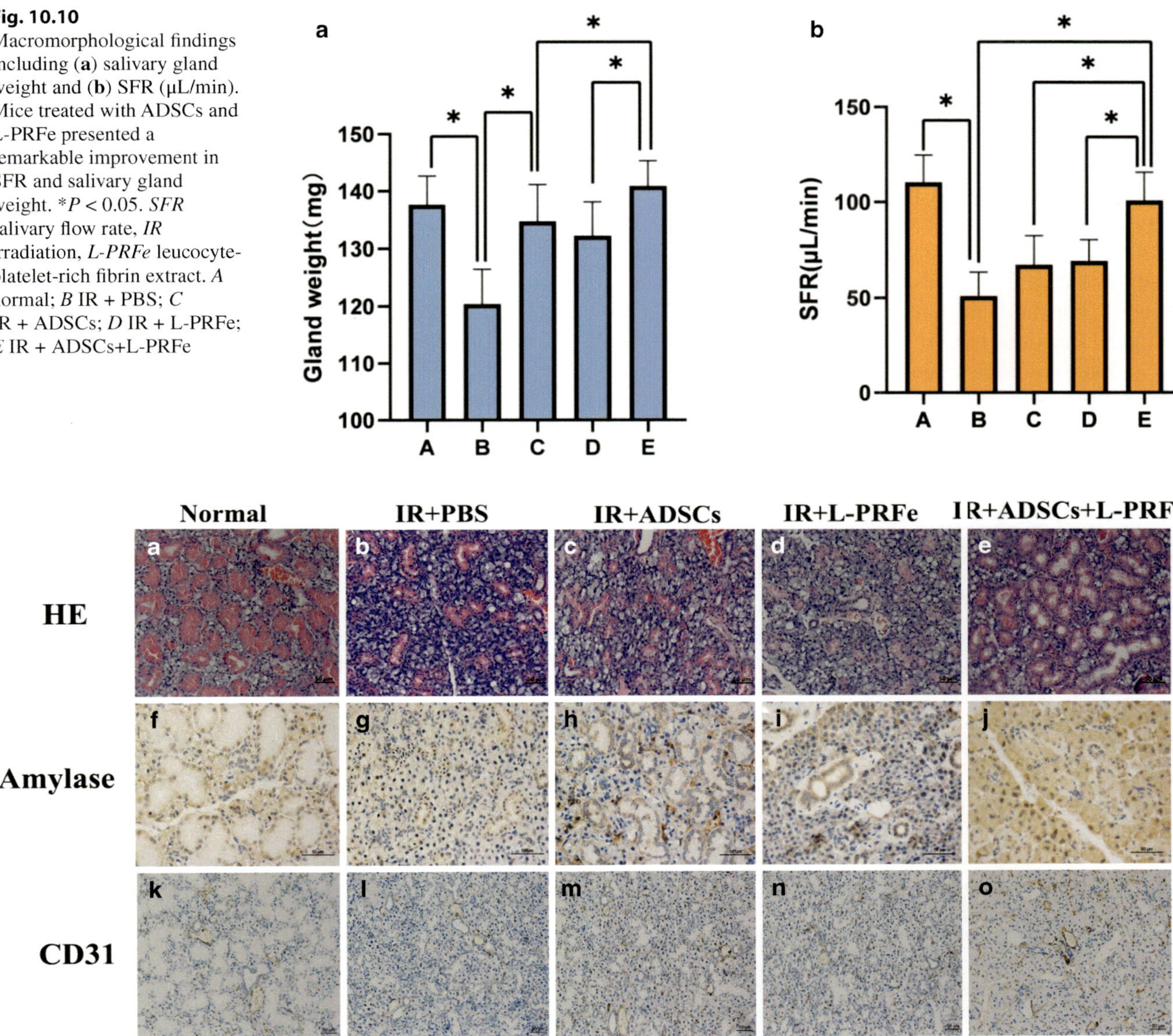

Fig. 10.10 Macromorphological findings including (**a**) salivary gland weight and (**b**) SFR (μL/min). Mice treated with ADSCs and L-PRFe presented a remarkable improvement in SFR and salivary gland weight. $*P < 0.05$. *SFR* salivary flow rate, *IR* irradiation, *L-PRFe* leucocyte-platelet-rich fibrin extract. *A* normal; *B* IR + PBS; *C* IR + ADSCs; *D* IR + L-PRFe; *E* IR + ADSCs+L-PRFe

Fig. 10.11 Micromorphological changes were observed by histological analysis. (*a–e*) H&E staining. (*f–j*) Amylase (AMY) production was remarkably improved when ADSCs combined with L-PRFe were transplanted. (*k–o*) The number of microvessels was also increased

agogues are the main treatment approaches at present. There is still no satisfactory treatment available to settle this fundamental issue. Thus, many therapeutic approaches have been developed to rehabilitate damaged salivary glands, such as stem cell therapy, gene therapy, and so on. Among them, BMSCs and ADSCs have been applied in tissue-engineered SGs to prevent or recover irradiation-induced SG damage. During the process of blood sample being centrifugated to prepare L-PRF, the supernatant, regarded as acellular or platelet-poor plasma (PPP), is proved to promote cell proliferation. Besides, L-PRF could improve the survival rate of transplanted adipose tissue, increase its potential of revascularization, and possess the ability to release growth factors slowly for 4 weeks in vitro. Thus, L-PRF extract (L-PRFe), obtained from L-PRF immersed in PPP, also had plenty of growth factors that can be used in the repair of damaged tissue. In our previous study, we placed the obtained L-PRF membrane fragments into microcentrifuge tubes containing PPP. And then these tubes were incubate at 37 °C for 1 week to allow growth factors discharged from L-PRF. Finally, the supernatant, which was considered as the L-PRFe, was harvested to be injected into C3H mice suffered from permanent SG damage induced by radiotherapy. At 12 weeks after transplantation, the implantation of ADSCs combined with L-PRFe significantly improved the salivary flow rate (SFR) (Fig. 10.10). Besides, fewer damaged acinar cells (Fig. 10.11) and higher α-amylase (AMY) levels in the L-PRFe combined ADSC-treated group as compared to the untreated irradiated

SGs. In summary, ADSC-combined L-PRFe presented satisfactory treatment results [28].

L-PRFe used alone could not be able to repair the damaged SG; ADSCs alone also failed to reconstruct the structure of SG, which demonstrated that ADSCs and L-PRFe seemed to present the synergistic effects to restore the function of damaged SG (Fig. 10.11).

By the way, concentrated growth factors (CGFs), prepared by low speed and low time of centrifugation compared to L-PRF, have also been introduced into oral surgeries, but the definite effect of the low speed on the biological functions of CGFs remains unclear. What is certain is that glass tubes would improve fibrin polymerization and help to produce a thicker and denser fibrinous fibrin clot as compared to plastic tubes during the preparation process of CGFs [29, 30]. Besides, slower centrifugation speeds and less centrifugation time (approximately 600–800 rpm for 3–6 min) have led to the formation of liquid PRF or named as injectable PRF (i-PRF) (Fig. 10.12) resulting to an upper plasma layer composed of liquid fibrinogen prior to buffy coat formation that remains in its liquid phase for 15 min before it was injected into targeted defect sites in vivo [31, 32]. Thus, liquid PRF not only could be used as an advanced local delivery system for biomolecules but also be considered as a potential carrier system for different types of cells that are beneficial for tissue regeneration for liquid PRF which also contains some regenerative growth factors. However, further studies are needed to perform to investigate how the properties of liquid PRF affect the carried various biomolecules and cells.

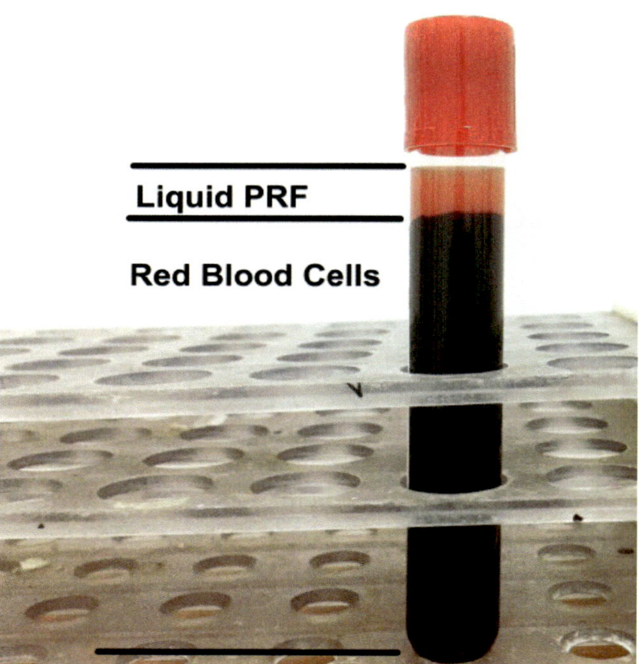

Fig. 10.12 Liquid PRF (injectable PRF, iPRF) prepared after the blood sample about 10 ml without anticoagulants was centrifugated at 700 rpm for 3 min. The upper layer of plasma contains leucocytes and growth factors. Red blood cells were concentrated at the bottom layer

10.8 The Preparation of Lyophilized Leucocyte-Platelet-Rich Fibrin (LL-PRF) and Its Effect on the Proliferative Capacity of BMSCs

As previously mentioned, L-PRF has been applied in bone defect repair, soft tissue repair, and oral implants, achieving satisfactory results. However, fresh L-PRF (FL-PRF) make it impossible to save and commercialize for a long time because it has to be used immediately after preparation. Many studies discussed the preparation of freeze-dried L-PRF and its potential applications. Freeze-drying could maintain the function of such essential proteins for a long time [33]. In our previous work, we discussed the preparation of lyophilized leucocyte-platelet-rich fibrin (LL-PRF) and investigated the effect of LL-PRF on the proliferative capacity of BMSCs [34].

10.8.1 Preparation of Lyophilized Leucocyte-Platelet-Rich Fibrin (LL-PRF)

In brief, The L-PRF clot was prepared and harvested according to the previous method, and the fresh L-PRF was considered as FL-PRF. Then half of FL-PRF was treated by lyophilization. Next, LL-PRF was harvested and stored at room temperature for more than 3 weeks. The collected FL-PRF and LL-PRF samples were processed for H&E staining and observation by SEM.

10.8.2 Characterization of LL-PRF and FL-PRF

The H&E staining views presented that FL-PRF was composed of numerous closely arranged, red-stained fiber bundles (Fig. 10.13a), whereas the LL-PRF fibrin network was loosely arranged (Fig. 10.13b). SEM views presented that fibers were arranged regularly and densely in the FL-PRF when compared with LL-PRF (Fig. 10.13c, d).

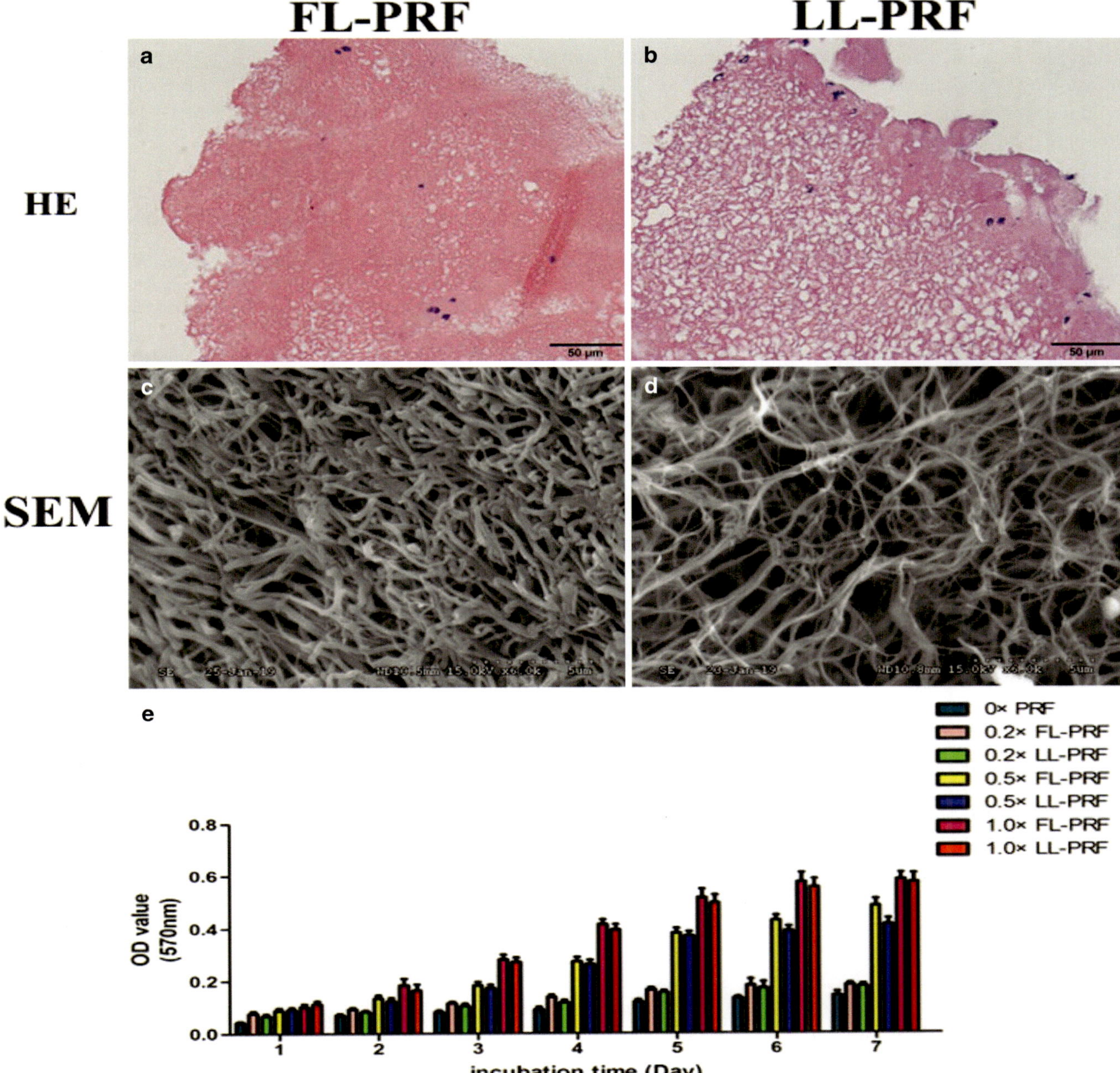

Fig. 10.13 Characterization of FL-PRF and LL-PRF. (**a**, **b**) H&E staining views presented that FL-PRF was composed of numerous closely arranged, red-stained fiber bundles whereas the LL-PRF fibrin network was loosely arranged. (**c**, **d**) SEM views presented that fibers were arranged regularly and densely in the FL-PRF when compared with LL-PRF. (**e**) MTT assays demonstrated that LL-PRF possessed a remarkable and dose-dependent effect on the proliferative potential of BMSCs

As displayed in Fig. 10.13e, the proliferative potential of BMSCs obviously increased as the concentrations of LL-PRF or FL-PRF increased. However, there is no conspicuous difference between the FL-PRF and LL-PRF groups. Such results demonstrated that LL-PRF possessed a remarkable and dose-dependent effect on the proliferative potential of BMSCs.

10.9 Conclusions

In view of the diversity of oral diseases, tissue regeneration and repair in defects of the oral and maxillofacial region remain a great challenge. Both the functional and aesthetical effects of the reconstructed tissues are required to be taken into consideration seriously. Platelet concentrates (PCs), including PRP and L-PRF, can be taken as a source of autologous growth factors and innovative biomaterials for tissue regeneration in stomatology. Many studies demonstrate that PRP and L-PRF could improve wound healing and accelerate bone formation, although there are some controversial concerns about the effectiveness of PCs in the treatment of different diseases. Especially L-PRF can be taken as an ideal tissue substitute for stimulated tissue regeneration naturally due to its function as biological active materials and scaffolds for cells, growth factors, and cytokine delivery. In summary, favorable effects on bone and soft tissue repair and reduction of postoperative complications were reported when PCs were used. Further studies are still needed to perform to address these controversial issues and help PCs, including PRP and L-PRF, to be applied in the oral and maxillofacial surgery.

References

1. Nesic D, Schaefer BM, Sun Y, Saulacic N, Sailer I. 3D printing approach in dentistry: the future for personalized oral soft tissue regeneration. J Clin Med. 2020;9(7):2238.
2. Mendelson A, Frank E, Allred C, Jones E, Chen M, Zhao W, Mao JJ. Chondrogenesis by chemotactic homing of synovium, bone marrow, and adipose stem cells in vitro. FASEB J. 2011;25(10):3496–504.
3. Zhao YH, Zhang M, Liu NX, Lv X, Zhang J, Chen FM, Chen YJ. The combined use of cell sheet fragments of periodontal ligament stem cells and platelet-rich fibrin granules for avulsed tooth reimplantation. Biomaterials. 2013;34(22):5506–20.
4. Castro AB, Meschi N, Temmerman A, Pinto N, Lambrechts P, Teughels W, Quirynen M. Regenerative potential of leucocyte- and platelet-rich fibrin. Part A: intra-bony defects, furcation defects and periodontal plastic surgery. A systematic review and meta-analysis. J Clin Periodontol. 2017;44(1):67–82.
5. Dohan Ehrenfest DM, Rasmusson L, Albrektsson T. Classification of platelet concentrates: from pure platelet-rich plasma (P-PRP) to leucocyte- and platelet-rich fibrin (L-PRF). Trends Biotechnol. 2009;27(3):158–67.
6. Dohan DM, Choukroun J, Diss A, Dohan SL, Dohan AJ, Mouhyi J, Gogly B. Platelet-rich fibrin (PRF): a second-generation platelet concentrate. Part I: technological concepts and evolution. Oral Surg Oral Med Oral Pathol Oral Radiol Endod. 2006;101(3):e37–44.
7. Choukroun J, Diss A, Simonpieri A, Girard MO, Schoeffler C, Dohan SL, Dohan AJ, Mouhyi J, Dohan DM. Platelet-rich fibrin (PRF): a second-generation platelet concentrate. Part IV: clinical effects on tissue healing. Oral Surg Oral Med Oral Pathol Oral Radiol Endod. 2006;101(3):e56–60.
8. Wang Z, Weng Y, Lu S, Zong C, Qiu J, Liu Y, Liu B. Osteoblastic mesenchymal stem cell sheet combined with Choukroun platelet-rich fibrin induces bone formation at an ectopic site. J Biomed Mater Res B Appl Biomater. 2015;103(6):1204–16.
9. Torabinejad M, Faras H. A clinical and histological report of a tooth with an open apex treated with regenerative endodontics using platelet-rich plasma. J Endod. 2012;38(6):864–8.
10. Lolato A, Bucchi C, Taschieri S, Kabbaney AE, Fabbro MD. Platelet concentrates for revitalization of immature necrotic teeth: a systematic review of the clinical studies. Platelets. 2016;27(5):383–92.
11. Padma R, Shilpa A, Kumar PA, Nagasri M, Kumar C, Sreedhar A. A split mouth randomized controlled study to evaluate the adjunctive effect of platelet-rich fibrin to coronally advanced flap in Miller's class-I and II recession defects. J Indian Soc Periodontol. 2013;17(5):631–6.
12. Zumaran CC, Parra MV, Olate SA, Fernandez EG, Munoz FT, Haidar ZS. The 3 R's for platelet-rich fibrin: a "super" tri-dimensional biomaterial for contemporary naturally-guided oro-maxillo-facial soft and hard tissue repair, reconstruction and regeneration. Materials (Basel). 2018;11(8):1293.
13. Tarallo F, Mancini L, Pitzurra L, Bizzarro S, Tepedino M, Marchetti E. Use of platelet-rich fibrin in the treatment of grade 2 furcation defects: systematic review and meta-analysis. J Clin Med. 2020;9(7):2104.
14. Sharma P, Grover HS, Masamatti SS, Saksena N. A clinicoradiographic assessment of 1% metformin gel with platelet-rich fibrin in the treatment of mandibular grade II furcation defects. J Indian Soc Periodontol. 2017;21(4):303–8.
15. Castro AB, Meschi N, Temmerman A, Pinto N, Lambrechts P, Teughels W, Quirynen M. Regenerative potential of leucocyte- and platelet-rich fibrin. Part B: sinus floor elevation, alveolar ridge preservation and implant therapy. A systematic review. J Clin Periodontol. 2017;44(2):225–34.
16. Wang Z, Hu H, Li Z, Weng Y, Dai T, Zong C, Liu Y, Liu B. Sheet of osteoblastic cells combined with platelet-rich fibrin improves the formation of bone in critical-size calvarial defects in rabbits. Br J Oral Maxillofac Surg. 2016;54(3):316–21.
17. Ortega-Mejia H, Estrugo-Devesa A, Saka-Herran C, Ayuso-Montero R, Lopez-Lopez J, Velasco-Ortega E. Platelet-rich plasma in maxillary sinus augmentation: systematic review. Materials (Basel). 2020;13(3):622.
18. Lemos CA, Mello CC, dos Santos DM, Verri FR, Goiato MC, Pellizzer EP. Effects of platelet-rich plasma in association with bone grafts in maxillary sinus augmentation: a systematic review and meta-analysis. Int J Oral Maxillofac Surg. 2016;45(4):517–25.
19. Zhang Y, Tangl S, Huber CD, Lin Y, Qiu L, Rausch-Fan X. Effects of Choukroun's platelet-rich fibrin on bone regeneration in combination with deproteinized bovine bone mineral in maxillary sinus augmentation: a histological and histomorphometric study. J Craniomaxillofac Surg. 2012;40(4):321–8.
20. Gassling V, Purcz N, Braesen JH, Will M, Gierloff M, Behrens E, Acil Y, Wiltfang J. Comparison of two different absorbable membranes for the coverage of lateral osteotomy sites in maxillary sinus augmentation: a preliminary study. J Craniomaxillofac Surg. 2013;41(1):76–82.
21. Choukroun J, Diss A, Simonpieri A, Girard MO, Schoeffler C, Dohan SL, Dohan AJ, Mouhyi J, Dohan DM. Platelet-rich fibrin (PRF): a second-generation platelet concentrate. Part V: histologic evaluations of PRF effects on bone allograft maturation in sinus lift. Oral Surg Oral Med Oral Pathol Oral Radiol Endod. 2006;101(3):299–303.
22. Eslami S, Faber J, Fateh A, Sheikholaemmeh F, Grassia V, Jamilian A. Treatment decision in adult patients with class III malocclusion: surgery versus orthodontics. Prog Orthod. 2018;19(1):28.
23. Munoz F, Jimenez C, Espinoza D, Vervelle A, Beugnet J, Haidar Z. Use of leukocyte and platelet-rich fibrin (L-PRF) in periodontally accelerated osteogenic orthodontics (PAOO): clinical effects on edema and pain. J Clin Exp Dent. 2016;8(2):e119–24.
24. Singh S, Jayan B. Comparative evaluation of periodontally accelerated osteogenic orthodontics (PAOO) versus conventional orthodontic tooth movement in adult patients with bimaxillary dentoalveolar protrusion. Int J Periodontics Restorative Dent. 2019;39(4):571–7.
25. Francisco I, Fernandes MH, Vale F. Platelet-rich fibrin in bone regenerative strategies in orthodontics: a systematic review. Materials (Basel). 2020;13(8):1866.
26. Liu B, Li L, Zhao J-H, Wang Z-F, Tan X-Y, Xu H-Y, Au R, Liu Y-P. Platelet-rich fibrin and adipose-derived stem cells improve the efficacy of fat transplantation and soft tissue repair. J Biomater Tissue Eng. 2015;5(4):275–82.

27. Liu B, Tan XY, Liu YP, Xu XF, Li L, Xu HY, An R, Chen FM. The adjuvant use of stromal vascular fraction and platelet-rich fibrin for autologous adipose tissue transplantation. Tissue Eng Part C Methods. 2013;19(1):1–14.
28. Wang Z, Xing H, Hu H, Dai T, Wang Y, Li Z, An R, Xu H, Liu Y, Liu B. Intraglandular transplantation of adipose-derived stem cells combined with platelet-rich fibrin extract for the treatment of irradiation-induced salivary gland damage. Exp Ther Med. 2018;15(1):795–805.
29. Tabatabaei F, Aghamohammadi Z, Tayebi L. In vitro and in vivo effects of concentrated growth factor on cells and tissues. J Biomed Mater Res A. 2020;108(6):1338–50.
30. Chen J, Jiang H. A comprehensive review of concentrated growth factors and their novel applications in facial reconstructive and regenerative medicine. Aesthet Plast Surg. 2020;44(3):1047–57.
31. Miron RJ, Zhang Y. Autologous liquid platelet rich fibrin: a novel drug delivery system. Acta Biomater. 2018;75:35–51.
32. Choukroun J, Ghanaati S. Reduction of relative centrifugation force within injectable platelet-rich-fibrin (PRF) concentrates advances patients' own inflammatory cells, platelets and growth factors: the first introduction to the low speed centrifugation concept. Eur J Trauma Emerg Surg. 2018;44(1):87–95.
33. Shi L, Li R, Wei S, Zhou M, Li L, Lin F, Li Y, Guo Z, Zhang W, Chen M, Shan G. Effects of a protective agent on freeze-dried platelet-rich plasma. Blood Coagul Fibrinolysis. 2019;30(2):58–65.
34. Wang Z, Han L, Sun T, Wang W, Li X, Wu B. Preparation and effect of lyophilized platelet-rich fibrin on the osteogenic potential of bone marrow mesenchymal stem cells in vitro and in vivo. Heliyon. 2019;5(10):e02739.

Application of Platelet-Rich Plasma in Other Aspects of Plastic and Aesthetic Surgery

11

Shikun Wei, LiWen Huang, and Biao Cheng

11.1 EPT in the Treatment of Male and Female Sexual Dysfunction

The treatment of sexual potential improvement is the fastest-growing and newest branch in the current medical profession. The treatment of sexual potential improvement includes various treatments and operations aimed at changing the aesthetic and functional aspects of male and female genitalia. With the rapid growth of the demand for sexual potential improvement, plastic surgery will also involve the treatment of sexual potential improvement. As a general term, genital plastic surgery, beauty, rejuvenation, and other terms have been widely used in medical literature. The treatment of sexual potential improvement is not only the plastic surgery of male and female sexual organs but also various treatment methods to improve sexual function for the purpose of treating sexual life disorder: no sexual desire, no arousal of sexual desire, no orgasm, sexual intercourse pain, etc.

At present, the main treatment methods of sexual dysfunction are surgery, hormone therapy, and psychotherapy. However, each therapy has its disadvantages. There are a lot of adverse events in hormone therapy. For patients with normal hormone levels or contraindications of hormone therapy and no indication for surgery, only psychotherapy is available. Enriched platelet is composed of many growth factors and active components. After the concentrated platelet is injected into the body, it interacts with the cells, matrix, and media around the injection site to promote the tissue regeneration at the injection site. The effects of enriched platelet on angiogenesis and tissue regeneration can be used to treat male and female sexual dysfunction. However, the scientific evidence supporting the therapeutic effect of enriched platelet on sexual function improvement needs to be further accumulated. At present, the efficacy of PRP in the improvement of sexual potential should be treated cautiously and scientifically, instead of flocking. Based on the current published literature, this paper will make a scientific analysis of the effect and possibility of enriched platelet treatment (EPT) in the treatment of male and female sexual dysfunction. It is expected that more evidence-based medical evidence will appear in the future.

11.1.1 EPT in the Treatment of Female Sexual Dysfunction

11.1.1.1 Female Sexual Dysfunction(FSD)

FSD is defined as the sexual condition and sexual health problems that make women suffer, which reduce their quality of life and their unwillingness to participate in interpersonal relationships. The prevalence of FSD varies in different races and countries [1]. Generally, sexual dysfunction is more common than male, but the research on FSD is not as good as male. Over the past few decades, women's understanding and expectations of sexual knowledge have improved. However, most women are reluctant to discuss the problems they encounter in their sexual life, so it is difficult to collect relevant data from the epidemiology of FSD. In 2017, Zhang [2] reported that a questionnaire survey was conducted among 25,446 women aged 20–70. The results showed that the prevalence of sexual dysfunction among women aged 20–70 in Chinese Mainland was estimated to be 29.7%. Among the prevalence rates, 21.6% were low desire, 21.6% were arousal disorders, 18.9% were lubrication disorders, 18.9% were orgasm disorders, and 14.1% were sexual intercourse pain.

At present, the main treatment methods for FSD are psychological intervention, behavioral intervention, hormone therapy, and psychopharmacological intervention. Due to the complexity and multifactor of FSD, the current treatment

S. Wei · L. Huang
Department of Burn and Plastic Surgery, General Hospital of Southern Theater Command, PLA, Guangzhou, China

B. Cheng (✉)
Department of Burn & Plastic Surgery, General Hospital of Southern Theater Command, Guangzhou, China

B. Cheng, X. Fu (eds.), *Platelet-Rich Plasma in Tissue Repair and Regeneration*, https://doi.org/10.1007/978-981-99-3193-4_11

may make some women suffer from sexual dysfunction without clinical improvement. Due to the complex factors of FSD and the different effects of existing treatment schemes, new safe and effective treatments need to be developed in this field [3]. In addition, A-level therapies can only choose psychotherapy and short-term testosterone treatment [4]. For those female patients with sexual dysfunction who have no surgical indications, normal hormone levels, or contraindications to hormone therapy, their A-level treatment can only choose psychological treatment [3]. While psychotherapy does help many women, there is no alternative to other A-level treatments.

Periurethral injection is an effective treatment for sexual dysfunction and urinary incontinence [5]. For example, periurethral injection of calcium hydroxyapatite crystals (CHAC) to treat urinary incontinence has been approved by FDA. However, such complications as urinary tract obstruction, infection, and granuloma caused by this treatment usually require surgical treatment [5, 6]. There are few reports about the improvement of sexual dysfunction before and after treatment. Graffiti spot is a controversial anatomical area of the anterior vaginal wall. People try to inject sodium hyaluronate (g-shot) into this area to improve orgasm. The American College of Obstetrics and Gynaecology has seriously questioned this treatment because of the possibility of granuloma at the site of hyaluronic acid injection [5]. The ability of autologous platelet concentrate to promote tissue regeneration and non-immunogenicity makes it possible to be recognized as an injection material.

11.1.1.2 EPT in the Treatment of FSD (Figs. 11.1, 11.2 and 11.3)

Research on the Improvement of Female Sexual Life Satisfaction by EPT

People are trying to find a simple, safe, and natural alternative therapy for FSD. In 2014, Runels [7] conducted a study on the therapeutic effect of injecting autologous platelet-rich

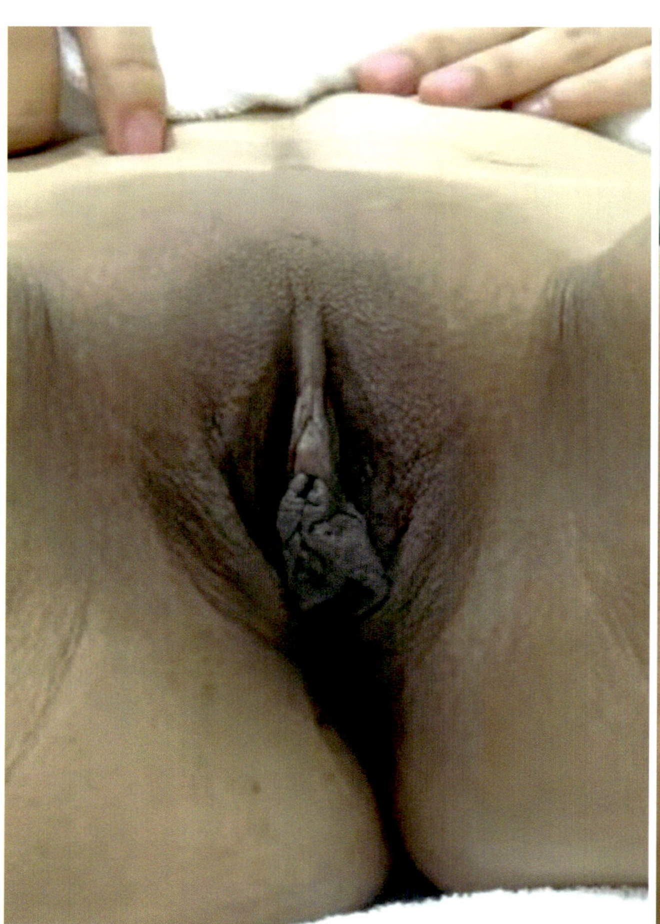

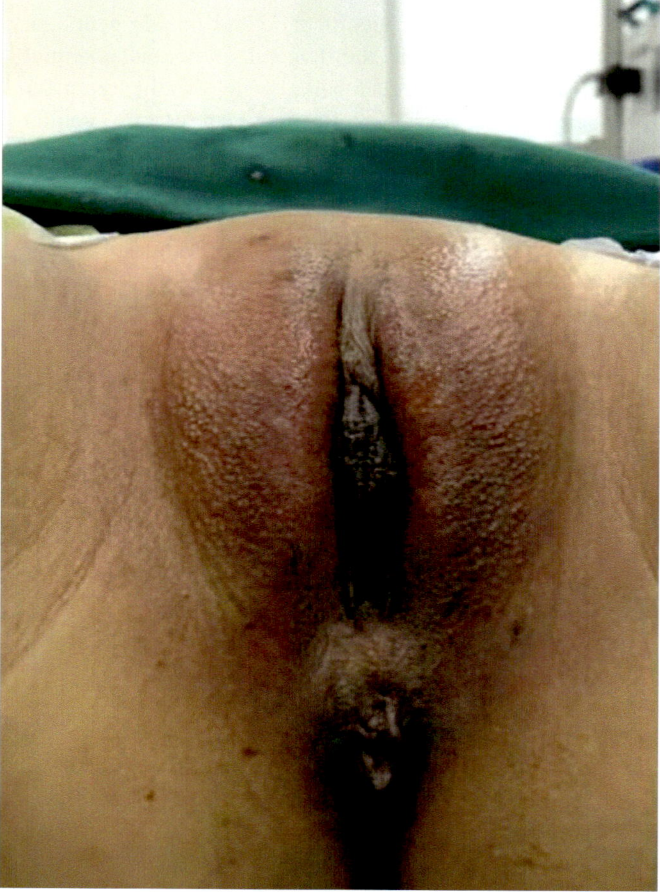

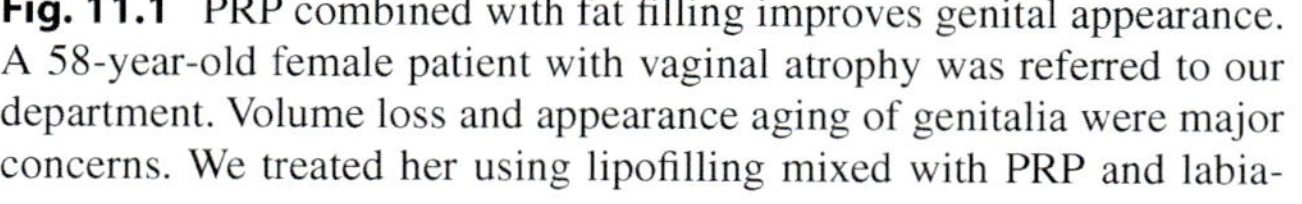

Fig. 11.1 PRP combined with fat filling improves genital appearance. A 58-year-old female patient with vaginal atrophy was referred to our department. Volume loss and appearance aging of genitalia were major concerns. We treated her using lipofilling mixed with PRP and labiaplasty surgery. A total of 50 c.c of autologous fat mixed with PRP was transferred to the labia majora and excessive minora skin was removed to improve appearance

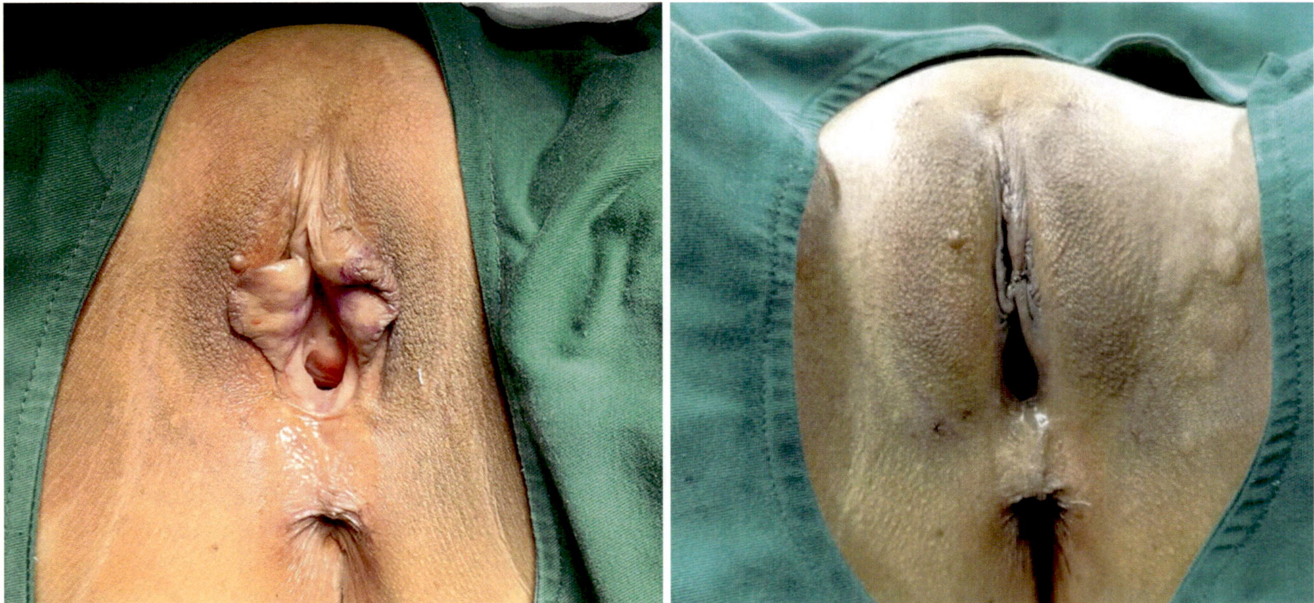

Fig. 11.2 PRP combined with fat filling improves genital appearance. A 47-year-old patient underwent labiaplasty minor plus PRP autogenous fat labia majora filling. Bilateral total 60 cc fat +4ccPRP. Preoperative and immediate postoperative photos

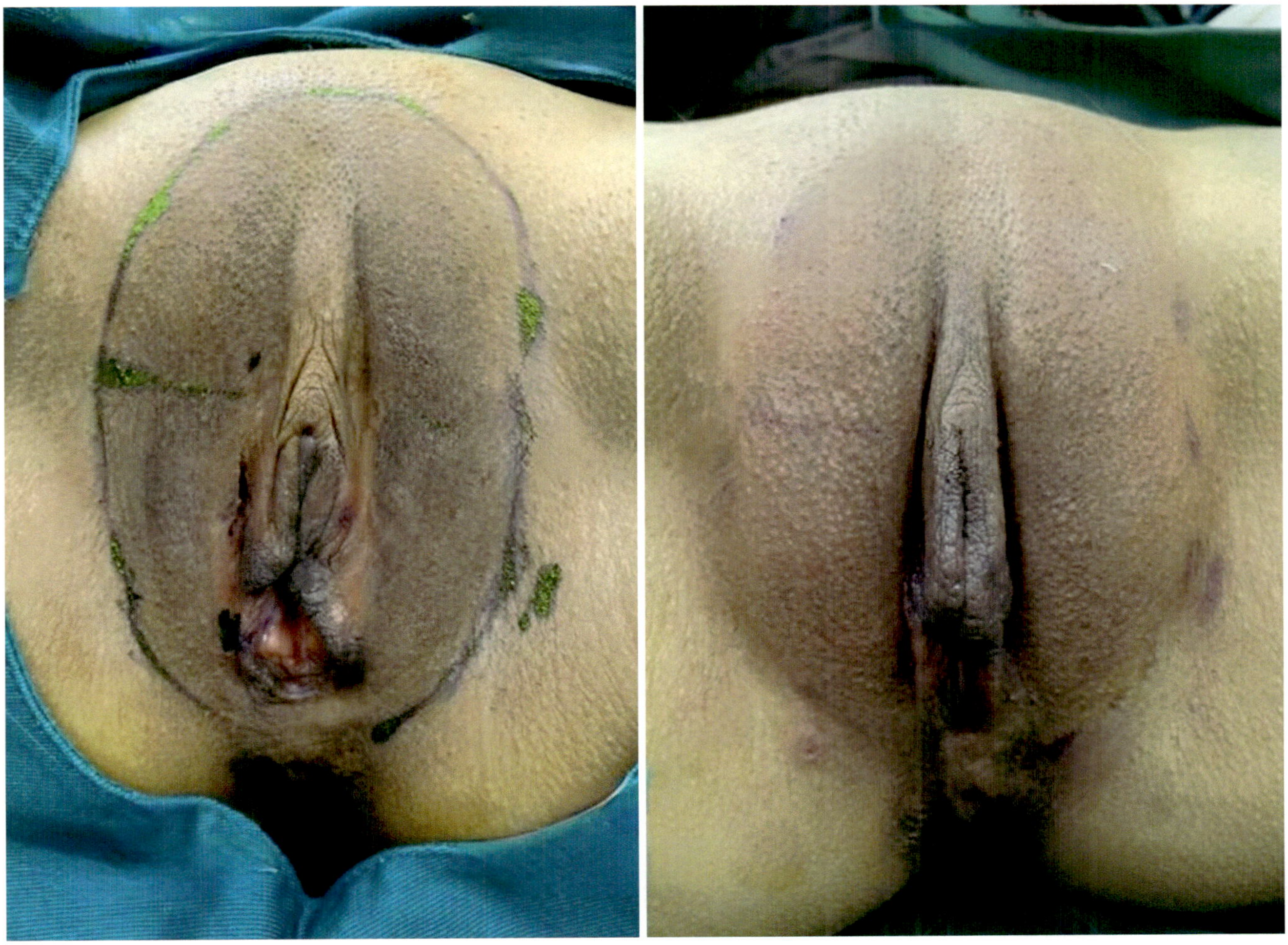

Fig. 11.3 PRP combined with fat filling improves genital appearance. A 42-year-old patient underwent ADM band vaginal tightening plus PRP autogenous fat labia majora filling. Bilateral total 50 cc fat +4ccPRP. Preoperative and immediate postoperative photos

plasma (PRP) into the clitoris and vagina on female patients with low desire or sexual intercourse pain. Before and after treatment, two standardized sexual function tests, namely, the efficacy of PRP which was tested by the female sexual function index (FSFI) and female sexual distress scale revised (FSDS-R), were conducted to measure the response to PRP treatment. The results showed that the average FSDS-R score decreased from 17 to 7 ($P = 0.04$), and the total FSFI score of 9 out of 11 women (82%) improved. Two patients (18%) did not improve. The improvement range of FSFI total score was 1.6–14.3. The difference between the average total number before and after treatment was 5.5 ($P = 0.01$). The average score of arousal increased by 1.2 points ($P = 0.009$), the average score of lubrication increased by 1.28 points ($P = 0.002$), the average score of desire increased by 0.82 points ($P = 0.06$), and the average score of climax increased by 1.08 points ($P = 0.05$). Two cases had extreme arousal, including urination arousal, persistent arousal, ejaculation orgasm, and spontaneous orgasm. These reactions lasted only 1–2 weeks and occurred in young patients undergoing surgery. The data showed that FSD improved to a certain extent, including the positive change of sexual difficulty and the decrease of sexual distress. The results show that PRP is effective in the treatment of FSD. But the researchers pointed out that the limited number of participants limited the conclusion.

In 2019, Sukgen [8] explored the impact of PRP injection on sexual function, orgasm, and sensation in FSD patients. Fifty two patients with FSD and orgasm disorder (FSFI ≤26, orgasmic score ≤ 3.75) were treated with PRP for four times. FSFI score, female genital self-image scale (FGSIS), FSDS-R, and Patient Global Impression of Improvement (PGI-I) were used to evaluate the treatment effect. The results showed that FSFI, FGSIS, and FSDS-R were improved after treatment ($P < 0.001$). The satisfaction rate of PGI-I was high. The results show that PRP is a minimally invasive, convenient, fast, and almost no adverse reaction treatment. Injection of PRP into the lower part of the anterior vaginal wall can improve female sexual life satisfaction.

Study on EPT Promoting Female Reproductive Organ Regeneration

In 2017, Neto [9] reported the safety, tolerability, and clinical efficacy of PRP injection in female clitoris, G-spot, and vaginal sensitive areas of women by measuring the responses of women to stress urinary incontinence, overactive bladder, lubrication, and sexual dysfunction (low libido, difficulty in sexual arousal, and difficulty in sexual intercourse). Fifty female patients aged 32–97 years (mean 62.8 years)were included in the study, containing 13 cases of stress urinary incontinence, 15 cases of overactive bladder, and 22 cases of mixed urinary incontinence, lack of lubrication, and sexual dysfunction (low libido, sexual arousal difficulty, sexual intercourse difficulty). All patients received PRP private injection therapy. After the first injection, they received the second treatment every 2 months, two times of treatment. The results showed that 94% of the 68 patients were satisfied and only 6% of the patients with overactive bladder had no improvement. The improvement of lubrication and sexual dysfunction (arousal, libido, dyspareunia, and anorexia) was subjectively reported through a questionnaire survey, and the effect became better after the second injection. There were 13 patients with stress urinary incontinence, and the remission rate was more than 90%. The remission rate of 15 patients with overactive bladder was 74%, and 6% (four cases) had no response. All 22 female patients with mixed urinary incontinence were satisfied with the results. Treatment was defined as subjective complete remission of urinary incontinence symptoms in patients with urinary incontinence (stress urinary incontinence, overactive bladder and mixed urinary incontinence). No extreme sexual arousal or ejaculation problems. There was no recurrence and serious side effects 6 months after the last treatment. One hundred percent of the patients were exposed to a burning sensation when injected through the urethra and clitoris. The regeneration of blood vessels and nerves in the vagina and clitoris can restore or enhance sexual response and sensitivity. The regeneration of collagen and sensory nerve can relieve sexual discomfort and improve vaginal sensitivity. For those with stress urinary incontinence and overactive bladder, this is a huge benefit, with the entire area around the urethra, the pubic cervical fascia, and the skein's gland rejuvenated for almost 1–2 years. This observation shows that PRP "O-shot" injection is a safe, effective, minimally invasive, and nonhormonal therapy for women with stress urinary incontinence, overactive bladder, lack of lubrication in sexual life, and sexual dysfunction (such as low libido, sexual arousal, or difficulty in sexual intercourse).

Among survivors of breast cancer, the incidence rate of one or more vulvovaginal atrophy (VVA) symptoms is about 50–70%. For postmenopausal breast cancer patients who cannot receive hormone therapy, autologous PRP combined with hyaluronic acid (A-PRP-HA) injection can be used as an alternative therapy. In 2018, Hersant [4] reported that the pretreatment vaginal health index (VHI) scores of 20 postmenopausal patients with VVA of breast cancer [in terms of vaginal pH, elasticity, fluid volume (secretion), epithelial integrity, and moisture] were all lower than 15 points. Vaginal injection of A-PRP-HA was performed at zero, one, three, and 6 months. The changes of vulvovaginal mucosa were evaluated by VHI score, and dyspareunia and sexual dysfunction were evaluated by FSD score. The results showed that the symptoms of vaginal dryness and difficult sexual intercourse were improved in all subjects. At the sixth month, the vaginal moisture and epithelial integrity were significantly improved, and the VHI score increased from 10.7 ± 2.12 before treatment to 20.75 ± 4.8 after treatment ($P < 0.0001$).

FSD score decreased significantly, from 36.35 ± 2.53 before treatment to 30.15 ± 2.47 after treatment ($P < 0.0001$). No adverse events occurred. A-PRP-HA vaginal injection therapy provides a new treatment for VVA patients who cannot receive hormone therapy. This therapy can increase the nutrition and hydration of vaginal mucosa in postmenopausal breast cancer patients.

The clinical study of EPT in the treatment of FSD is shown in Table 11.1.

11.1.1.3 Summary

Some FSD is mainly manifested in decreased libido, disorder of sexual arousal, insufficient lubrication during sexual intercourse, and disorder of orgasm, which can be treated by injecting autologous platelet concentrate into the Skene's gland and clitoris. Because the platelet concentrate comes entirely from its own blood, there is no additive, so there is no immune response [10]. Autologous concentrated platelets have no antigen reaction. A large number of existing evidences show that autologous concentrated platelet injection therapy is safe.

Other studies have shown that platelet concentrates induce new tissue regeneration by activating pluripotent stem cells inherent in most parts of the body. Growth factor produced by activated platelets can stimulate cells to differentiate into various types of tissues [6]. Therefore, when activated platelet concentrate is injected into human tissues and releases growth factors and cytokines, it may promote the differentiation of pluripotent stem cells; promote angiogenesis, fibroblast growth, gland (Skene's gland) proliferation, and new neuron growth; and improve physiological response. The recovery of blood flow and nerve regeneration in the vagina and clitoris will enhance female sexual response and sensitivity, especially for FSD caused by vaginal atrophy. Collagen and sensory nerve regeneration can also relieve sexual discomfort and enhance vaginal sensitivity. The improvement of clitoral blood flow can also promote sexual arousal and improve orgasm.

11.1.2 EPT in the Treatment of Male Sexual Dysfunction

11.1.2.1 Erectile Dysfunction(ED)and Peyronie's Disease(PD)

ED is a kind of male erectile weakness or erectile instability and unable to have sex pathological state. Scholars from Boston University School of Medicine reported the relationship between male age and ED: 22% of men under the age of 40 have ED, and 49% of men under the age of 70 have ED. The Global Online Sexual Behavior Survey shows that ED patients tend to be younger, and the prevalence of ED is on the rise [11].

The pathogenesis of ED is complex. Moreland [12] reported that the pathogenesis of ED is related to the destruction of penile smooth muscle. The larger the area of the destroyed smooth muscle in the total penile tissue, the more serious is ED. Oxidative stress can also lead to degradation

Table 11.1 Clinical study of EPT in the treatment of FSD

Types of diseases	PRP production method	PRP usage	The role of PRP	Experimental defect	Author [Ref.]
FSD	Regen® or truPRP® system	PRP was injected into the anterior wall of the vagina and clitoris between the vagina and urethra	FSDS-R score decreased from 17 to 7 ($P = 0.04$). The difference between the average total number of FSFI before and after treatment was 5.5 ($P = 0.01$)	The sample size of patients is too small	Runels [7]
FSD	3200 rpm/8 min	PRP was injected into one-third of the anterior vaginal wall. PRP was injected every 4 weeks for four times	FSF, FGSIS, and FSDS-R were improved ($P < 0.001$). The satisfaction rate of PGI-I was high	There was no placebo control group or other treatment groups	Sukgen [8]
FSD	No data	PRP "O-shot" injection: 2 mL was injected into pubic cervical fascia (G-spot); 0.5 mL of Skene's gland (female paraurethral gland) and 1 mL of clitoral area (button part of clitoris) were injected. After the first injection, the second treatment was carried out every 2 months	The remission rate of stress urinary incontinence was more than 90%. The remission rate of overactive bladder was 74%. All female patients with mixed urinary incontinence were satisfied with the results	There was no placebo control group or other treatment groups	Neto [9]
FSD	1500G/5 min	Intravaginal injection of a-PRP-ha was performed at zero, one, 3, and 6 months, respectively	The VHI score increased from 10.7 2.12 to 20.75 4.8; FSD decreased from 36.35 ± 2.53 to 30.15 ± 2.47 before treatment	No placebo control group or other treatment groups (such as PRP injection group and HA injection group)	Hersant [4]

Note: *FSD* female sexual dysfunction

of collagen types I, III, and IV [13]. The expression of p42/44 mitogen-activated protein kinase increased with age; TGF-β(TGF-b1) can promote collagen deposition and penile fibrosis [14].

Studies have shown that ED not only affects patients' sexual function but also affects patients' health. The meta-analysis of Guo [15] showed that compared with normal people, ED patients have a higher risk of coronary events ($P < 0.001$). Prostate cancer prevention trial data show that cardiovascular events (including myocardial infarction death) in ED patients are twice as high as that in normal men [16]. However, most ED patients only want to have a satisfactory normal sexual life, and they are not aware of these potential health risks [17]. Today, PRP can be used as a non-surgical treatment for ED patients.

PD is an abnormal disease of the penis characterized by fibrosis, pain, and deformity of the tunica albuginea [18], ED (40–60%) [19], or distress [18]. Publications from 1965 to 2015 showed that the prevalence of PD in some populations ranged from 0.5% to 20.3%. PD is a disease caused by multiple factors. Its pathogenesis is still unclear. Its manifestations are genetic susceptibility and penile tissue inflammation [20]. PD is associated with Dupuytren contracture. Their genes are the same as those of myofibroblasts in differentiation and plaque formation [21]. Recently, people have focused on the cytokine TGF-β 1; TGF-β 1 can affect extracellular matrix and induce penile leukoplakia fibrosis [22].

American Urological Association guidelines for conservative treatment of PD with injection of verapamil or interferon α-2B can produce many side effects. Pain relief can be achieved through extracorporeal shock wave therapy. There are many studies on the treatment of collagenase clostridium histolyticum (CCH) injection, and there are also many clinical uses [18]. However, CCH only destroys plaques through fermentation and has no effect on inflammation and regeneration of penile tissue [23].

PDGF, VEGF, FGF, EGF, IGF-1, TGF-β1, and other growth factors and mediators can promote angiogenesis. Therefore, it is assumed that PRP has a therapeutic effect on sexual dysfunction [24]. Platelets are in contact with endothelial cells. α-Particles release growth factors that can promote tissue repair, such as enhancing chemotaxis, promoting cell proliferation, promoting neovascularization, and promoting extracellular matrix regeneration [25]. Increased platelets in damaged tissues will lead to the release of more bioactive factors, thus promoting the healing process [26]. In addition, mRNA transcription in cells is stimulated to activate a new cascade pathway, further promoting angiogenesis, endothelialization, and collagen formation and thus promoting tissue regeneration [27].

The main observation index of ED clinical research is to evaluate erectile function through electrical stimulation (such as sponge body pressure and penile histopathological analysis). The main clinical indicators of ED were the results of duplex Doppler ultrasound and international erectile function index (IIEF-5). Pathological analysis of the penis is the main observation index in preclinical study of PD. Bifunctional Doppler ultrasound, Peyronie's disease questionnaire (PDQ), and IIEF-5 were used in clinical study.

11.1.2.2 Treatment of Male Sexual Dysfunction with EPT

Study on EPT in the Treatment of ED

From 2013 to 2015, Epifanova [28] conducted a clinical trial to evaluate the safety and efficacy of PRP in the treatment of ED. They developed and optimized the RPP production process. Quantitative and qualitative components of aFGF, bFGF, PDGF-AA, PDGF-BB, VEGF, and VEGF-D in inactive PRP before and after freezing were evaluated. The subjects were randomly divided into three groups: 30 patients in the first group received PRP injury treatment activated by 10% CaCl2 solution; in the second group, 30 patients were treated with 10% $CaCl_2$ solution activated PRP and PDE-5 inhibitor; and in the third group, 15 patients were treated with activated PRP. PRP was injected once a week for three times. EF improvement was recorded 28 days after treatment. In the first group, statistically significant improvements were observed in peak systolic velocity (PSV) ($P = 0.005$), resistance index (RI) ($P = 0.001$), IIEF-5 ($P = 0.046$), and sexual contact (SEP) scores ($P = 0.001$). In the second group, PSV ($P = 0.028$), RI ($P = 0.129$), IIEF-5 ($P = 0.046$), and SEP ($P < 0.05$) were improved. There were significant differences in IIEF-5, Sep ($P = 0.005$), PSV, and RI ($P > 0.05$) in the third group. According to the measurement by endopat vascular endothelial detection system, the endothelial function of all groups at 6 months was significantly improved compared with baseline ($P < 0.018$) [29]. The researchers believe that PRP therapy can release growth factors, which is safe and effective without adverse reactions [28, 29]. Although this study confirmed that EF was improved at the end of the experiment, there were still limitations in this study, such as the lack of placebo group and other treatment groups and the lack of long-term follow-up.

In 2018, Matz [30] made a study on the safety and feasibility of platelet-rich fibrin matrix (PRFM) in the treatment of common urinary system diseases. The patient received 1–8 injections of PRFM with a volume of 4–9 mL each time. On average, each person received 2.1 injections of PRFM. No adverse reaction occurred or aggravated after a 15-month follow-up. Men's IIEF-5 increased by an average of 4.14 points. At the end of the experiment, the researchers stressed that more subjects need to be studied to confirm the safety of PRFM, and the evaluation of the efficacy of PRFM needs to use objective research methods rather than just questionnaire surveys.

In 2018, Ruffo [31] reported that 60 patients with mild and severe ED were randomly assigned to group A or group B. Group A received low intensity shock wave (LISW) every 6 weeks (1500 times/time), and group B received LISW +6 PRP injections every 6 weeks (once every 2 weeks). The results showed that in group A, IIEF-5 was improved from 11 cases to 18 cases, SEP-Q2 from 48% to 62%, SEP-Q3 from 28% to 48%, IIEF-5 from 10 cases to 22 cases, SEP-Q2 from 52% to 75%, and SEP-Q3 from 30% to 62%. The results showed that LISW+PRP combined therapy was effective in the treatment of ED. However, there is no standardized scheme for the preparation and application of PRP and the standard method for the evaluation results, and further research is needed.

In 2021, Taş [32] reported that 31 ED patients received penile cavernous PRP injection for 3 times in 15 days. Erectile function (EF) was assessed by the international erectile function index (IIEF-EF) at one, three, and 6 months after treatment. The average IIEF-EF was 18 before treatment and 20 at 1, 3, and 6 months after treatment ($p < 0.001$). However, the median IIEF-EF value was still within the range of mild to moderate classification, and the increase was not significant. The score of sexual satisfaction after treatment was significantly higher than that before operation ($p = 0.002$). At the first follow-up after the third injection, a 4 mm-diameter fibrotic plaque was observed on the ventral side of the middle trunk of the penis. However, the patient did not notice the plaque, and there were no symptoms of pain, penis shortening, thinning, or bending. There is still a short board in this experiment, which lacks the placebo group, and the sample size of patients is too small.

In 2021, Ma [33] reported that 30 patients with premature ejaculation were injected with micronized acellular dermal matrix (MADM) particles + PRP into the buck fascia. The curative effect was evaluated by vaginal ejaculation latency (scale), stopwatch, and diagnostic tool of premature ejaculation. The satisfaction of sexual partners and adverse events were also recorded. The results showed that all patients recovered well without infection or allergy. The average latency of vaginal ejaculation was 0.72 ± 0.28 min before operation and 2.41 ± 0.54 min, 2.64 ± 0.41 min, 2.79 ± 0.25 min, and 2.89 ± 0.35 min after 4, 8, 16, and 20 weeks, respectively. After treatment, both the diagnostic tools for premature ejaculation and the satisfaction of sexual partners were significantly improved. The results showed that MADM granule combined with PRP injection was safe, effective, and simple in the treatment of premature ejaculation.

Study on EPT in the Treatment of PD

In 2014, Virag [34] treated 13 PD patients with an average age of 57.5 years with hyaluronic acid (HA) + PRP four times within 2 months. HA + PRP was used under local anesthesia in the treatment of leukoplakia. During a mean follow-up of 9 months, ten patients (77%) had a 30% decrease in penile curvature, and seven patients (53%) had a decrease in penile plaque density, and size IIEF-5 scores were improved. Although the authors believed that HA could prolong the effect of PRP, the composition of PRP was not analyzed [29]; additional PRP and HA monotherapy groups should be established. The limitation of the experiment is that there is no placebo group or other commonly used treatment groups.

Virag [24] continued his research on this basis and published his research results on 90 PD patients in 2017. The course of treatment was injection once every 15 days, a total of 4 times. Before injection, 22G or 18G needle was used to puncture fibrous plaque or calcified plaque. According to the research results, the curvature angle of the penis can be reduced to 6.54–10.51 °, and the thickness of the tunica albuginea can be reduced to 1.11–0.52 mm. Calcification persisted, but the density of calcification decreased in six cases. According to PDQ and IIEF-5 questionnaire, there was significant improvement. The incidence of hematoma and ecchymosis was 10% and 6.7%, respectively. The defect of the experiment is that the author did not analyze the composition of PRP [24]. The limitation of the experiment is that there is no placebo group or other commonly used treatment groups.

Marcovici [35] reported a case of PD treated with PRP. PRP therapy was injected twice at the point of maximum curvature of the penis. Then use the penis pump daily. The penile curvature angle decreased significantly after two months [35]. In order to better describe the effect, Marcovici [35] scanned the penis with ultrasound and recorded whether there was calcification. PDQ and IIEF-5 were used for evaluation.

Matz [30] reported the effect of PRFM injection therapy on PD. IIEF-5 score increased by 4.14 points compared with baseline, penile curvature angle decreased in 80% of patients, and pad use rate decreased by 50% in a female patient with stress urinary incontinence [30]. Patients with the same disease had different injection treatment times. In addition, the author believes that placebo has therapeutic effect and emphasizes that the placebo treatment group should be added to the follow-up study. The limitation of this study is that the sample size of patients is too small.

The clinical study of EPT in the treatment of ED and PD is shown in Table 11.2.

11.1.2.3 Summary

The pathogenesis of ED and PD is complex. The pathogenesis of ED is related to the destruction of penile smooth muscle. PD is characterized by fibrosis of the tunica albuginea and inflammation of penile tissue with ED. Autologous PRP can release a variety of active substances, such as PDGF-AA,

Table 11.2 Clinical study of EPT in the treatment of ED and PD

Types of diseases	PRP production method	PRP usage	The role of PRP	Experimental defect	Author [Ref.]
ED	6000 rpm/6 min	The patient received 1–8 injections of PRFM with a volume of 4–9 mL each time. On average, each patient received 2.1 injections of PRFM	Men's IIEF-5 increased by an average of 4.14 points	There was no placebo group and the sample size was too small	Matz [30]
ED	No data	PRP should be treated within the injury. PRP was injected once a week for three times	PRP has therapeutic effect and no adverse reactions	There was no placebo group or other treatment groups, and there was no long-term follow-up	Epifanova [28]
PD	No data	PRP was injected into plaques every 15 days for 4 times. Before injection, 22G or 18G needle was used to puncture fibrous plaques or calcified plaques	According to PDQ and IIEF-5 questionnaire, there was significant improvement	No analysis of PRP composition and no placebo control group or other treatment groups (e.g., CCH injection)	Virag [24]
ED	6000 rpm/6 min	The patient received 1–8 injections of PRFM with a volume of 4–9 mL each time. On average, each patient received 2.1 injections of PRFM	Men's IIEF-5 increased by an average of 4.14 points	There was no placebo group and the sample size was too small	Matz [30]
ED	No data	HA + PRP was injected into the white film for four times	The curvature decreased by 30% in 77% of the patients, and the density and size of plaque decreased in 53% of the patients	There were no PRP or HA monotherapy group and no placebo group or other commonly used treatment methods (such as CCH injection)	Virag [34]
ED	No data	PRP was injected twice at the point of maximum curvature of penis, 1 mL each time, once every four weeks	After two months, the penile curvature angle decreased significantly	Case report	Marcovici [35]
ED	2800 rpm/8 min and then 3500 rpm/10 min	PRP was injected into the cavernous body of penis, 3 mL each time, once every 15 days, 3 times in total	The mean IIEF-EF was 18 before treatment and 20 at 1, 3, and 6 months after treatment ($P < 0.001$). The score of sexual satisfaction after operation was significantly higher than that before operation ($P = 0.002$)	There was no placebo group and the sample size was too small	Taş [32]

Note: *ED* erectile dysfunction, *PD* peyronie's disease

PDGF-BB, VEGF, VEGF-D, FGF, and so on. These active substances can regulate angiogenesis, inflammatory process, apoptosis, fibrosis, and muscle regeneration and can promote tissue regeneration.

Platelet concentrates were injected into the lesions of ED and PD; the active substances in platelets can promote angiogenesis, muscle regeneration, fibroblast growth, and nerve regeneration. Vascular and muscle regeneration can improve ED, fiber regeneration can slow down the process of fibrosis, and nerve regeneration can improve the sexual sensitivity and EF recovery of ED and PD patients.

11.1.3 EPT in the Treatment of Lichen Sclerosus of Perineum in Men and Women

11.1.3.1 Lichen Sclerosus

Vulvar lichen sclerosus (LS) is a chronic inflammatory skin disease. Vulvar scar and sexual dysfunction are its main clinical symptoms. LS can occur in any part of the body of male and female patients, but mainly in the female anogenital epithelium. Male genital lichen sclerosus (MGLSC) is mostly glans and medial prepuce. Other common complications include hypopigmentation, erythema, infiltration and mossization, and penis organic diseases such as phimosis, balanoprepucial adhesions, meatal stenosis, and naviculomeatal valve insufficiency. The main clinical symptom was difficulty in sexual intercourse, which seriously affected the quality of life (QOL). The main clinical symptoms of female LS were whitening and atrophy of the vulva, perineum, and perianal skin in the shape of "8." Inflammation can lead to scarring and structural changes, such as clitoral phimosis, labial adhesions, crevices, and rectal strictures. The most common clinical symptom is vulvar pruritus. Some patients will also have burning sensation and difficulty in sexual intercourse. The incidence rate of LS is unknown. A recent report from the Netherlands showed that the histologically confirmed female LS incidence rate increased from 7.4 cases per 100,000 women to 14.6 cases between 1991 and 2011. The increased awareness of the disease and the increased rate of biopsy and diagnosis have led to an increase in the incidence rate [36]. However, the actual incidence rate will certainly be higher, because this study excluded those patients who had a clinical diagnosis of LS but did not have a biopsy or whose pathology was not clear.

Although the symptoms of LS have been described in the literature more than a century ago, the pathogenesis, histological diagnosis, and treatment of LS are still not completely clear. There is evidence that LS is a genetic and autoimmune disease. Studies have shown that 12% of the first-class female relatives of 1000 female patients with vulvar LS have LS, indicating that the family history of LS is positive [37]. LS is assumed to be an autoimmune disease in female patients. Some features of LS are similar to other autoimmune diseases, such as high prevalence and correlation with other autoimmune diseases in women [38].

Although LS cannot be completely cured, there are many treatments that can alleviate and prevent the development of the disease. The purpose of LS treatment is to reduce itching and pain symptoms, prevent anatomical structure and appearance changes caused by scars, and prevent malignant transformation. Conventional treatment methods include topical corticosteroids, local calcineurin inhibitors, photodynamic therapy (PDT), high-intensity-focused ultrasound (HIFU) and fractional CO2 laser (fxco2), vulvar adhesiolysis, and perineal plasty. Current international treatment guidelines recommend topical steroids to reduce clinical symptoms and increase disease-free intervals [39]. However, postmenopausal women need to continue to take corticosteroids, which has hormone side effects, and there is also the possibility of vulvar atrophy and deterioration. PRP is the newest treatment for advanced and difficult VLS [40].

11.1.3.2 Treatment of Lichen Sclerosus in Men and Women with EPT

In 2020, Navarrete [41] reported a study on the safety and effectiveness of autologous PRP (TPRP) in the treatment of MGLSC that failed to respond to conventional treatment. Five patients with sclerosing lichen of male genitalia who had been treated for six months but had no effect received subcutaneous injection of TPRP sclerosing area at a dose of 0.1 mL/cm^2, 2–3 mL each time. The patients were evaluated at one day, one week, and four weeks after operation. The second TPRP was performed eight weeks after operation, whether there are complications such as bleeding, hematoma, and infection in each follow-up record. The assessment methods included taking photos, IGA (Investigator's Global Assessment) scale (0–5), symptom scale (0–5), and DLQI (Dermatology Life Quality Index). The results show that baseline means that the IGA of five patients was 3.6 ± 0.57. Four patients completed 18 months of follow-up, with a baseline mean IGA of 3.63 ± 0.73. The mean IGA at six months was 3.13 ± 0.84. The mean IGA at 12 months was 3.25 ± 0.63. The mean IGA at 18 months was 3.25 ± 0.49. The mean baseline pain at erection was 1 ± 1.3 (range: 0–3); after 10 months, all patients were 0; the baseline mean value of pruritus was 0.8 ± 0.96 (range: 0–2); after seven months, all patients were 0; the baseline mean value of acupuncture sensation was 0.8 ± 1.14 (range: 0–3); after ten months, all patients were 0: patients without pain at rest. The baseline mean DLQI was 6 ± 3.51. The baseline mean DLQI of the 4 patients who completed the follow-up was 6.25 ± 4.48 and 4.5 ± 5.63 at 6 months and 1.25 ± 2.45 after 12 months.

In 2021, Tedesco [42] reported that six female patients with LS received PRP injection therapy to treat LS, and video thermography (VTG) was used to evaluate the treatment effect. PRP was injected into the vulva at 0, 15, and 30 days, respectively, and VTG was evaluated at 7 and 30 days after injection. The results showed that the average temperature of the vulva and perineum was between 33.7 and 36.3 °C, and each patient had at least one low temperature zone. There were significant differences between patients. There was a thermal difference of 2.2–1.2 °C in low-temperature area. The results show that PRP is effective in the treatment of VLS. Video thermography is a useful clinical monitoring method to identify and track VLS.

In 2021, Tedesco [43] reported that 40 patients with LS (24 males and 16 females) were divided into two groups on average. AD-SVF and AD-SVF + PRP were injected subcutaneously into the sclerotic area. Before treatment and six months after treatment, the treatment effect was evaluated by clinical evaluation and DLQI. All patients were able to tolerate the two operations, and no side effects occurred during and after the operation. Analysis based on disease stage showed that the clinical score of early-stage patients was significantly higher than that of late-stage patients (early stage, 2.2 ± 0.8; late stage, 1.6 ± 1.0, $p = 0.046$). A separate analysis of the two study groups showed that there was a significant difference in AD-SVF PRP (early, 2.6 ± 0.7; late, 1.3 ± 1.0, $p = 0.011$), while there was no difference in AD-SVF treatment group (early, 2.0 ± 0.8; late, 2.0 ± 0.9, $p = 0.77$). In addition, independent analysis of male and female patients did not prove any relevant difference in clinical scores ($f = 2.0 \pm 1.1$; $m = 1.79 \pm 0.9$, $p = 0.52$). Based on the analysis of disease stage, the DLQI questionnaire in the AD-SVF + PRP group was significantly higher than that in the late LS group (− 4.7 ± 2.8 vs − 1.7 ± 2.2; $P < 0.05$ and 0.036), but AD-SVF + PRP can increase the adverse clinical outcomes of advanced patients. The results showed that AD-SVF + PRP had a synergistic effect in early LS patients. It is suggested that the combination therapy should be given priority, but it is not recommended to use AD-SVF and PRP in late LS patients.

Tedesco [44] reported in 2020 that male and female patients with LS treated with PRP had different treatment effects. Forty-three male patients with LS and 51 female patients with LS were treated by injecting about 4 mL (range 2–4 mL) of PRP into the posterior labial frenulum (2 wheals), clitoral prepuce (2 wheals), and left and right labia minora (2 wheals) with a 27-gauge needle. Male patients were injected subcutaneously at four points in the base of sclerotic area. It was injected once every 15 days, 3 times in total. The patients were followed up and evaluated by DLQI six months after the last treatment. The results showed that all patients had a good tolerance to PRP, and the symptoms were significantly relieved after six months of treatment. The pain and burning sensation of male and female LS patients were relieved obviously, but the female patients were more obvious. There was no difference in the relief of pruritus between male and female patients, and the relief of sexual intercourse difficulties was different between male and female patients. The remission of dyspareunia was obvious in men, but not in women. The results showed that PRP had a good effect on the treatment of LS and improve QOL and sexual function of male and female LS patients.

In 2019, some scholars conducted a randomized, placebo-controlled, double-blind clinical trial of PRP for the treatment and follow-up of LS [45]. Pathologists evaluated the inflammatory infiltration of biopsy tissue before and after treatment. "Clinical Scoring System (CSS) for LS" can evaluate the severity of LS according to the symptoms of patients and the impression of researchers. It is a proven and effective evaluation method. There was no significant difference in the results of inflammatory reaction. The difference in the mean score of CSS was −7.74 in the PRP group and − 9.44 in the placebo group. The results of this study show that PRP is not effective in the treatment of vulvar LS but the experimental sample size is too small [45].

The clinical study of EPT in the treatment of LS and VLS is shown in Table 11.3.

11.1.3.3 Summary

The primary goal of vulvar LS treatment is to reduce inflammation. PRP therapy is based on the release of high levels of growth factors that can regulate the proliferation of mesenchymal cells and the synthesis of extracellular matrix to promote tissue regeneration. PRP can effectively promote tissue regeneration in the treatment of venous ulcer, diabetes foot ulcer, and tendon disease.

Although many trials have confirmed that PRP can reduce the clinical symptoms of VLS, the sample size of PRP in the treatment of VLS is still too small, many trials have no placebo control group, and the preparation process of PRP is not the same. Moreover, some studies have carried out two kinds of interventions at the same time, that is, PRP combined with other injection materials, such as adipose-derived mesenchymal cells, and cannot determine which component plays a major role. Other studies showed that histopathology showed no significant difference between the two groups.

We need a large number of trials to confirm the effectiveness of PRP in the treatment of VLS.

11.1.4 Summary

In conclusion, the limitations of available data on platelet concentration for the treatment of sexual dysfunction are noteworthy. Before the regulatory authorities approve the use of platelet concentrate for clinical treatment, more high-quality preclinical studies and animal studies, as well as related studies approved by ethics or registered in clinical trials, are needed to better understand the safety, mechanism of action, and clinical effect of platelet concentrate [46, 47].

There are some design defects in the existing research of EPT in the treatment of male and FSD, such as small sample size and no placebo group and control group. Moreover, there is a defect in the number of times of platelet concentration treatment, because many effects are achieved through paracrine and autocrine mechanisms. Therefore, platelet concentration therapy needs a course of treatment and repeated stimulation, and its cumulative effect is based on the treatment time. In addition, what are the relative and absolute contraindications of platelet concentration therapy?

The problems to be solved in the future include the effective concentration and frequency of injection. If the amount of one injection cannot reach the necessary concentration of growth factor, it will be difficult to maintain the cascade of repair reactions. Platelet concentrates can promote inflammation [48], regeneration, repair, anti-inflammatory [49], and neuroprotective and neurotrophic effects of growth fac-

Table 11.3 Clinical study of EPT in the treatment of LS and VLS

Types of diseases	PRP production method	PRP usage	The role of PRP	Experimental defect	Author [Ref.]
LS	No data	The sclerotic area was subcutaneously injected with TPRP at a dose of 0.1 mL/cm², 2–3 mL each time. Another TPRP was performed at eight weeks	The mean IGA and DLQI were decreased after operation. Erectile pain, itching, and tingling were relieved, and QOL was improved	The number of patients is small and the follow-up time is short. It cannot improve the aesthetic appearance of the penis	Navarrete [41]
VLS	No data	About 4 mL (range 2–4 mL) of PRP per treatment was injected into the posterior fourchette (2 wheals), into the hood (2 wheals), and into the left and right labia minor (2 wheals) with a 27-gauge needle. One infiltration every 15 days for 3 times	Video thermography showed at least one hypothermia area in all patients. The average temperature of the vulva and perineum was between 33.7 and 36.3 °C. there was a large difference between patients. There was a thermal difference of 2.2 to 1.2 °C in low-temperature area	The number of patients enrolled for the study is small. Moreover, not many patients are administered with PRP injections and, above all, no standardized technique as yet exists for this therapy, for its mechanisms of precise action and for the variable interpatient response to it	Tedesco [42]
LS	No data	AD-SVF + PRP (15 mL AD-SVF mixed with 4 mL PRP) was injected subcutaneously in sclerotic area once every four months for two times	Early LS patients combined with AD-SVF and PRP have synergistic effect; it is recommended to give priority to combination therapy, but it is not recommended to use AD-SVF and PRP combination therapy for late LS patients	There was no placebo control group or other treatment groups	Tedesco [43]
LS	(C.Punt-biomed system and SELPHYL®, Cascade medical enterprises, UK, ltd., Plymouth, UK)extraction kit	About 4 mL (range 2–4 mL) of PRP per treatment was injected into the posterior fourchette (2 wheals), into the hood (2 wheals), and into the left and right labia minor (2 wheals) with a 27-gauge needle. One infiltration every 15 days for 3 times	The results showed that PRP had a good effect in the treatment of LS and could improve QOL and sexual function of male and female patients with LS	The sample size is small and the follow-up time is short	Tedesco [44]
LS	No data	The treatment group was subcutaneously injected with PRP, and the control group was subcutaneously injected with normal saline	Histopathological examination showed no significant difference in inflammation between placebo group and PRP group	Small sample size	Goldstein [45]

Note: *LS* lichen sclerosus, *VLS* vulvar lichen sclerosus

tors [50], realize its therapeutic potential, and influence the key factors of FSD, ED, PD, LS, and VLS. There is a positive correlation between the growth factors released by α-particles and the platelet concentration in the final cell product. How to make the best use of degranulation activation technology [26, 28, 29]?

EPT is safe, but it is still in the experimental stage for FSD, ED, PD, and LV. Since the exact mechanism of platelet concentration has not been elucidated, it is speculated that platelet concentration may realize its therapeutic potential through the regeneration of endothelial cells, smooth muscle cells, and connective tissue. But it still needs a large sample, placebo-controlled, multicenter study to make up for the lack of existing data, parallel system of information biology analysis, and functional testing. Finally, the safety and effectiveness of platelet concentration in sexual potential were obtained [51].

11.2 Application of EPT in Lip Plastic Surgery

11.2.1 Application of EPT in Improving Nasolabial Groove

Deep facial wrinkles such as nasolabial grooves are due to insufficient volume caused by atrophy of subcutaneous tissue. Injectable dermal filler is usually used for treatment. The disadvantages of absorbable fillers are that they are non-permanent and have foreign body reactions. Although there are some injectable soft tissue fillers (such as poly-L-lactic acid) that promote tissue proliferation through tissue fibrosis, these fillers still belong to non-biological implant materials. Clinically, there is a need for an autologous filler that can promote tissue proliferation.

In 2010, Sclafani [52] reported that injection of PRFM can improve deep nasolabial sulcus. Fifteen patients with moderate to severe nasolabial sulcus were treated. After the successful production of PRFM, No. 30 and No. 27 needles were used for intradermal or subcutaneous injection under the nasolabial sulcus. The injection methods were mainly linear injection and continuous puncture injection. The scope of nasolabial sulcus correction is complete correction from the fold of nasal alar to the junction of the oral cavity. Follow-up was performed 1, 2, 6, and 12 weeks after treatment. The severity of nasolabial sulcus was assessed by wrinkle assessment score (WAS) and global aesthetic improvement scale [53]. Take photos before and after treatment and keep them. The results showed that the WAS increased by 2.17 ± 0.56 immediately after treatment. The smallest improvement was in the first week. The WAS increased by 0.65 ± 0.68, but it still improved compared with that before treatment. At the second, sixth, and 12th week, WAS scores increased significantly, which were 0.97 ± 075, 1.08 ± 0.59, and 1.13 ± 0.72, respectively ($p < 0.001$ at all time points). The WAS after treatment was significantly improved compared with that before treatment. There was no significant difference in WAS at 2, 6, and 12 weeks of follow-up. The results confirmed that the single treatment of autologous PRFM was well tolerated and could significantly correct the deep nasolabial sulcus without excessive fibrosis or foreign body reaction. Unlike other subcutaneous fillers (e.g., poly-L-lactic acid), PRFM works rapidly.

In 2015, Xu et al. [54] reported that fat-derived SVF combined with PRP injection to improve nasolabial groove therapy can significantly improve nasolabial groove depression in middle-aged and elderly patients without using exogenous filling materials, which has a very good application prospect. The improvement effect of nasolabial groove was the best seven days after operation, which may be related to local swelling. The improvement effect began to decline after seven days. It remained stable 1–6 months after operation, but the effect was significantly better than that before treatment. The performance after seven days may be due to the absorption of serum components of the injection mixture and the improvement of swelling. Under the action of later cytokines, mesenchymal stem cells can differentiate into fibroblasts and secrete type II collagen, so as to maintain a certain tissue capacity in nasolabial sulcus. However, the specific mechanism is not clear, which is the problem to be solved by future research. No recurrence of nasolabial groove was found during the longest nine-month follow-up. In addition, there were no adverse reactions and complications during injection and follow-up, and the safety of treatment was reliable. More detailed and comprehensive treatment results need to be observed and discussed based on expanding the sample size.

11.2.2 Application of EPT in Cleft Lip and Palate Surgery

Cleft lip and palate are one of the most common congenital diseases in children. It will seriously affect children's appearance and cause children's psychological and social burdens. Scar management after cleft lip and palate plasty is very important. It often requires years of follow-up treatment to prevent postoperative scar hyperplasia. Plastic surgeons are still exploring various treatment methods to reduce postoperative scars. PRP is rich in many cytokines and growth factors, helping to regenerate damaged tissue and improve scar appearance. PRP is effective in the treatment of muscle injury, chronic wounds, and atrophic and contractile scars by restoring skin tissue and texture.

In 2020, Refahee et al. [55] reported that the improved Millard technology combined with PRP injection in the treatment of congenital cleft lip can effectively improve the healing of skin and muscle wounds and reduce the formation of scar tissue. Twenty-four patients with nonsyndromic complete unilateral cleft lips were randomized to repair surgery at the age of 3–6 months. In the experimental group, 12 patients with unilateral cleft lip were treated with modified Millard operation. PRP was injected into the muscle and skin around the wound immediately after the wound was sutured. In the control group, 12 patients with cleft lip only received modified Millard operation. After six months, the muscle scar width was evaluated by ultrasonography, and the skin surface scar width was evaluated by photos. The results showed that the scar width in the treatment group was significantly improved compared with that in the control group. It is proved that autologous PRP injection can effectively improve the healing of skin and muscle wounds and reduce the formation of scar tissue.

11.2.3 Application of EPT in Correcting Lip Defect

Lips are divided into red lips and white lips, which have obvious color differences. Because of this structural characteristic of lip tissue, the method of repairing lip defect is more difficult than that of other parts. The common repair methods of lip defects are as follows:

1. The residual lip tissue increases. It can be filled with autologous tissue transplantation, such as autologous dermis transplantation, myofascial transplantation, autologous fat transplantation, etc.
2. Repair with surrounding lip tissue. The defect site is usually repaired with contralateral lip tissue. For small-scale defects, local "V-Y" flap is generally used for repair; for a wide range of lip defects, local pedicled flap and cross lip flap were used to repair the upper lip tissue defects.

3. Buccal axial membrane and lingual axial membrane flap. It is mainly used for the repair of lip red defects. If peripheral lip tissue or buccal axial membrane and lingual axial membrane tissue are selected to repair lip defects, there is not only the risk of flap necrosis but also insufficient correction due to insufficient amount of local transferred tissue. The operational risk is high, and it also destroys the shape of the contralateral natural lip. Due to the need for short-term lip and tongue braking after operation, there is mouth opening disorder and eating difficulty, which makes the patient more painful and has the disadvantages of sensory disorder, dryness in the repair area, and the need for stage II surgical repair. In recent years, some scholars have used skin fillers to repair lip defects or implant prostheses. However, in addition to their unsatisfactory biocompatibility, these biomaterials also have great differences between their biomechanical properties and lip tissues. After implantation, they are locally hard and feel bad. Patients have obvious discomfort and even affect their functions.

As an important component of soft tissue, adipose tissue has been widely used in the treatment of facial soft tissue depression. When repairing lip soft tissue defect, the texture of the filled tissue is similar to that of lip tissue, and autologous adipose tissue transplantation is an ideal treatment. However, due to the lip and other active parts, the fat particles will be damaged and absorbed in varying degrees after transplantation, the survival rate is low, and the volume of surviving fat changes greatly, so the results after transplantation are difficult to predict. PRP is a platelet concentrate obtained by whole blood centrifugation, which is four times higher than that of whole blood. After activated, its platelets can release a variety of growth factors. These growth factors promote the division and proliferation of adipose stem cells and the vascularization of transplanted fat through mutual synergy.

Therefore, some studies have used PRP to improve the survival rate of lip transplantation fat particles. In 2013, Wang Xin et al. [56] reported that filling lip soft tissue defects with autologous PRP fat particles can improve the survival rate of transplanted fat, reduce the absorption of fat particles, and have a definite appearance effect. There were 12 cases of lip soft tissue defect, including 7 cases of red lip defect and 5 cases of red and white lip defect. There were five cases of secondary deformity after unilateral cleft lip operation, two cases of traumatic and infectious deformity, and five cases of residual deformity after hemangioma treatment. The filling methods are as follows:

1. For patients with congenital lip hypoplasia, autologous PRP fat particles were injected into the deformity site at multiple levels and sites.
2. Injection volume of each part ≤10 mL/time is generally about 20%. The remaining PRP fat particles were stored in a refrigerator at a deep low temperature (−25 °C). one to two months after operation, whether to use modified filling again was determined according to the lip shape. If necessary, PRP can be extracted again in 3–6 months or fat suction injection can be performed.
3. Lip soft tissue defects caused by lip trauma, lip surgery, radiotherapy, freezing, and sclerotherapy are often accompanied by paralysis scar adhesion between soft tissue and deep tissue. Autologous PRP fat particles can be injected while loosening the paralysis scar. The injection method and the time of reinjection are the same as before. Antibiotics were applied for 5–7 days after operation. The donor area was bandaged with abdominal belt changed dressing 24 h later, and the suture was removed ten days later. The recipient area was gently massaged and shaped after operation, and the special adhesive tape was pasted and fixed for one week and then removed. Avoid improper massage and external pressure. The results showed that the appearance of lip defects in 12 patients was natural after filling, and there was no obvious fat absorption. Followed up for 6–12 months, the treatment effect was stable and both doctors and patients were satisfied.

The advantages of PRP in PRP fat granule transplantation are the following:

1. No immunogenicity. The lips were filled with autologous adipose tissue and autologous platelets, and no rejection occurred.
2. The lip is relatively thin and soft. It is located in the active part of the face. It has high requirements for the biocompatibility and biomechanical properties of the implanted materials. If bad implants are used, the activity function of the lip may be affected. PRP fat particles are autologous tissue. After filling in the receiving area, they feel good and the patients have no discomfort. They are especially suitable for smokers or patients who make a living with their lips (such as divers, musical instrument players, etc.).
3. The supply area is guaranteed. The abdomen is the main donor area, and its fat reserves are enough to meet the clinical needs; platelets are taken from peripheral blood and generally do not exceed 100 mL.
4. Reoperation rate is low. PRP improves the survival rate of fat transplantation; reduces the liquefaction, necrosis, and absorption of transplanted fat; and reduces the risk of multiple operations.
5. It is especially suitable for parts with poor blood supply. Due to the poor blood supply of lip soft tissue defects left after radiotherapy, sclerosis, trauma, and other operations,

Table 11.4 Clinical study of EPT in lip plastic surgery

Types of diseases	PRP production method	PRP usage	The role of PRP	Experimental defect	Author [Ref.]
NLFs	1100 rpm/6 min	Intradermal or subcutaneous injection under nasolabial sulcus is mainly linear injection and continuous puncture injection	The WAS was significantly higher than that before operation ($P < 0.001$ at all time points)	Too few patient samples	Sclafani [52]
NLFs	160G/10 min and then 400G/10 min	The deep dermis and subcutaneous tissue of human nasolabial sulcus were injected by linear injection method	The WAS was significantly higher than that before operation ($P < 0.001$ at all time points)	Too few patient samples	Xu [54]
Cleft lip	250G/10 min and then 1000G/10 min	Following muscle closure, approximately 0.25 mL of PRP was injected on each side along the suture line of the muscle layer, and another 0.25 mL of PRP was injected on each side along the suture line of the dermis layer	Scar width showed a significant improvement in the study group	No placebo control group or other treatment groups	Refahee [55]
Lip soft tissue defect	2500 rpm/10 min and then 2500G/10 min	The ratio of PRP to fat particles is 1:3	PRP can improve the survival rate of transplanted fat and reduce the absorption of fat particles, and the appearance effect is accurate	No placebo control group or other treatment groups	Wang [56]

Note: *NLFs* deep nasolabial folds

it is difficult to survive the transplantation of fat. However, platelets in PRP can release growth factors in a variety of proportions close to the normal physiological concentration in the body, so as to play the best synergistic effect between them and promote the division of various types of tissue cells in the body. Proliferation and neovascularization are more conducive to the survival of transplanted fat.

6. Good cell biological effect. Exogenous growth factor has a single component, limited source, and high price, and there is a certain risk of immune rejection and disease transmission. PRP is an autologous platelet, which contains the same proportion of growth factors as human growth factors. It optimizes the repair and regeneration of adipose tissue through synergistic promotion. Moreover, the action time of platelets in vivo is 5–7 days, which is much longer than that of exogenous growth factors (a few hours). It can slowly release growth factors for a long time. It maintains a high concentration of growth factor in the receptor area and makes it play a better role in tissue repair. It is an ideal growth factor library for clinical application.
7. No tumorigenicity. A large number of growth factors released by platelet activation attach to the surface of target cell membrane on the receptor axis and activate cell membrane receptors. These membrane receptors induce intrinsic signal proteins and stimulate the normal gene sequence expression of cells. Therefore, the growth factor released by PRP does not enter the target cells, which will not change the genetic properties of the target cells but only accelerate the process of normal healing.

The lip soft tissue defect caused by congenital hypoplasia can be directly filled with fat particles and PRP. After operation, the lip is soft and has good continuity with the surrounding normal tissue, and the curve is soft and natural. For the defect caused by trauma, first completely loosen the deep paralysis mark adhesion, and at the same time, carry out the compound filling of fat particles and PRP, which can not only treat the depression deformity but also prevent the re-paralysis mark adhesion between the skin and deep tissues. Before filling the soft tissue depression after sclerotherapy of hemangioma, it is necessary to determine whether the lesion itself is consolidated. If there is venous sinus, fat particles cannot be filled; otherwise it is easy to cause fat embolism and serious complications. Before consolidation, even with other methods (such as dermal adipose tissue flap filling), there is a risk of excessive intraoperative bleeding and low postoperative tissue survival rate. In conclusion, although PRP can improve the survival rate of fat transplantation, it is still observed that some patients with fat transplantation will have postoperative absorption and local slight asymmetric deformity. Therefore, storing an appropriate amount of fat particles can be used for fine-tuning filling of local tissues. In addition, the biggest risk of adipose tissue transplantation is infection. If infection occurs, fat liquefaction and necrosis are easy to occur. Antibiotics are recommended for 5–7 days to prevent infection.

The clinical study of EPT in lip plastic surgery is shown in Table 11.4.

11.3 Application of EPT in Ear Plastic Surgery

11.3.1 Basic Research of EPT in Ear Plastic Surgery

11.3.1.1 Protective Effect of EPT on Ear Skin Cartilage Complex Transplantation

Composite transplantation has the advantages of good skin color, low incidence of donor site complications, good skin texture, and simple operation. However, composite transplantation has some limitations, such as it can only be used to treat small defects and the survival rate is uncertain. PRP contains a large number of growth factors and is widely used in tissue regeneration.

In 2014, Jeon et al. [57] reported that PRP as an adjuvant can improve the survival rate of cartilage skin composite grafts. Cartilage skin composite grafts were implanted into the ears of 20 New Zealand white rabbits. The graft is then rotated and returned to its original position, thereby destroying the original circulation at the bottom of the graft. Each ear was randomly divided into two groups: experimental group ($n = 20$, PRP group) and control group ($n = 20$, control group). The experimental group was injected with 1.0 mL PRP around the composite skin graft, and the control group was injected with normal saline. The therapeutic effect was evaluated by graft survival, skin blood flow, CD31 stained vessels, and vascular endothelial growth factor protein levels. The results showed that the graft survival rate and blood perfusion volume of the experimental group were higher than those of the control group 12 days after operation. The number of CD31+ blood vessels and the expression of vascular endothelial growth factor were significantly increased in the experimental group. The results showed that the application of PRP in the rabbit ear model of cartilage skin composite transplantation could improve the graft survival rate and graft blood flow. PRP can increase the number of blood vessels and VEGF expression. These results suggest that PRP may increase neovascularization and improve the survival rate of cartilage skin composite transplantation.

In 2014, Choi et al. [58] also confirmed that RPR can increase the neovascularization of cartilage skin composite grafts and improve the survival rate. Moreover, they further confirmed the optimal injection time of PRP. Twenty-four rabbits were randomly divided into four groups. In group 1, autologous PRP was injected into the recipient site three days before transplantation, three days after transplantation in group 2, and three days after transplantation in group 3. Group 4 in the control group was not injected with PRP. The median survival rate and microvessel density of grafts were evaluated by naked eye photos and immunofluorescence staining on the 21st day of transplantation. In group 1, the survival rate of transplanted plants was 97.8%, that of the second group was 69.2%, that of the third group was 55.7%, and that of the control group was 40.8%. Group 1 mean vessel count was 34 (weekly) × 200 HPF, the average vessel count in group 2 was 24.5, the average vessel count in group 3 was 19.5, and the average vessel count in the control group was 10.5. Studies have shown that PRP can increase the viability of cartilage skin composite grafts. The survival rate and microvessel density of the experimental group were higher than those of the control group. The graft survival rate and revascularization rate of the preinjected PRP group were the highest. PRP treatment has the characteristics of minimally invasive, rapid, easy to apply, and low price, which provides a potential clinical approach for larger composite transplantation.

However, Bulam et al. [59] reported that autologous PRP was injected into the capsule for cartilage graft after dorsal cartilage transplantation in rabbits. The cartilage transplantation group injected with PRP subcutaneously after operation obtained less weight loss rate and higher histopathological score, but the results were not statistically significant. Further studies are needed to explore the different application modes and longer-term results of PRP treatment.

11.3.1.2 Basic Study on the Protective Effect of EPT in Ear Reconstruction Tissue Engineering

EPT Can Reduce the Inflammatory Reaction or Immune Rejection of Scaffold Materials in Tissue Engineering

Total external ear reconstruction is still a difficult point in ear reconstruction surgery. The ability of cartilage regeneration is low. Autologous costal cartilage is still the first choice for ear reconstruction surgery. However, autogenous costal cartilage reconstruction of external ear still has some disadvantages, such as donor site deformity, long operation time, poor rib plasticity, and different hardness from ear cartilage. The key of this technique is to plant the obtained and cultured autologous chondrocytes on the scaffold and implant them into the subcutaneous defect area. In recent years, scientists have developed many biodegradable cartilage tissue engineering scaffold biomaterials, such as hydrogels (such as collagen, fibrin, collagen, agarose, or sodium alginate) and solid polymer scaffolds (such as polyglycolic acid (PGA), polylactic acid (PLA), and their copolymers). However, biodegradable materials still have some disadvantages, such as uncontrollable degradation rate and difficult to maintain the appearance of tissue-engineered cartilage. Moreover, these natural or synthetic materials are still exogenous and may produce serious inflammatory reaction or immune rejection after transplantation.

In 2017, Liao et al. [60] reported that the addition of PRP to PLGA (poly(lactic-co-glycolic acid)) membrane encapsulated cut cartilage has a protective effect. Cartilage grafts were obtained from one ear of ten New Zealand rabbits. The experiment was divided into three groups: bare cartilage slice transplantation group, PLGA membrane-wrapped cartilage slice transplantation group, and PRP mixed cartilage slice and PLGA membrane-wrapped cartilage slice transplantation group. Three subcutaneous bags were made on the back of the rabbit, and then the grafts were implanted into the subcutaneous bags. After three months, all rabbits were killed and specimens were collected. The sections were stained with hematoxylin and eosin, toluidine blue, and type II collagen by immunohistochemistry. The biomechanical properties of the grafts were evaluated. The results showed that the PLGA membrane samples met the current biological evaluation standards for medical devices. After three months, in the PLGA membrane-wrapped cartilage slice transplantation group, moderate absorption of the grafts was observed, while the cut cartilage mixed with PRP had no obvious macro absorption, and the histological section also showed the same results. The stress-strain curve of compression test showed that the elastic modulus of nude cartilage slice transplantation group was 7.65 ± 0.59 MPa. In PLGA membrane-wrapped cartilage slice transplantation group, the pressure was 5.98 ± 0.45 MPa; in the PRP mixed cartilage section and PLGA membrane-wrapped cartilage section transplantation group, the pressure was 7.48 ± 0.55 MPa. The results showed that PRP could reduce the absorption of PLGA membrane-wrapped cartilage grafts and foreign body inflammation, increase the production of type II collagen, and increase the compression modulus. PRP can improve the survival rate of transplanted cartilage.

EPT Can Improve the Survival Rate of Cartilage in Tissue Engineering

Plastic surgery requires various forms of cartilage grafts to repair tissue defects or reconstruct a part of the body. Bare or wrapped, crushed, or cut is the main form of cartilage transplantation. In addition to teorhinoplasty and reconstruction, cartilage transplantation is also used for cranioplasty, lower eyelid reconstruction, orbital repair, zygomatic expansion, and nipple reconstruction. The shape and quality of cartilage grafts are very important to maintain the surgical effect, but cartilage grafts are often absorbed and reduced in volume. The calcification, hardness increase, and deformation of the grafts are caused by the decreased activity of the transplanted cartilage. Exposing the graft contour under the skin may lead to asymmetric surgical results. Absorbed cartilage grafts may also disengage from the fixed suture, resulting in graft displacement or dislocation. Treatment failure or reoperation will reduce patient satisfaction. Sometimes it is necessary to take new cartilage again, which will cause damage to the patient again. Improving the survival of cartilage grafts is very important for clinical effect.

In 2017, Wang et al. [61] reported that a nondegradable porous polyurethane scaffold with complex PRP gel could be used as a potential substitute for ear cartilage. Porous scaffolds with specific details were prepared by rapid prototyping technology using elastic polyurethane with good biocompatibility, high safety, and nondegradability. PRP containing fibrin and abundant autologous growth factor can be used as a cell carrier to expand cells in vitro. Polyurethane/PRP/autologous chondrocyte composites were successfully prepared by crosslinking polyurethane skeleton, PRP, and cells and implanted subcutaneously in the back of nude mice. The results showed that this method made the cell distribution more uniform and the cell density higher, promoted the proliferation of chondrocytes, induced the high-level expression of aggrecan and type II collagen genes, increased the content of glycosaminoglycan, and promoted the regeneration of cartilage tissue. This cartilage tissue engineering is a promising method for external ear reconstruction.

In 2020, Wang et al. [62] randomly divided 48 New Zealand white rabbits into 4 groups: PRP group, vascularization (VES) group, PRP + VES group, and control group. Rabbit auricle cartilage was cut into 2 mm pieces and injected into tissue engineering chambers (TECs). At the eighth week, the cartilage structures were collected and measured for histomorphology, immunohistochemical staining, and mechanical strength. The results showed that the PRP + VES structure presented a white cartilage-like appearance, and the cartilage volume increased by 600% compared with the original volume, from 0.30 to 1.8 ± 0.1789 mL. Histological staining showed proliferation of marginal chondrocytes in PRP group and PRP + VES group. Mechanical strength showed that the cartilage structure of PRP + VES group showed similar mechanical properties to that of normal cartilage. After PRP- and TEC-induced vascularization of rabbit auricular cartilage fragments, the volume of cartilage tissue increased significantly. Adding PRP to TEC can greatly reduce the incidence of complications.

Application of EPT in Three-Dimensional Printing of Ear Tissue Engineering

External ear reconstruction of congenital microtia is still a difficult problem in plastic surgery. The hallmark of successful auricle reconstruction is that the external ear has good three-dimensional contour, biomechanics, and mobility. Autologous costal cartilage transplantation, prosthesis reconstruction, and polymer implants are the three main surgical methods at present. The perfect graft should be able to meet the function while maintaining the shape and certain mobility. However, none of the existing surgical methods can meet this condition. Costal cartilage has certain compliance, but its mobility is not good, and the carving process is difficult. Removal of costal cartilage may result in hemopneumothorax and chest wall insufficiency. Plastic surgeons should have good carving skills and three-dimensional consciousness to carve a suitable auricle cartilage graft. The use of Medpor (Stryker) can avoid the complications of cutting the autologous costal cartilage. However, Medpor is too hard, and there is a risk of prosthesis exposure due to long-term friction and compression with the skin. The development of tissue engineering provides hope for the repair of tissue defects. Cartilage tissue engineering can provide anatomical auricles for auricle reconstruction. However, there are also many problems in ear tissue engineering, such as the shape and size of ear cartilage carvings are difficult to maintain the initial state after transplantation, the transplanted scaffold cannot change into autologous tissue, and the cultured auricle will be deformed due to skin contraction after transplantation. Cartilage fragment transplantation is often used in rhinoplasty and has good cosmetic effect. However, cartilage fragment grafts have no support and cannot maintain a specific shape. Therefore, cartilage fragment grafts are not suitable for ear reconstruction. Three-dimensional printing technology has been widely used in tissue engineering, which can print exactly the same graft as required and can control the adhesion and proliferation of three-dimensional porous and complex internal structure cells in the printing process.

In 2019, Liao et al. [63] reported that a porous and hollow polyamide auricle mold filled with sliced cartilage and PRP was prepared by using three-dimensional printing technology. Three-dimensional printed ear grafts have appropriate biomechanics, shape retention, good chondrocyte activity, and extracellular matrix formation ability. Three-dimensional porous hollow auricle mold is designed by Materialise Magics v20.03 software. Ten molds were prepared by selective laser sintering of polyamide. Cartilage grafts were obtained from the ears of New Zealand rabbits, and blood was extracted for centrifugation to produce PRP. The ear cartilage was cut into small pieces of 0.5–2.0 mm and weighed and mixed with PRP, and then the mixture was put into a hollow mold. Then the composite graft was implanted into the back of rabbits ($n = 10$) and evaluated after four months. The shape and composition were evaluated histologically, and the hardness was tested biomechanically. The results showed that the three-dimensional printing auricle mold was 0.6 mm thick, with communication between the inner and outer surfaces and circular pores of 0.1–0.3 cm. After four months, the fused shape of the excised cartilage was highly consistent with that of the human auricle. The weight of cartilage was 5.157 ± 0.230 g ($p > 0.05$). Histological staining showed that chondrocytes had high activity and produced cartilage matrix components such as type II collagen and glycosaminoglycan. Hardness test shows that the rigidity of auricle is 0.158 ± 0.187 n/mm, which is similar to that of human auricle. The results showed that three-dimensional printed bone grafts had good biomechanical properties and shape retention properties, and chondrocytes had good viability and produced extracellular matrix.

The basic research of EPT in ear plastic surgery is shown in Table 11.5.

11.3.2 Clinical Study of EPT in Ear Plastic Surgery

11.3.2.1 Clinical Application of EPT in Replantation of Severed Ear

When microsurgery is unable to anastomose blood vessels to reconstruct blood supply, completely severed ears can be replanted without microsurgery. However, simple replantation of completely severed ears has complications such as poor perfusion leading to partial or complete necrosis. The development of postoperative adjuvant therapy such as hyperbaric oxygen treatment (HBOT), aspirin, prostaglandin, dextran-40, and leech has improved the survival rate of severed ear replantation. However, the success rate of replantation of severed ears without microvascular reconstruction is rare.

In 2017, Lee et al. [64] reported a case of successful ear replantation after non-microsurgery. Postoperative adjuvant treatment included local HBOT, PRP injection, and polydeoxyribonucleic acid (PDRN) injection. A 76-year-old man with left ear completely severed for 1 h went to the emergency department. Put the severed ear in a normal saline container. After admission, physical examination showed that the auricle was broken in the sagittal plane. No suitable vessel (vessel diameter > 0.5 mm) for microsurgical vascular reconstruction was found at the incision edge. After informing the patient that there may be partial or total necrosis in broken ear replantation, it was decided to try the treatment scheme of continuous local HBOT after broken ear replantation. Minimal debridement of broken ears is necessary and anatomical reduction must be done as much as possible. After the operation, the external auditory canal was filled with gauze balls; the disposable paper cup was cut according to the patient's auricle and fixed on the skin around the ear and sealed with transparent film (Tegaderm film, 3 M, Hutchinson) to prevent oxygen leakage. Provide pure oxygen with a flow rate of 2 L/min to the paper cup cavity through the rubber tube. Tegaderm membrane covering the cup cavity can indirectly observe whether the oxygen is positive pressure. To prevent air leakage, replace the paper cup cover every two days. Local HBOT is carried out for the first 24 hours after surgery and then repeated for five days before discharge. On the second day after operation, congestion in the vein of the entire replanted auricle was observed. Injection of PRP and PDRN increased the perfusion of the composite transplanted tissue. For every three days, 3 mL of PRP was injected into the intact ear near the injury site (1 mL

Table 11.5 Basic research of EPT in ear plastic surgery

Animal type	EPT manufacturing method	EPT usage	Animal model	Role of EPT	Author[Ref.]
New Zealand white rabbits	160 g/10 min and 400 g/10 min	PRP was injected evenly into the surrounding skin of the composite graft	Ear cartilage skin complex transplantation	PRP may increase neovascularization and improve the survival rate of cartilage skin composite grafts	Jeon [57]
New Zealand white rabbits	1000 rpm/10 min and 5000 rpm/10 min	Autologous PRP was injected into the recipient sites three days before grafting in group 1, on the day of grafting in group 2, and three days after grafting in group 3	Ear cartilage skin complex transplantation	The survival rate and revascularization rate of preinjected PRP grafts were the highest	Choi [58]
New Zealand white rabbits	Regen-ACR (Regenlab, Switzerland) PRP preparation kit	PRP was injected into the pockets in which the cartilage grafts were placed	Ear cartilage skin complex transplantation	Although less weight loss rates and higher histopathologic scores were obtained in subcutaneously PRP injected cartilage graft groups, these results were not statistically significant	Bulam [59]
New Zealand white rabbits	The solution of 3.8% sodium citrate was used to prevent coagulation. The entire serum component and the upper 6–8 mm of blood cell component is pipetted into a sterile vacurette without citrate. This material is again centrifuged at 2000 rpm for 5 minutes	Diced cartilage blended with PRP and wrapped with PLGA membrane	Ear cartilage skin complex transplantation	PRP can reduce the absorption of PLGA membrane encapsulated cut cartilage grafts. PRP can reduce the foreign body inflammatory reaction in PLGA membrane-encapsulated cartilage, increase the production of type II collagen, and increase the compression modulus	Liao [60]
New Zealand white rabbits	1800 rpm/10 min and 3600 rpm/10 min	Polyurethane/ platelet-rich plasma/ autologous chondrocyte composites	Polyurethane/ platelet-rich plasma/ autologous chondrocyte composites was transplanted subcutaneously	This cartilage tissue engineering method may be a promising method for external ear reconstruction	Wang [61]
New Zealand white rabbits	215 g/10 min and 863 g/10 min	Rabbit auricle cartilage/ PRP/vascularized tissue engineering complex	Rabbit auricle cartilage/PRP/ vascularized tissue engineering complex was transplanted subcutaneously	A large number of engineered cartilage can be obtained by adding autologous ear cartilage fragments mixed with PRP in tissue engineering	Wang [62]
New Zealand white rabbits	The solution of 3.8% sodium citrate was used to prevent coagulation. The entire serum component and the upper 6–8 mm of blood cell component is pipetted into a sterile vacurette without citrate. This material is again centrifuged at 1228 g for 5 min	Diced cartilages were mixed with PRP and placed into the mold, completely filling the mold	The graft was inserted inside the subcutaneous skin pocket	Three-dimensional printed grafts have appropriate biomechanical properties and shape retention characteristics. Chondrocytes have good vitality and produce chondrocyte extracellular matrix	Liao [63]

at three points, 1 cm apart) for nine days. PDRN (PLACENTEX Intergro, mastelli SRL, Sanremo, Italy) was injected at six points of replanted ears in an even double dose (3 mL, 5.625 mg) every two days for ten days. The symptoms improved significantly on the ninth day after operation. On the 14th day after operation, the transplanted ears almost completely survived (except for 2 small eschar). The eschar was smeared with antibacterial ointment, and the eschar completely fell off and the wound healed 18 days after operation. The patient was discharged 19 days after operation.

After discharge, continue to apply antibiotic ointment to the wound. The replanted ears almost completely healed 53 days after operation. Local continuous HBOT combined with local injection of PRP and PDRN may improve the survival rate of severed ear replantation. However, further studies are needed to confirm the effectiveness of PRP plus hyperbaric oxygen therapy.

11.3.2.2 Clinical Application of EPT in the Treatment of Ear Keloid

Keloid is a benign fibroproliferative disease, which can occur spontaneously or is caused by minor trauma or skin injury. Keloid is a hard, uplifted, often shiny mass. Some keloid skin has pigmentation, which usually invades adjacent normal tissues. Keloids can grow in any part of the body, but they are best found in the chest, upper arms, shoulders, and face. Itching, folliculitis, infection, and unsightly appearance seriously affect the life and work of patients. The pathogenesis of keloid is not clear, and its treatment is difficult and the effect is poor. In the past, surgical resection of keloid has always been the basis of treatment. However, the recurrence rate of simple surgical resection is very high. Therefore, surgeons often choose to explore multimodal comprehensive treatment, such as compression, freezing, corticosteroid injection, radiotherapy, laser, silica gel tablets, verapamil, 5-fluorouracil, bleomycin, interferon, botulinum toxin A, and colchicine. It is now confirmed that PRP has the ability to promote wound healing, angiogenesis, tissue regeneration, and recovery. However, there is still not enough literature to report its role in the treatment of keloid.

In 2017, Jones et al. [65] reported that a comprehensive therapy of local scar resection, autologous PRP at the wound site, and indoor superficial radiotherapy after operation has a good effect on ear scar. Forty-nine patients with ear keloid underwent local scar resection, and then autologous PRP was applied at the wound site, and indoor superficial radiotherapy (SRT) was performed after operation. Patients were instructed to apply cream (specially designed for the treatment of keloid) for nursing after operation. The cream contains silica gel, vitamin E, antioxidants, and 0.5% hydrocortisone. The usage is twice a day for three months. The patients were followed up 10 days, 1 month, 3 months, 6 months, 9 months, and 12 months after operation. The results showed that the success rate of a two-year follow-up was 94%. The results showed that the combined therapy was an effective alternative therapy for the treatment of ear keloid. The trial also has the disadvantages of small cost and short average follow-up time (two years). In the future, two groups of randomized control group should be designed to further compare the efficacy.

In 2018, Azzam et al. [66] reported a comprehensive treatment of ear scars with local scar resection, intraoperative cryotherapy, and autologous PRP at the wound site. Fifty patients with ear keloid underwent local scar resection, and then 2–3 mL PRP was injected into the wound bed, under the skin flap, skin, and incision. Finally, a handheld liquid nitrogen device (elbocreo leather company in Lyon, France) was used to treat the wound. Different probes were used for different sizes of scars. According to the size of the wound and the specification of the cryoprobe, perform 1–8 times of freezing to completely freeze the wound. The surface area of the frozen area is calculated from the surface area of the frozen probe used. The freezing treatment is always controlled by an impedance meter (cryomoneur Erbe, Lyon, France), and the freezing strength can be known. The freezing time is the time required to make the impedance value reach 1000 K Ω, and it takes about 30 seconds to form a 3–5 mm freezing halo. Only one freeze-thaw cycle is performed for each treatment. Follow up once a month after treatment, measure scars, and take photos. All keloids were assessed by Vancouver Scar Scale (VSS) score before treatment and 12 months after treatment by 2 researchers. The treatment effect was evaluated by an independent observer using four scales according to the reduction of scar: (1) "main flattening" (including complete flattening) which corresponds to the reduction of scar surface by 80–100%, (2) "significant" reduction of 50–80%, (3) "medium" between 30% and 50%, (4) "treatment failure" which reduced the scar surface by <30%. Recurrence was defined as the recurrence of scars or beyond the scope of the original operation. The results showed that 37 (74%) of the 50 keloids achieved the treatment effect, 30 completely flattened, and 7 significantly flattened 1 year after the follow-up. Thirty-four cases (68%) of fifty cases of keloid were treated with resection, cryotherapy, and PRP. The average follow-up was one year without recurrence. Three patients with keloid (15%) needed triamcinolone acetonide injection. After a one-year follow-up, the keloid was basically or completely flattened without recurrence. Treatment failed in 13 cases (26%) (keloid area decreased by <30%). Temporary pain and local hypoesthesia were the main postoperative complications. The results showed that the combined therapy had low recurrence rate, good cosmetic effect, good tolerance, and no obvious complications.

The clinical study of EPT in ear plastic surgery is shown in Table 11.6.

Table 11.6 Clinical study of EPT in ear plastic surgery

Types of diseases	PRP production method	PRP usage	The role of PRP	Experimental defect	Author [Ref.]
Replantation of severed ears without blood vessels	150 g/15 min;400 g/10 min	PRP was injected on the second day after operation. 3 mL of PRP was injected into the complete ear near the injury site every three days (at three points, 1 mL at each point, with an interval of 1 cm) for nine days	PRP can improve the viability of composite grafts	Case report	Lee [64]
Ear keloids	The harvest SmartPrep system platelet concentrate (PC) procedure packs	PRP was placed directly on the wound bed and under the flap and then closed using a standardized subcutaneous suture method to promote aesthetics. The additional PRP was then applied directly to the closed incision and allowed to dry	PRP can promote wound healing, regulate inflammation, and regulate collagen production	No control group, small sample size, and short follow-up time	Jones [65]
Ear keloids	None	2–3 cubic centimeters of PRP were injected into the wound bed and under the flap, and then PRP was injected into the skin and incision site	PRP can promote wound healing, regulate inflammation, and regulate collagen production	No control group, small sample size, and short follow-up time	Azzam [66]

11.4 Application of EPT in Orbital Lightening

The skin of eyelid is the thinnest skin of the human body. The dermis is thin and the eyelids are almost transparent, so it is easy to produce wrinkles. The eyebrows, upper and lower eyelids, inter eyebrow area, and inner canthus area form the orbital subunit structure. Periorbital region is one of the earliest aging regions. The aging process is influenced by genetic and environmental factors. Rough, wrinkled, uneven texture, dryness, and pigmentation are the characteristics of aging skin around the eyes.

Infraorbital dark circles refer to the dark skin in the infraorbital area below the lower eyelid. The dark circles under the orbit seriously affect the aesthetics. People try to find a variety of good treatments. The incidence of suborbital dark circles is regardless of gender, age, and race. Moreover, with the increase of age, skin relaxation, and the change of subcutaneous fat distribution, the dark circles under the orbit will continue to deteriorate. Hyperpigmentation, translucent orbicularis oculi muscle of the lower eyelid, loose skin, and shadow of lacrimal groove are all the causes of treatment. Because infraorbital dark circles are caused by many factors, the treatment must vary according to the etiology. For hyperpigmentation dark circles, local bleach, chemical peeling, and laser are effective.

PRP contains a variety of growth factors that promote wound healing. More than 95% of pre-synthetic growth factors will be endocrine within 1 hour and attached to the receptors of grafts, flaps, or wound cells. PRP has been widely used in plastic surgery, such as facial beauty, neck lifting, various breast operations, autologous fat transplantation, and lip augmentation. The combined application of PRP and CO_2 laser can promote wound healing, promote the formation of collagen fiber bundles, and reduce complications.

In 2014, Mehryan et al. [67] evaluated the therapeutic effect of PRP injection therapy on infraorbital dark circles and crow's feet. The subjects were ten Fitzpatrick III and IV patients with dark circles. Each patient had a history of at least one year of infraorbital dark circles and/or mild periocular skin wrinkles. The treatment method was subcutaneous injection of 1 mL PRP at both sides of the suborbital dark circles and 0.5 mL PRP at the crow's feet. No ice was applied to the injection site after operation. The patients were followed up and evaluated at one week, one month, and three months after treatment. The effects of melanin content, color uniformity, hydration of cuticle, wrinkle volume, and visibility index were evaluated at the three-month follow-up. The overall evaluation of doctors, the satisfaction survey of participants, and the evaluation of side effects were also carried out. The results showed that the improvement of color uniformity of infraorbital skin was statistically significant ($p = 0.010$), but the results of other indicators showed no significant difference. The satisfaction score of participants and the overall evaluation score of doctors were 2.2 and 1.7, respectively, using a 0–3 score system. The results showed that subcutaneous injection of PRP could improve the dark circles under the orbit but had no obvious effect on crow's feet. Large sample size-controlled clinical trials and longer follow-up are also needed.

In 2014, Al Shami [68] reported that PRP was used to treat periorbital hyperpigmentation (POH). Fifty patients with POH received PRP injection. Treatment frequency is once a month, three times in total. The evaluation time points were before injection, one month after each injection, and three months after the last injection. The efficacy was evaluated by standardized digital photography. The results showed that at 3 months after the last treatment, 2 patients (4%) had excellent improvement, 6 patients (12%) had significant improvement, 23 patients (46%) had moderate improvement, and 19 patients (38%) had slight improvement. The results showed that PRP is an effective method for the treatment of periorbital pigmentation, but it still needs to be compared with other methods.

In the improvement of infraorbital circles and lacrimal groove deformities, Neinaa [69] reported in 2020 that the effects of platelet-depleted plasma (PPP) gel and PRP on orbital subjuvenation were reported. Sixty-eight female patients with dark circles or lacrimal groove deformities were injected with 1.0 mL PRP in the left suborbital area and 1.0 mL PPP gel in the periosteal area of the right suborbital area. Then the message was gently conveyed to fit the outline of the surrounding tissue. It was done once every two weeks, a total of three times. After treatment, the patients were followed up three times a month. Clinical symptom evaluation and dermatoscopy were performed before treatment and at the end of follow-up. The results showed that the clinical symptoms, pigmentation, and tear mark scale of the two groups were significantly improved. Compared with group B, the improvement of clinical and dermoscopy in group A was more significant. The results confirm that PPP gel and PRP are effective methods to improve the aesthetic appearance of the infraorbital area. PRP seems to be less effective than PPP gel. The limitations of this study are small sample size, lack of male control group, and short follow-up time.

In 2021, Diab and others [70] reported the efficacy of PPP gel and PRP in orbital aging. A total of 40 female patients with orbital wrinkles and/or dark circles were injected with PRP in the right periorbital area with 26 g of scalp. Plasma gel was injected into the left orbital region with a 22G needle. Each patient received treatment once every four weeks, a total of two times. Patients were assessed by subjective [followed up by global aesthetic improvement score (GAIS) and patient satisfaction (Likert scale)] and objective [antera three-dimensional camera] manner two weeks after each treatment (weeks 2 and 6) and 12 weeks after the last treatment (week 16). The results showed that after the second treatment, the two methods significantly improved the wrinkles around the orbit, and the effect of plasma gel injection side was better. However, the effect achieved by these two methods cannot last for three months. In addition, objective evaluation could not prove any improvement in periorbital pigmentation. The deficiency of this study is the assessment of the impact of photoaging, and the average age of the assessment object is too young.

In 2018, Nofal et al. [71] reported the comparison of carboxylation therapy and PRP in the treatment of POH. One side of the face of 30 patients with POH was treated with carboxylation and the other side with PRP. Test side: 1 ml PRP was injected into the periorbital space, twice a week, seven times in total. Control side: 5 mL carbon dioxide was injected into the lateral third of each eyelid with No. 30 needle at the rate of 50 mL/min, once a week, seven times in total. Three months after treatment, it was evaluated by the evaluation of investigators, the visual analog scale of patients and doctors, and the satisfaction of patients. The results showed that all patients completed the course of treatment on the carboxyl side. Ten patients on the treatment side of PRP did not complete the whole course of treatment because they could not bear the pain and side effects. POH was significantly improved on both sides ($P \leq 0.0001$). There was no significant difference between the two therapies. The side effects of carboxyl treatment were tolerable and mild, while the side effects of PRP were relatively severe and lasted for several days. The results show that the two methods are effective in the treatment of POH, and the curative effects of the two methods are equivalent. Carboxylation therapy is simpler, more effective, and better tolerated than PRP. However, a large number of trials and comparative studies are still needed. In order to better evaluate the treatment response, objective evaluation methods are also needed.

In 2021, Asilian et al. [72] reported the comparison of carboxylation therapy and PRP in the treatment of POH. One side of the face of 21 patients with POH was treated with carboxylation and the other side with PRP. Test side: 1 mL PRP was injected into the periorbital space, once a week, six times in total. Control side: 5 mL carbon dioxide was injected into the lateral third of each eyelid with No. 30 needle at the rate of 50 mL/min, once every two weeks, three times in total. Patients and dermatologists assessed periorbital darkness using visual analogue scale (VAS) before and eight weeks after operation. Use a digital camera to assess skin vessels and pigmentation. The results showed that there was no significant difference in preoperative and postoperative photo analysis, including vascular and pigmentation scores, between the two facial evaluation sides; therefore, neither carboxylation therapy nor PRP can successfully improve periocular pigmentation. Dermatology department considered that VAS score was not improved after carboxylation therapy and PRP therapy. However, the VAS score after carboxylation therapy and PRP therapy was improved compared with that before operation (P-value of both methods <0.001), but there was no significant difference between the two methods (P-value = 0.85). Surgery-related side effects showed that the incidence of inflammation/edema was significantly higher after carboxyl treatment ($P < 0.05$), while the incidence of ecchymosis and pain was higher after PRP treatment (*P*-value = 0.02). The results showed that the efficacy of the two methods in the treatment of POH was not significant. The authors believe that the insignificant effect is due to the technology, material quality or preparation process, and patient selection. More evaluation, longer follow-up time, and new experimental design are also needed.

The clinical study of EPT in orbital lightening is shown in Table 11.7.

Table 11.7 Clinical study of EPT in orbital lightening

Types of diseases	PRP production method	PRP usage	The role of PRP	Experimental defect	Author [Ref.]
Infraorbital dark circles and crow's feet wrinkles	1600–1800 g/6 min and 2000 g/5 min	1 mL PRP was injected subcutaneously into each side of the infraorbital black eye and 0.5 mL PRP was injected subcutaneously at the crow's feet	Subcutaneous injection of PRP can improve the dark circles under the orbit, but it has no obvious effect on crow's feet	No control group, small sample size, and short follow-up time	Mehryan [67]
POH	1600 rpm/10 min and 4000 rpm/10 min	PRP was injected into the selected area using a 32G needle for superficial microinjections via the mesotherapy technique, and the injections were administered into the papillary dermis (1.5–2.0 mm deep), once a month, three times in total	PRP is a useful treatment for POH	Lack of control group	Al-Shamil [68]
Infraorbital dark circles and tear trough deformity	3000 rpm/105 min and 1500 rpm/5 min	The left side was injected intradermally with 1.0 mL of PRP into the infraorbital area using 1 mL insulin syringe. Right side was injected with a small depot of PPP gel supraperiostealy by push technique in the tear trough deformity of infraorbital area using a 1 mL insulin syringe and then messaged gently to conform to the contour of the surrounding tissues	PPP gel and PRP are both effective methods to improve the aesthetic appearance of the infraorbital area. PPP gel seems to be more effective than PRP	Small sample size, lack of male control, short follow-up (only three months), and lack of statistical data on monthly clinical and dermoscopic results	Neinaa [69]
Periorbital wrinkles and/or dark circles recruited	320 g/5 min and 1000 g/5 min	PRP was injected intradermally using 26G needles in the Rt-sided periorbital area, while plasma gel was injected subdermally in the left (Lt) side using 22G needles. Each patient received two treatment sessions four weeks apart	Both modalities yielded a significant improvement of periorbital wrinkles after the second session, with significantly better results on the plasma gel injected side. Besides, objective assessment could not prove any improvement in POH	The study lacks the evaluation of the impact of photoaging, and the average age of the study population is relatively young	Diab [70]
POH	150–200 g/10 min and1500–2000 g/15 min	Test side: 1 mL of PRP was immediately injected into periorbital areas preferably in loose skin of both lids as superficial microinjections via the mesotherapy technique: 0.2–0.3 mL of PRP was injected into the papillary dermis (1.5–2.0 mm deep); two injections were performed in each eye lids with 1 cm space between injections, once every two weeks, seven times in total. Control side: Carbon dioxide gas was intradermally injected at the lateral one-third of each eye lid (5 cc gas in each puff according to standardized flowmetry) using 30G needle, with infusion velocity 50 mL/min, once every week, seven times in total	Both PRP and carboxytherapy are relatively effective and their efficacy is comparable in treatment of POH. Carboxytherapy is simple and slightly more effective modality and well tolerated than PRP	Few cases and short follow-up time	Nofal [71]

(continued)

Table 11.7 (continued)

Types of diseases	PRP production method	PRP usage	The role of PRP	Experimental defect	Author [Ref.]
POH	150–200 g/10 min and 1500–2000 g/15 min	Test side: 1 mL of PRP injected in periorbital space, once a week, six times in total Control side: The amount of 5 cc of CO_2 was intradermally injected at the one-third lateral part of each eyelid using a 30-gauge needle with a velocity of 50 cc per minute, once every two weeks, three times in total	The insignificant efficacy of the two approaches for the POH treatment	High cost, few cases, and short follow-up time	Asilian [72]

11.5 Application of EPT in Improving Facial Skin Texture

Skin aging is a cellular change caused by internal and external factors and the change of dermal extracellular matrix protein, especially the degeneration of connective tissue. The regeneration of aging skin requires extracellular matrix remodeling. Activated fibroblasts play an important role in the process of extracellular matrix remodeling. Various growth factors and cell adhesion molecules in PRP may play a role in activating the synthesis of fibroblasts, collagen, and cell matrix, so as to make the skin younger. However, the number of PRP-related studies on facial rejuvenation is very small.

Concentrated platelet can promote skin and wound healing and healing. In order to further understand the potential role of PRFM subcutaneous injection in the treatment of cosmetic, facial plastic and reconstructive surgery, attention has been paid to its biological effects on the tissues and cells of the skin. In 2012, Sclafani et al. [10] reported that subcutaneous injection of PRF can induce the formation of skin collagen, blood vessels, and fat in the human skin. Four healthy adult volunteers received PRFM injection into the deep dermis and lower dermis. Full-thickness skin biopsy specimens were collected from the treatment area within ten weeks for histological evaluation. The results of histological examination supported soft tissue enhancement, which was the same as the clinical observation. From seven days after treatment to the end of the experiment, obvious activated fibroblasts and new collagen were observed. Neovascularization was observed within 19 days after treatment, and intradermal aggregation of adipocytes and stimulation of subcutaneous adipocyte formation were also found. During the whole experiment, new blood vessels and adipocytes were found, but fibroblast proliferation was not obvious. Only a very slight chronic inflammatory reaction was observed at the earliest time point of the study, and no abnormal mitosis was observed throughout the study. The results confirmed that PRFM injection into the deep dermis and subcutaneous injection can stimulate the changes of skin cells, which are conducive to the recovery of the skin. Histological and cytological changes confirmed the potential role and use of subcutaneous PRFM therapy in cosmetic, facial plastic, and reconstructive surgery.

In 2014, Yuksel et al. [73] reported the effect of PRP treatment on anti-aging of the human facial skin. Ten healthy patients were treated with PRP. Apply PRP to the patient's forehead, cheekbones, and chin with derma roller, and then inject it into the crow's feet with No. 27 syringe. Before operation and three months after the last PRP treatment, the overall facial appearance, skin laxity, wrinkle condition, and pigmentation disorder were evaluated, and the score range was 0–5. When volunteers evaluated their faces, three different dermatologists evaluated them simultaneously with the same five-point scale. The results showed that there were significant differences in the overall appearance, skin relaxation, sagging, and wrinkles of the patients. Dermatologists evaluated that there was only statistically significant difference in skin relaxation, and no side effects were observed. The results show that PRP can be used as an effective method for facial skin rejuvenation.

In 2020, Hassan et al. [74] evaluated the effect of injectable platelet-rich fibrin (i-PRFM) for injection on facial skin regeneration. Eleven patients received subcutaneous injection of i-PRFM on the face. The specific parts were bilateral zygomatic area intradermal injection (1 mL each), nasolabial groove injection (0.5 mL each), and upper lip skin injection above the red lip margin (1 mL). 0.1 mL injection with an interval of 5 mm was injected, once a month, three times in total. Efficacy was assessed by objective skin analysis (via) and subjective patient-reported outcome (face-q) at baseline and three months after the last treatment. The results showed that after three months of treatment, the skin surface spots ($P = 0.01$) and pores ($P = 0.03$) were significantly improved.

Skin texture, wrinkles, UV spots, and porphyrins show quantitative improvement. The appearance satisfaction measured by face-q scale was significantly improved compared with the baseline, including skin satisfaction ($p = 0.002$), facial appearance satisfaction ($p = 0.025$), cheek satisfaction ($p = 0.001$), lower part and mandibular line satisfaction ($p = 0.002$), and mouth and lip satisfaction ($p = 0.04$). No major adverse reactions occurred. Improvements in skin analysis parameters and patient self-assessment scores demonstrate that i-prfm injection can restore facial skin rejuvenation.

In 2019, Maisel Campbell et al. [75] evaluated the safety and efficacy of PRP in the treatment of skin aging symptoms based on existing literature evidence. Search the literature before March 2019 in the Cochrane Library, MEDLINE (PubMed), EMBASE, and Scopus. The prospective trial of PRP treatment for skin aging evaluation involves at least ten patients. Finally, 24 studies were included in the experimental study, including 8 randomized controlled trials (RCTs). The total number of patients receiving PRP was 480. The overall assessment of doctors showed that PRP injection alone could temporarily improve the appearance, texture, and wrinkles of the facial skin, as well as the fine lines and pigmentation around the orbit. PRP adjuvant therapy can accelerate skin healing after laser surgery. Although the improvement is less than 50%, the patient satisfaction is high. Due to the lack of standardization in the preparation, administration route, and evaluation index of PRP, the treatment results have certain limitations. PRP injection is beneficial and safe in the treatment of skin aging. Studies have confirmed that PRP is the most effective in improving facial skin wrinkles. However, it is not clear how long the treatment effect can last. More high-quality trials and adequate follow-up are needed to optimize the treatment plan.

The research of EPT in improving facial skin texture is shown in Table 11.8.

Table 11.8 Clinical research of EPT in improving facial skin texture

Types of diseases	PRP production method	PRP usage	The role of PRP	Experimental defect	Author [Ref.]
Normal skin	1100 rpm/6 min. The platelets were then resuspended in the supernatant plasma by gently inverting the tube ten times, and the resulting mixture was transferred sterilely to a second tube containing a regulated amount of calcium chloride	At specified time points after treatment between 30 minutes and 10 weeks, 5 mm full-thickness skin biopsy specimens were taken from each injection site and the wounds closed with 3–0 chromic sutures	PRFM can stimulate the formation of blood vessels, fat, and collagen	Lack of control group and the number of cases is small	Mehryan [10]
Facial skin	PRP preparation kit, details unknown	PRP was applied thrice at two-week intervals on the face of ten healthy volunteers. It was applied to individual's forehead, malar area, and jaw by a dermaroller and injected using a 27-gauge injector into the wrinkles of crow's feet	PRP can improve the general appearance, sagging, and wrinkle of the facial skin	Lack of control group, the number of cases is small, and short follow-up time	Yuksel [73]
Facial skin	PRF® PROCESS system technology (700 rpm for 3 min, 60 g RCF)	i-PRFM was injected subcutaneously at bilateral zygomatic areas (1 mL each), nasolabial sulcus (0.5 mL each), and upper lip skin above the red lip margin (1 mL). 0.1 mL injection was injected at an interval of 5 mm	Subcutaneous injection of i-PRFM can improve facial spots and large pores, with high patient satisfaction and no complications	Lack of control group, the number of cases is small, and short follow-up time	Hassan [74]

References

1. Du J, Ruan X, Gu M, et al. Prevalence of and risk factors for sexual dysfunction in young Chinese women according to the female sexual function index: an internet-based survey. Eur J Contracept Reprod Health Care. 2016;21(3):259–63.
2. Zhang C, Tong J, Zhu L, et al. A population-based epidemiologic study of female sexual dysfunction risk in mainland China: prevalence and predictors. J Sex Med. 2017;14(11):1348–56.
3. Buster J, Kingsberg S, Kilpatrick C. Practice bulletin no.119: female sexual dysfunction. The American College of Obstetricians and Gynecologists. Pract Bull. 2011;117(4):996–1007.
4. Hersant B, SidAhmed-Mezi M, Belkacemi Y, et al. Efficacy of injecting platelet concentrate combined with hyaluronic acid for the treatment of vulvovaginal atrophy in postmenopausal women with history of breast cancer: a phase 2 pilot study. Menopause. 2018;25(10):1124–30.
5. Benshushan A, Brzezinski A, Shoshani O, et al. Periurethral injection for the treatment of urinary incontinence. Obstet Gynecol Surv. 1998;53(6):383–8.
6. Alijotas-Reig J. Foreign-body granuloma after injection of calcium hydroxylapatite for treating urinary incontinence. Obstet Gynecol. 2011;118(5):1181–2.
7. Runels C, Melnick H, Debourbon E, et al. A pilot study of the effect of localized injections of autologous platelet rich plasma (PRP) for the treatment of female sexual dysfunction. J Women's Health Care. 2014;3(4):1000169.
8. Sukgen G, Ellibeş Kaya A, Karagün E, et al. Platelet-rich plasma administration to the lower anterior vaginal wall to improve female sexuality satisfaction. Menopause. Turk J Obstet Gynecol. 2019;16(4):228–34.
9. Neto JB. O-shot: PRP female privacy treatment. J Women's Health Care. 2017;6(5):1000395.
10. Sclafani AP, McCormick SA. Induction of dermal collagenesis, angiogenesis, and adipogenesis in human skin by injection of platelet-rich fibrin matrix. Arch Facial Plast Surg. 2012;14(2):132–6.
11. Shaeer O, Shaeer K, Fode M, et al. The global online sexuality survey (GOSS) 2015: erectile dysfunction among english-speaking internet users in the United States. Hum Androl. 2017;7:111–9.
12. Moreland RB. Is there a role of hypoxemia in penile brosis: a viewpoint presented to the Society for the study of impotence. Int J Impot Res. 1998;10(2):113–20.
13. El-Sakka AI. Reversion of penile fibrosis: current information and a new horizon. Arab J Urol. 2011;9:49–55.
14. Castela Â, Soares R, Rocha F, et al. Erectile tissue molecular alterations with aging—differential activation of the p42/44 MAP kinase pathway. Age. 2011;33(2):119–30.
15. Guo W, Liao C, Zou Y, et al. Erectile dysfunction and risk of clinical cardiovascular events: a meta-analysis of seven cohort studies. J Sex Med. 2010;7(8):2805–16.
16. Loprinzi PD, Nooe A. Erectile dysfunction and mortality in a national prospective cohort study. J Sex Med. 2015;12(11):2130–3.
17. Colson MH, Cuzin B, Faix A, et al. La dysfonction érectile, une présence active. Theol Sex. 2018;27(1):9–17.
18. Nehra A, Alterowitz R, Culkin DJ, et al. Peyronie's disease: AUA guideline. J Urol. 2015;194(3):745–53.
19. Campbell J, Alzubaidi R. Understanding the cellular basis and pathophysiology of Peyronie's disease to optimize treatment for erectile dysfunction. Transl Androl Urol. 2017;6(1):46–59.
20. Bivalacqua TJ, Purhoit SK, Hellstro WJG. Peyronie's disease: advances in basic science and pathophysiology. Curr Urol Rep. 2000;1(4):297–301.
21. Bilgutay AN, Pastuszak AW. Peyronie's disease: a review of etiology, diagnosis, and management. Curr Sex Health Rep. 2015;7(2):117–31.
22. Culha MG, Erkan E, Cay T, et al. The effect of platelet-rich plasma on Peyronie's disease in rat model. Urol Int. 2019;102(2):218–23.
23. Abdel Raheem A, Johnson M, Ralph D, et al. Collagenase clostridium histolyticum: a novel medical treatment for peyronie's disease. Minerva Urol Nefrol. 2018;70(4):380–5.
24. Virag R, Sussman H, Lambion S, et al. Evaluation of the benefit of using a combination of autologous platelet rich-plasma and hyaluronic acid for the treatment of peyronie's disease. Sex Health. 2017;1:1–8.
25. Sclafani AP. Applications of platelet-rich fibrin matrix in facial plastic surgery. Facial Plast Surg. 2009;25(4):270–6.
26. Middleton KK, Barro V, Muller B, et al. Evaluation of the effects of platelet-rich plasma (PRP) therapy involved in the healing of sports-related soft tissue injuries. Iowa Orthop J. 2012;32:150–63.
27. Scarcia M, Maselli FP, Cardo G, et al. The use of autologous platelet rich plasma gel in bulbar and penile buccal mucosa urethroplasty: preliminary report of our first series. Arch Ital Urol Androl. 2016;88(4):274–8.
28. Epifanova MV, Chalyy ME, Krasnov A. Investigation of mechanisms of action of growth factors of autologous platelet-rich plasma used to treat erectile dysfunction. Urologiia. 2017;15(4):46–8.
29. Chalyj ME, Grigorjan VA, Epifanova MV, et al. The effectiveness of intracavernous autologous platelet-rich plasma in the treatment of erectile dysfunction. Urologiia. 2015;4:76–9.
30. Matz EL, Pearlman AM, Terlecki RP. Safety and feasibility of platelet rich fibrin matrix injections for treatment of common urologic conditions. Investig Clin Urol. 2018;59(1):61–5.
31. Ruffo A, Stanojevic N, Iacono F, et al. Treating erectile dysfunction with a combination of low-intensity shock waves (LISW) and platelet-rich plasma (PRP) injections. J Sex Med. 2018;15(7):S318–9.
32. Taş T, Çakıroğlu B, Arda E, et al. Early clinical results of the tolerability, safety, and efficacy of autologous platelet-rich plasma administration in erectile dysfunction. Sex Med. 2021;9(2):100313.
33. Ma Z, Li M, Wang XS, et al. Application of micronised acellular dermal matrix for primary premature ejaculation: a preliminary study. Andrologia. 2021;53(4):e13994.
34. Virag R, Sussman H, Lobel B. A new treatment of LaPeyronie's disease by local injections of plasma rich platelets (PRP) and hyaluronic acid. Preliminary results. E-Mém Acad Natl Chir. 2014;13:96–100.
35. Marcovici I. PRP and correction of penile curvature (Peyronie's disease). Am J Cosmetic Surg. 2019;36(3):117–20. https://doi.org/10.1177/0748806818798280.
36. Bleeker MC, Visser PJ, Overbeek LI, et al. Lichen sclerosus: incidence and risk of vulvar squamous cell carcinoma. Cancer Epidemiol Biomarkers Prev. 2016;25:1224–30.
37. Sherman V, McPherson T, Baldo M, et al. The high rate of familial lichen sclerosus suggests a genetic contribution: an observational cohort study. Eur Acad Dermatol Venereol. 2010;24(9):1031–4.
38. Krapf JM, Mitchell L, Holton MA, et al. Vulvar lichen Sclerosus: current perspectives. Int J Women's Health. 2020;12:11–20.
39. Kirtschig G, Cooper S, Aberer W, et al. Evidence-based (S3) Guideline on (anogenital) Lichen scle-rosus. Eur Acad Dermatol Venereol. 2017;31:e81–3.
40. Tedesco M, Pranteda G, Chichierchia G, et al. The use of PRP (platelet-rich plasma) in patients affected by genital lichen sclerosus: clinical analysis and resultsEur Acad Dermatol Venereol. 2019;33(2):e58–9.
41. Navarrete J, Echarte L, Sujanov A, et al. Platelet-rich plasma for male genital lichen sclerosus resistant to conventional therapy: first prospective study. Dermatol Ther. 2020;33(6):e14032.
42. Tedesco M, Garelli V, Elia FU, et al. Usefulness of video thermography in the evaluation of platelet-rich plasma effectiveness in vulvar lichen sclerosus: preliminary study. Dermatolog Treat. 2021;32(5):568–71.

43. Tedesco M, Bellei B, Garelli V, et al. Adipose tissue stromal vascular fraction and adipose tissue stromal vascular fraction plus platelet-rich plasma grafting: new regenerative perspectives in genital lichen sclerosus. Dermatol Ther. 2020;3(6):e14277.
44. Tedesco M, Garelli V, Bellei B, et al. Platelet-rich plasma for genital lichen sclerosus: analysis and results of 94 patients Are there gender-related differences in symptoms and therapeutic response to PRP? Dermatolog Treat. 2020;06:1–5.
45. Goldstein AT, Mitchell L, Govind V, et al. A randomized double-blind placebo-controlled trial of autologous platelet-rich plasma intradermal injections for the treatment of vulvar lichen sclerosus. Am Acad Dermatol. 2019;80(6):1788–9.
46. Burnett AL, Nehra A, Breau RH, et al. Erectile dysfunction: AUA guidline. J Urol. 2018;200(3):633–41.
47. EAU. European Association of Urology Guidelines. 2018th ed. Copenhagen: EAU; 2018.
48. Chen N-F, Sung C-S, Wen Z-H, et al. Therapeutic effect of platelet-rich plasma in rat spinal cord injuries. Front Neurosci. 2018;12:252.
49. Zhang J, Middleton KK, Fu FH, et al. HGF mediates the anti-inflammatory effects of PRP on injured tendons. PLoS One. 2013;8(6):e67303.
50. Wu CC, Wu YN, Ho HO, et al. The neuroprotective effect of platelet-rich plasma on erectile function in bilateral cavernous nerve injury rat model. J Sex Med. 2012;9(2):2838–48.
51. Epifanova MV, Gvasalia BR, Durashov MA, et al. Platelet-rich plasma therapy for male sexual dysfunction: myth or reality? Sex Med Rev. 2020;8(1):106–13.
52. Sclafani AP. Platelet-rich fibrin matrix for improvement of deep nasolabial folds. J Cosmet Dermatol. 2010;9(1):66–71.
53. Lemperle G, Holmes RE, Cohen SR, et al. A classification of facial wrinkles. Plast Reconstr Surg. 2001;108:1735–50.
54. Xiang X, Haibin W, Zhongsheng S, et al. Clinical study on improving nasolabial groove by fat derived SVF combined with PRP injection. Chin J Cosmet Plast Surg. 2015;26(2):72–5.
55. Refahee SM, Aboulhassan MA, Abdel Aziz O, et al. Is PRP effective in reducing the scar width of primary cleft lip repair? A randomized controlled clinical study. Cleft Palate Craniofac J. 2020;57(5):581–8.
56. Xin W, Xiaoping C, Jinde L, et al. Clinical observation of autologous platelet rich plasma fat particles filling in the correction of lip soft tissue defects. Chin J Cosmet Plast Surg. 2012;23(9):544–7.
57. Jeon YR, Kang EH, Yang CE, et al. The effect of platelet-rich plasma on composite graft survival. Plast Reconstr Surg. 2014;134(2):239–46.
58. Choi HN, Han YS, Kim SR, et al. The effect of platelet-rich plasma on survival of the composite graft and the proper time of injection in a rabbit ear composite graft model. Arch Plast Surg. 2014;41(6):647–53.
59. Bulam H, Ayhan S, Yilmaz G, et al. The effect of subcutaneous platelet-rich plasma injection on viability of auricular cartilage grafts. J Craniofac Surg. 2015;26(5):1495–9.
60. Liao JL, Chen J, He B, et al. Viability and biomechanics of diced cartilage blended with platelet-rich plasma and wrapped with poly (lactic-co-glycolic) acid membrane. J Craniofac Surg. 2017;28(6):1418–24.
61. Wang Z, Qin H, Feng Z, et al. Platelet-rich plasma gel composited with nondegradable porous polyurethane scaffolds as a potential auricular cartilage alternative. J Biomater Appl. 2016;30(7):889–99.
62. Wang M, Chen G, Li G, et al. Creating cartilage in tissue-engineered chamber using platelet-rich plasma without cell culture. Tissue Eng Part C Methods. 2020;26(7):375–83.
63. Liao J, Chen Y, Chen J, et al. Auricle shaping using 3D printing and autologous diced cartilage. Laryngoscope. 2019;129(11):2467–74.
64. Lee SK, Lim YM, Lew DH, et al. Salvage of unilateral complete ear amputation with continuous local hyperbaric oxygen, platelet-rich plasma and polydeoxyribonucleotide without microrevascularization. Arch Plast Surg. 2017;44(6):554–8.
65. Jones ME, McLane J, Adenegan R, et al. Advancing keloid treatment: a novel multimodal approach to ear keloids. Dermatol Surg. 2017;43(9):1164–9.
66. Azzam EZ, Omar SS. Treatment of auricular keloids by triple combination therapy: surgical excision, platelet-rich plasma, and cryosurgery. J Cosmet Dermatol. 2018;17(3):502–10.
67. Mehryan P, Zartab H, Rajabi A, et al. Assessment of efficacy of platelet-rich plasma (PRP) on infraorbital dark circles and crow's feet wrinkles. J Cosmet Dermatol. 2014;13(1):72–8.
68. Al-Shami SH. Treatment of periorbital hyperpigmentation using platelet-rich plasma injections. Am J Dermatol Venereol. 2014;3(5):87–94.
69. Neinaa YME, Hodeib AAE, Morquos MM, et al. Platelet-poor plasma gel vs platelet-rich plasma for infraorbital rejuvenation: a clinical and dermoscopic comparative study. Dermatol Ther. 2020;33(6):e14255.
70. Diab HM, Elhosseiny R, Bedair NI, et al. Efficacy and safety of plasma gel versus platelet-rich plasma in periorbital rejuvenation: a comparative split-face clinical and antera 3D camera study. Arch Dermatol Res. 2021;1:1.
71. Nofal E, Elkot R, Nofal A, et al. Evaluation of carboxytherapy and platelet-rich plasma in treatment of periorbital hyperpigmentation: a comparative clinical trial. J Cosmet Dermatol. 2018;17(6):1000–7.
72. Asilian A, Amiri A, Mokhtari F, et al. Platelet-rich plasma versus carboxytherapy for the treatment of periocular hyperpigmentation; which approach is superior? Dermatol Ther. 2021;34(4):e14980.
73. Yuksel EP, Sahin G, Aydin F, et al. Evaluation of effects of platelet-rich plasma on human facial skin. J Cosmet Laser Ther. 2014;16(5):206–8.
74. Hassan H, Quinlan DJ, Ghanem A, et al. Injectable platelet-rich fibrin for facial rejuvenation: a prospective, single-center study. J Cosmet Dermatol. 2020;19(12):3213–21.
75. Maisel-Campbell AL, Ismail A, Reynolds KA, et al. A systematic review of the safety and effectiveness of platelet-rich plasma (PRP) for skin aging. Arch Dermatol Res. 2020;312(5):301–15.

12 The Application of PRP in Fat Transplantation

Biao Cheng, Yuan Gao, Yunmin Zhu, Panshi Jin, and Qiao Pan

12.1 Introduction

The technology of autologous fat transplantation was developed in the early twentieth century. Fat transplantation, as soft tissue filler, has been widely applied in plastic surgery such as breast augmentation surgery, scar depression, and facial remodeling. However, fat transplantation can only be used to fill deep tissue as fat particles are quite large in diameter. In recent years, the application of nanofat and Svf-gel has been widely applied in treatment of facial aging. During fat transplantation, mechanical injury caused by injection force and ischemic injury reduce the survival rate of grafts, which lead to a series of complications such as fat liquefaction and necrosis, thus leading to the 20–80% absorption of fat graft. Therefore, tremendous efforts should be taken to improve the survival rate of fat transplantation. Platelet-rich plasma (PRP), as platelet concentrates obtained from the whole blood, can release a host of growth factors, cytokines, chemokines, microRNA, and other bioactive substances. PRP is a safe treatment and has been widely used to repair tendon, ligament, and cartilage injury, accelerate wound healing, and improve facial aging. Studies showed that PRP can provide the nutrition for fat tissue and secrete growth factors to facilitate the proliferation and differentiation of adipose-derived stromal cells (ADSCs). Furthermore, PRP can increase the survival rates of autologous fat transplantation or decrease the fibrosis and cyst of fat grafts [1, 2].

B. Cheng (✉)
Department of Burn & Plastic Surgery, General Hospital of Southern Theater Command, Guangzhou, China

Y. Gao · Y. Zhu · P. Jin · Q. Pan
Department of Burn and Plastic Surgery, General Hospital of Southern Theater Command, PLA, Guangzhou, Guangdong, China

12.2 The Basic Research of PRP in Fat Transplantation

12.2.1 The Research of PRP in ADSCs

ADSCs obtained by liposuction have the potential of self-renewal, proliferation, and multidirectional differentiation. ADSCs can secrete a certain amount of cytokines to achieve the effect of anti-inflammatory, anti-oxidation, and resistance to oxygen-free radical damage. The cytokines with high expression levels include hepatocyte growth factor (HGF), transforming growth factor-β (TGF-β), and vascular endothelial growth factor (VEGF). Fibroblast growth factor-2 (FGF-2) and angiopoietin-1 (ANG-L) have a moderate expression and angiopoietin-2 (ANG-2) has a low expression. ADSCs can differentiate into various cell lines, including mesodermal bone cells, adipocytes, chondrocytes, endothelial cells, nerve cells, and pancreatic islet cells, which contributed to repair damaged tissues and organs.

PRP contains a host of angiogenic growth factors such as platelet-derived growth factor (PDGF), TGF-β, epidermal growth factor (EGF), VEGF, and fibroblast growth factor (FGF), which can promote the proliferation of ADSCs and improve the overall survival rate of fat grafts as well. Studies have shown that suppression of VEGF impairs fat graft retention and the differentiation of adipose tissue [3, 4]. FGF-2 obviously promotes the adipogenic differentiation of human ASCs [5]. EGF and PDGF are shown to inhibit the transformation of adipocyte due to reduced *PPAR-γ* transcription. Growth factors in PRP can promote cell proliferation and inhibit ASC differentiation by downregulating the expression of BMPRIA and FGFR1 that are the key receptors to mediate adipogenesis [6, 7].

Fukaya et al. [8] found that PRP could inhibit the fat precursor cell apoptosis, thus promoting fat survival. Cervelli [9] believed that PRP could not promote ADSC adipogenesis alone but combined with insulin could promote ADSC adi-

B. Cheng, X. Fu (eds.), *Platelet-Rich Plasma in Tissue Repair and Regeneration*, https://doi.org/10.1007/978-981-99-3193-4_12

pogenesis. Xu et al. [10] believe that activated platelets can promote the proliferation and osteogenesis of ADSCs. Atashi et al. [11] believed that unactivated platelets could promote ADSC proliferation more than activated platelets. Tobita et al. [12] believed that RPP contained various growth factors and mediated multiple pathways of tissue repair. The experiments showed that PRP showed the efficacy on the ADSC proliferation. At present, the specific mechanism of PRP on the ADSC proliferation remains elusive. The mechanism may be that PRP can regulate the secretion of proteins related to inflammatory response and angiogenesis, inhibit the expression levels of inflammatory factors such as IL-6 and IL-8, and thus promote the proliferation and differentiation of ADSCs [13, 14].

The optimal concentration of PRP to promote the ADSC proliferation seems to be controversial. Kakudo et al. [15] believed that both 1% and 5% were more appropriate, and greater than 5% PRP would inhibit the proliferation of ADSCs. Amable et al. [16] used 1–30% concentration of PRP to culture adipose stem cells and believed that 10% concentration of PRP was the best concentration to promote the adipose stem cell proliferation. Liu [17] studied the culture of ADSCs with 5–15% PRP and found that 12.5% PRP could promote the ADSC proliferation. Willemsen [18] retained the adipogenic characteristics of ADSCs cultured with PRP and lost the characteristics of differentiation into myofibroblasts and proangiogenic factors. Fifteen percent may be an appropriate concentration, as too high has an inhibitory effect on ADSCs. Cervelli et al. [19] believed that 1–50% concentration PRP had an ideal effect. Van et al. [20] believed that 20% PRP had the best effect on promoting ADSC proliferation. Li [21] compared the mixed transplantation effect of 0%, 10%, 20%, and 30% volume fractions of PRP and ADSCs. The results showed that 20% PRP significantly increased the survival rate of fat, while no significant difference was found between 20% and 30% groups. Therefore, it was suggested that 20% had the best effect of promoting the proliferation of ADSCs. Amable [22] evaluated the dose-dependent manner of 1–30% PRP on the ADSC proliferation. The results showed that 1% PRP has a similar effect as 10% FBS and 10% PRP on promoting the ADSC proliferation. Together, aforementioned studies indicate that PRP can obviously increase fat graft retention by ASC proliferation when cells were cultured in an adipogenic environment.

12.2.2 The Animal Research of PRP in Fat Transplantation

In animal experiments, Seyhan et al. [23] randomly divided 344 mice into 4 groups and found that PRP combined with ADSCs had the lowest absorption rate of fat transplantation, and histopathology showed that the number of fat survival, the number of blood vessels, and the level of growth factor were the highest in this group. Rodriguez-Flores [24] mixed rabbit inguinal fat extract and PRP in a 1:1 ratio and injected mixture under the subcutaneous skin. Four months later, adipocytes and angiogenesis were not different between the PRP + ADSC group and the control group, but the inflammatory response and cyst formation in the PRP + ADSC group were lower than that in the control group. Pires Fraga [25] evaluated the effect of PRP on fat graft survival in a rabbit model. Fat grafts were collected from the dorsal scapular area and mixed with the same volume of PRP activated by $CaCl_2$ and thrombin. The mixtures of PRP and fat were transplanted into the subcutaneous of rabbit. The results showed that the mixture significantly increase the number of viable adipocytes and promote angiogenesis in the PRP group; however, the control group showed an obviously increased necrotic area and inflammation area. Oh [26] mixed human fat and PRP activated by thrombin and CaCl2 at a volume ratio of 7:2 and then transplanted the mixture on the scalps of nude mice. The results showed that PRP had a higher volume and weight of fat grafts than that in the control group after treatment for 10 weeks.

In our previous study, we took the waist and abdominal fat of healthy women who had received liposuction surgery (Fig. 12.1), extracted the nanometer fat from the adipose tissue by emulsifying and centrifuging, and then extracted PRP and fully activated PRP by calcium gluconate solution. 0.5 mL mixture of PRP and nanofat, 0.5 mL mixture of PRP and adipose tissue, 0.5 mL mixture of saline and nanofat, and 0.5 mL mixture of saline and adipose tissue were randomly injected into the dorsal of nude mice at an interval of 3 cm and 2 cm, respectively, all injections at a ratio of 1:4 to form a self-control study. Scanning electron microscopy (SEM) showed that the vascular composition and structure of extracellular matrix

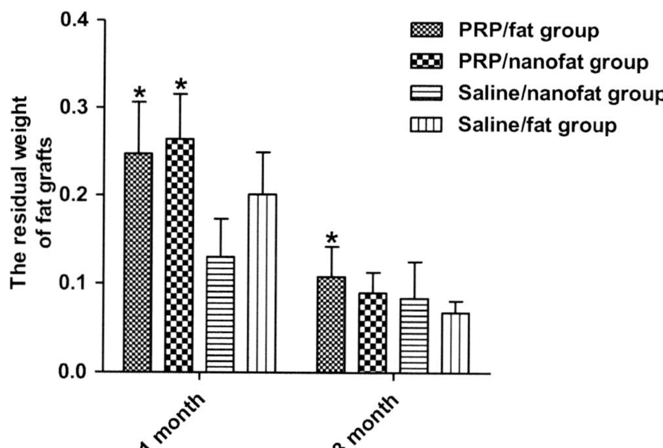

Fig. 12.1 The comparison of residual weight of grafts among the four groups at one and 3 months after grafting. * $p < 0.05$ represent the significant significance between the saline/nanofat group and saline/fat group

(ECM) remained intact in the nanofat. One and 3 months after transplantation, the residual weight of graft in the PRP/nanofat group and the PRP/fat group was significantly higher than that of the groups of saline/fat group and saline/nanofat. The PRP/nanofat group had more neovascularization and less surrounding fibrous tissue encapsulation.

In conclusion, activated PRP can maintain viable adipocytes, promote angiogenesis, and reduce inflammation response and the formation of cyst.

12.3 The Clinical Application of PRP in Fat Transplantation

12.3.1 The Application of PRP and Fat in Breast Implant

Gentile [27] evaluated the effect of PRP on the survival rate of fat grafts in breast reconstruction surgery. One hundred patients were divided into two groups: half was treated with PRP/fat graft and the other half was treated by PRP alone. PRP was activated by calcium. The maintenance rate of contour repair after 1 year was 69% in the PRP + fat group and 39% in the fat only group. We used PRP combined with fat filling breast augmentation (Fig. 12.2). Remove fat from the thighs. Then, PRP was injected into the chest.

12.3.2 The Application of PRP and Fat in Facial Contour

Cervelli [28] showed that the optimal rate of PRP and fat graft is 40%, which maintain fat grafts up to 50 weeks. The local injection of insulin after treated with 40% PRP/fat for 7 and 15 days further increased the restoration of soft tissue after 12 weeks compared to fat alone.

In another study, 14 patients who underwent facial fat transplantation with PRP were included in this study. Outcomes were determined by differences in the preoperative and postoperative FACE-Q modules. This module is designed as a tool for reporting the measurement outcome of patients who undergo facial plastic surgery. The survey contents include facial appearance satisfaction module, cheek satisfaction module, skin satisfaction module, psychological function module, social function module, aging appearance evaluation module, and result satisfaction module. All patients were followed up for at least 9 months. The FACE-Q satisfaction and quality of life in patients showed significant improvement postoperative [29].

Our group observed 58 patients who wanted to undergo autologous fat granule transplantation from May 2017 to July 2018; they were randomly divided into experimental group and control group (Fig. 12.3). The control group was treated with autologous fat transplantation alone, while the experimental group was treated with PRP combined with autologous fat transplantation. Three months after treatment, the facial subcutaneous fat thickness and the improvement of color spots were compared between the two groups, and the therapeutic effect was evaluated by the patients themselves according to the observation indicators. After 3 months of treatment, the thickness and stain of facial depression in the two groups were improved compared with those before treatment. PRP combined with autologous fat transplantation has a good chemotherapy effect, lasting efficacy, and high acceptance and satisfaction of patients and is suitable for clinical promotion (Fig. 12.4).

In conclusion, the combined application of PRP and fat transplantation can improve the survival rate and retention time of fat grafts, increase clinical treatment satisfaction, and maintain a longer therapeutic effect.

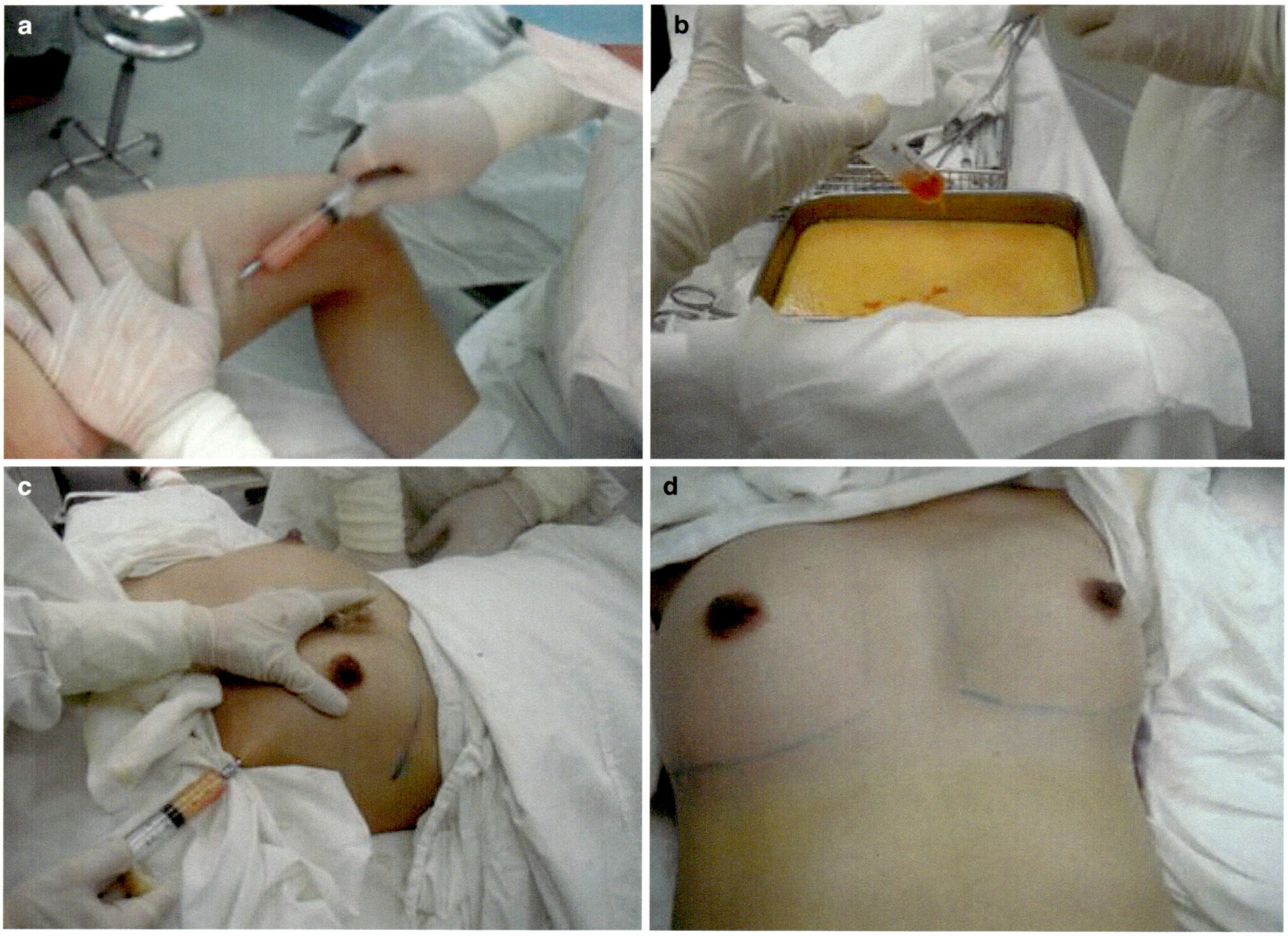

Fig. 12.2 PRP combined with fat filling breast augmentation (**a**) Remove fat from the thighs. (**b**) The prepared PRP is mixed with fat. (**c**) Particulate fat containing PRP is injected into the chest. (**d**) Immediately after fat with PRP is injected into the chest

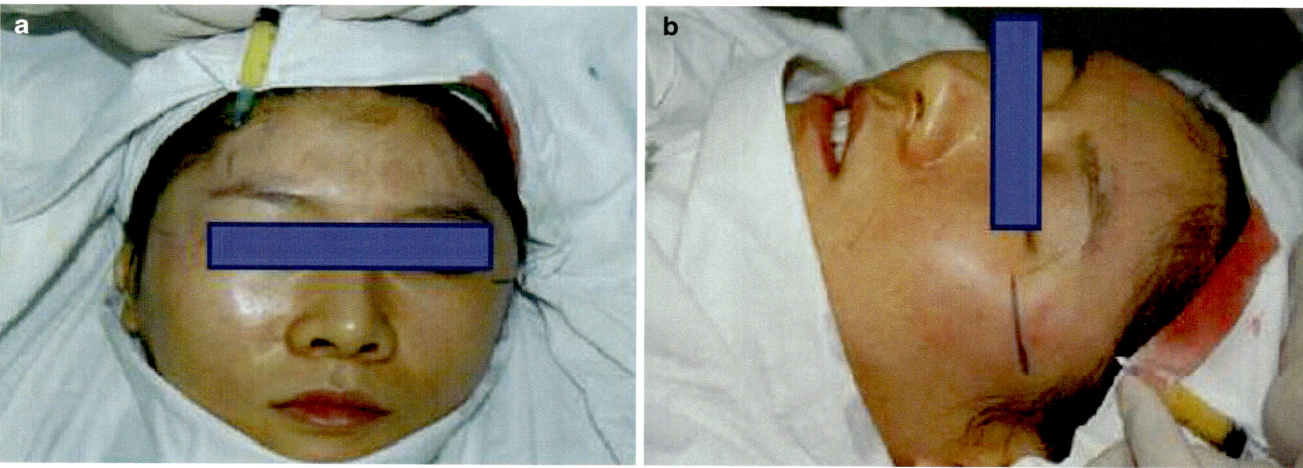

Fig. 12.3 PRP and fat fill the temporal area. (**a**) Fat mixed with PRP was injected into the right temporal region. (**b**) An equal amount of fat mixed with PRP was injected into the left temporal region

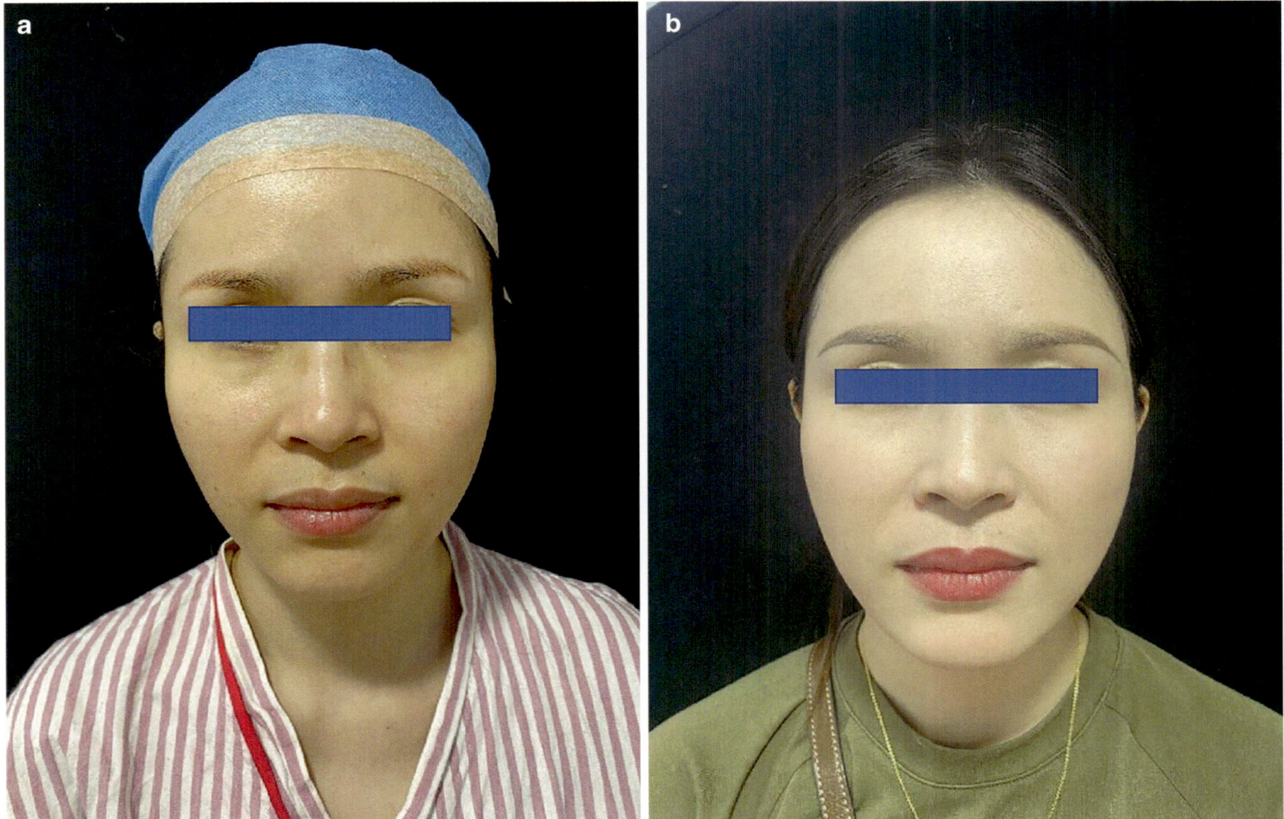

Fig. 12.4 PRP and fat fill face, preoperation and 3 months after fat mixed with PRP. (**a**) pre-operation; (**b**) postoperation

12.4 The Therapeutic Method and Notice of PRP and Fat Transplantation

12.4.1 Therapeutic Method

12.4.1.1 Selection of Supply Areas

Subcutaneous fat in the abdomen, buttocks, thighs, upper arms, back, side breasts, and calves is a good source of living cells. However, some studies suggest that lipoprotein enzyme activity in adipose tissue of different parts of the human body is different, and the survival rate of adipose tissue with high activity is higher after transplantation. The study found that lipoprotein enzyme activity was highest in the thighs and buttocks. The second is the lower abdomen. Therefore, it is better to choose the lower part of the trunk as the donor area for fat transplantation.

12.4.2 Collection Method

Swelling anesthesia is an important part of liposuction, and the main components of local anesthetics are lidocaine and epinephrine. These two drugs inhibit glucose transfer, lipolysis, and proliferation of adipocytes, requiring the fat granules to be rinsed before transplantation. After swelling anesthesia, most doctors collect fat by means of syringe connected with trocar. For large amount of fat collection, special negative pressure liposuction machines can be used to adjust the negative pressure, such as hydrodynamic liposuction machines, which can collect and purify fat while liposuction, greatly improving the efficiency of collection. Liposuction needles for fat collection have also been improved, and gentle manipulation of fat during liposuction minimizes damage to fat cells. There is no significant difference between syringe extraction and liposuction machine extraction. The negative pressure generated by the syringe is about −0.6 ATM, while the negative pressure of liposuction machine is generally about −0.9 ATM. There is no difference of order of magnitude, and there is no obvious difference in the physical damage of fat.

12.4.3 Purification Method

1. **Rinse.** The damaged cells and their released free fatty acids and blood cells are removed by rinsing, which are

inflammatory stimulants that aggravate the inflammatory response after fat transplantation and thus accelerate the degradation of fat cells.
2. **Centrifugal purification.** Centrifugal purification can not only effectively remove impurities and purify fat particles but also greatly increase the fat content in the injection volume of the same volume of graft and indirectly improve the surgical effect and efficiency.
3. **Additional bioactive substances.** PRP is added to the aspirated fat granules; the activated plasma can release a lot of bioactive substances, which can promote cell metastasis, proliferation, growth, and angiogenesis.
4. **Injection method.** The extracted fat particles should be injected as soon as possible after purification. The longer the waiting time is, the greater influence on the activity of adipocytes is. Generally speaking, fresh fat be in isolation for more than 4 h, the fat survival rate will be greatly reduced. A smaller amount of fat can be placed in each tunnel through which the needle passes by using a thinner needle, so that each group of fat particles have more opportunities to contact the vascular bed. When the larger fat particles pass through, they have to bear the greater mechanical extrusion pressure on the needle wall, which will cause destructive damage to the fat particles.

At present, 13–17G needle is in common use, in addition to less damage to fat particles; injection resistance is small, easy to operate, and not easy to penetrate small blood vessels to inject fat into the blood vessels. During the injection, multi-level and multi-tunnel injection was used to evenly disperse the fat particles in the tissue space as far as possible, so that most of the fat cells could obtain nutrition from the recipient area.

12.4.3.1 Risks and Complications

1. **Infection.** Infection usually appears 5–7 days after the operation, with local redness, swelling, heat, and pain. In severe cases, local skin is flushed and blue or the pinhole does not heal and is purulent. The symptoms of infection should be treated in a timely manner to the hospital.
2. **Hematoma.** Hematoma may form during liposuction and injection. In general, severe hematomas do not occur.
3. **Skin ecchymosis.** Skin ecchymosis is caused by blood exudation. Skin ecchymosis usually does not require special treatment and can be resolved in 2–3 weeks.
4. **Skin necrosis.** Most of the skin necrosis occurred in the liposuction area. Once skin necrosis occurs, seek medical advice as soon as possible to reduce the occurrence of obvious scarring.
5. **Local skin uneven.** 3–6 months after surgery, the body itself can adjust; most can be restored to flat; if it is still uneven, there is a need to go to the hospital for correction.
6. **Lipoma formation.** Granular fat injected subcutaneously may aggregate or stimulate host cells to increase lipoma formation. After the formation, only go to the hospital through the way of excision.
7. **Liquefaction of fat.** Excessive injection of adipose tissue or the adipose tissue naturally aggregates after injection, resulting in the failure of the injected fat to survive, resulting in necrosis and liquefaction of fat. When fat liquefaction occurs, need to go to the hospital puncture fluid or negative pressure drainage.

12.4.3.2 Recovery Time

Autologous fat granule injection graft for wrinkle removal generally does not require hospitalization. After 1–2 weeks, the swelling can be reduced and normal work and life can be achieved. If one injection cannot achieve a satisfactory effect due to absorption problems with fat graft, two or three injections may be required.

12.4.3.3 Notices

1. Stop taking aspirin and other nonsteroidal anti-inflammatory drugs for 2 weeks before surgery, no smoking for 2 weeks before surgery. Female patients should avoid menstruation during surgery.
2. Take a bath before surgery and keep clean.
3. Reduce postoperative activities as much as possible to facilitate recovery and detumescence, but do not need to rest in bed.
4. Apply elastic bandages as far as possible to avoid hematoma and help tighten the skin within half a month after surgery.

References

1. Jin R, Zhang L, Zhang YG. Does platelet-rich plasma enhance the survival of grafted fat? An update review. Int J Clin Exp Med 2013;6(4):252–258.
2. Oh DS, Cheon YW, Jeon YR, et al. Activated platelet-rich plasma improves fat graft survival in nude mice: a pilot study. Dermatol Surg. 2011;37(5):619–25.
3. Yamaguchi M, Matsumoto F, Bujo H, Shibasaki M, Takahashi K, Yoshimoto S, et al. Revascularization determines volume retention and gene expression by fat grafts in mice. Exp Biol Med (Maywood). 2005;230:742.
4. Fukumura D, Ushiyama A, Duda DG, Xu L, Tam J, Krishna V, et al. Paracrine regulation of angiogenesis and adipocyte differentiation during *in vivo* adipogenesis. Circ Res. 2003;93:e88.
5. Kakudo N, Shimotsuma A, Kusumoto K. Fibroblast growth factor-2 stimulates adipogenic differentiation of human adipose-derived stem cells. Biochem Biophys Res Commun. 2007;359(2):239–44.
6. Kumar A, Ruan M, Clifton K, Syed F, Khosla S, Oursler MJ. TGF-β mediates suppression of adipogenesis by estradiol through connective tissue growth factor induction. Endocrinology. 2012;153:254.

7. Camp HS, Tafuri SR. Regulation of peroxisome proliferator-activated receptor gamma activity by mitogen-activated protein kinase. J Biol Chem. 1997;272:10811.
8. Fukaya Y, Kuroda M, Aoyagi Y, et al. Platelet-rich plasma inhibits the apoptosis of highly adipogenic homogeneous preadipocytes in an in vitro culture system. Exp Mol Med. 2012;44(5):330–9.
9. Cervelli V, Scioli MG, Gentile P, et al. Platelet-rich plasma greatly potentiates insulin-induced adipogenic differentiation of human adipose-derived stem cells through a serine/threonine kinase Akt-dependent mechanism and promotes clinical fat graft maintenance. Stem Cells Transl Med. 2012;1(3):206–20.
10. Xu FT, Li HM, Yin Q, et al. Effect of activated autologous platelet-rich plasma on proliferation and osteogenic differentiation of human adipose- derived stem cells in vitro. Am J Transl Res. 2015;7(2):257–70.
11. Atashi F, Jaconi ME, Pittet-Cuenod B, et al. Autologous platelet-rich plasma: a biological supplement to enhance adipose- derived mesenchymal stem cell expansion. Tissue Eng Part C Methods. 2015;21(3):253–62.
12. Tobita M, Tajima S, Mizuno H. Adipose tissue- derived mesenchymal stem cells and platelet-rich plasma: stem cell transplantation methods that enhance stemness. Stem Cell Res Ther. 2015;6:215.
13. Andia I, Rubio-Azpeitia E, Maffulli N. Platelet-rich plasma modulates the secretion of inflammatory/angiogenic proteins by inflamed tenocytes. Clin Orthop Relat Res. 2015;473:1624–34.
14. Liao HT, James IB, Marra KG, et al. The effects of platelet-rich plasma on cell proliferation and Adipogenic potential of adipose-derived stem cells. Tissue Eng Part A. 2015;21(21–22):2714–22.
15. Kakudo N, Minakata T, Mitsui T, et al. Proliferation-promoting effect of platelet-rich plasma on human adipose-derived stem cells and human dermal fibroblasts. Plast Reconstr Surg. 2008;122:1352.
16. Amable PR, Teixeira MV, Carias RB, et al. Mesenchymal stromal cell proliferation, gene expression and protein production in human platelet-rich plasma-supplemented media. PLoS One. 2014;9(8):e104662.
17. Liu HY, Wu AT, Tsai CY, et al. The balance between adipogenesis and osteogenesis in bone regeneration by platelet-rich plasma for age-related osteoporosis. Biomaterials. 2011;32:6773.
18. Willemsen JC, Spiekman M, Stevens HP, et al. Platelet-rich plasma influences expansion and paracrine function of adipose- derived stromal cells in a dose-dependent fashion. Plast Reconstr Surg. 2016;137(3):554e–65e.
19. Cervelli V, Scioli MG, Gentile P, et al. Platelet-rich plasma greatly potentiates insulin-induced adipogenic differentiation of human adipose-derived stem cells through a serine/threonine kinase Akt-dependent mechanism and promotes clinical fat graft maintenance. Stem Cells Transl Med. 2012;V1N3:206–20.
20. Van Pham P, Bui KH, Ngo DQ, et al. Activated platelet-rich plasma improves adipose- derived stem cell transplantation efficiency in injured articular cartilage. Stem Cell Res Ther. 2013;4(4):91.
21. Li F, Guo W, Li K, Yu M, et al. Improved fat graft survival by different volume fractions of platelet-rich plasma and adipose- derived stem cells. Aesthet Surg J. 2015;35(3):319–33.
22. Amable PR, Teixeira MVT, Carias RBV, Granjeiro JM, Borojevic R. Mesenchymal stromal cell proliferation, gene expression and protein production in human platelet-rich plasma-supplemented media. PLoS One. 2014;9:e104662.
23. Seyhan N, Alhan D, Ural AU, et al. The effect of combined use of platelet-rich plasma and adipose- derived stem cells on fat graft survival. Ann Plast Surg. 2015;74(5):615–20.
24. Rodriguez-Flores J, Palomar-Gallego MA, Enguita-Valls AB, et al. Influence of platelet-rich plasma on the histologic characteristics of the autologous fat graft to the upper lip of rabbits. Aesthet Plast Surg. 2011;35(4):480–6.
25. Pires Fraga MF, Nishio RT, Ishikawa RS, ,et al. Increased survival of free fat grafts with platelet-rich plasma in rabbits. J Plast Reconstr Aesthet Surg2010,63(12):e818–e822.
26. Oh DS, Cheon YW, Jeon YR, Lew DH. Activated platelet-rich plasma improves fat graft survival in nude mice: a pilot study. Dermatol Surg. 2011;37(619):619.
27. Gentile P, Di Pasquali C, Bocchini I, Floris M, Eleonora T, Fiaschetti V, Floris R, Cervelli V. Breast reconstruction with autologous fat graft mixed with platelet-rich plasma. Surg Innov. 2013;20(370):370.
28. Cervelli V, Scioli MG, Gentile P, Doldo E, Bonanno E, Spagnoli LG, Orlandi A. Platelet-rich plasma greatly potentiates insulin-induced adipogenic differentiation of human adipose-derived stem cells through a serine/threonine kinase Akt-dependent mechanism and promotes clinical fat graft maintenance. Stem Cells Transl Med. 2012;1(206):206.
29. Ozer K, Colak O. Micro-autologous fat transplantation combined with platelet-rich plasma for facial filling and regeneration: a clinical perspective in the shadow of evidence-based medicine. J Craniofac Surg. 2019;30(3):672–7.

Basic Research on the Effect of PRP on Cell Biological Function

13

Xi Yu, Hongchen He, Lei Zhang, and Biao Cheng

The platelet-rich plasma and its related products have been reported to be involved in the repair of skin wounds and the improvement of facial rejuvenation, which must interact with related functional cells. This chapter reviews the effects of platelet-rich plasma on cell biological functions, including cell proliferation, cell migration, autophagy, and apoptosis, so as to reveal the possible reasons for its function at the cellular level.

PRP obtained by centrifuge of whole blood is characterized with the supraphysiological platelet concentrations and the promising experimental and clinical results. It has been confirmed that over hundreds of bioactive molecules secreted from platelet α-granules in platelet contributed to the injured tissue regeneration and repair [1]. PRP can be regarded as a bioactive niche of multiple growth factors (GFs) and cytokines. Among the platelet-derived bioactive factors, platelet-derived growth factor (PDGF), basic fibroblast growth factor (bFGF), vascular endothelial growth factor (VEGF), insulin-like growth factor-1 (IGF-1), transforming growth factor-β (TGF-β), and others may act as signal mediators of cell-cell/cell-extracellular matrix (ECM) crosstalk and regulators of multiple tissue regeneration processes [2, 3]. The bioactive molecules from PRP have been demonstrated in numerous studies that they displayed fundamental biomolecular functions in tissue regeneration [4]. Those molecules can integrate with transmembrane receptors and initiate cascaded repair and regeneration process inducing cell proliferation, migration, and ECM regulation [5]. Although the underlying mechanism of interaction between PRP and targeted tissue remains unclear, in this chapter, we intended to gather recent basic studies about the effects of PRP on cell biological functions.

X. Yu · H. He (✉)
Department of Rehabilitation Medicine, West China Hospital, Sichuan University, Chengdu, China

L. Zhang
Department of Plastic Surgery, Hangzhou Meilai Medical Hospital, Hangzhou, Guangdong, China

B. Cheng
Department of Burn & Plastic Surgery, General Hospital of Southern Theater Command, Guangzhou, China

13.1 Promote Cell Proliferation

The renewal of injured tissue lays the foundation for tissue regeneration and repair. During tissue regeneration process, cell proliferation is the basic key to the neo-tissue formation. In general, despite the diverse PRP preparation procedures, it has been confirmed that a concentration of $1–1.5 \times 10^6/\mu L$ platelet count is the most appropriate, and a majority of studies have reported the facilitation effects of PRP on proliferation ability of different key cell types.

In order to evaluate the effective application condition of PRP, different PRP concentrations were achieved by varying the PRP-to-media ratio (Vol/Vol) in which the cells were cultured. Amaral et al. found that at specific concentrations, PRP enhanced cell proliferation and induced angiogenesis. Two percent PRP matched human umbilical vein endothelial cell (HUVEC) proliferation both in basal and growth control medium [6]. Cho et al. also reported that 2% PRP-treated human skin fibroblasts (HDFs) had stimulated cell proliferation and increased the expression of human procollagen I alpha 1, elastin, and matrix metalloproteinases, for example, MMP-1 and MMP-2, which would promote the wound healing [7]. 5% [6, 8] and 10% PRP [6, 9] were tested, and reported favorable results induced greater human mesenchymal stromal cells (hMSCs) and human dermal fibroblast proliferation while with human keratinocyte cell line (HACAT). Furthermore, Wang and his colleagues found an increase in proliferation of mesenchymal stem cells (MSCs) when incubated with 10% PRP while a decrease when 20% PRP was used [9]. Similarly, Amable et al. found that 10% PRP could contribute to increased cell proliferation of hMSCs from the bone marrow, adipose tissue, and Wharton's jelly while higher volume ratio PRP inversely inhibited the cell proliferation [10]. For nerve regeneration, Zheng et al. exposed

B. Cheng, X. Fu (eds.), *Platelet-Rich Plasma in Tissue Repair and Regeneration*, https://doi.org/10.1007/978-981-99-3193-4_13

Schwann cells (SCs) to different concentrations of PRP (e.g., 40%, 20%, 10%, 5%, and 2.5%) and found that 5–20% PRP significantly stimulated SC proliferation but not high PRP concentrations (40%) [11]. The studies from Berndt et al. [12] and Atashi et al. [13] both reported that 20% PRP would be efficient for adipose-derived mesenchymal stem cells and human fibroblasts. Moussa et al. displayed that the effect of PRP on cell proliferation of osteoarthritis (OA) chondrocytes was concentration-dependent and significant enhancements on cell proliferation with 10% and 20% PRP [14].

To further explore and study the positive reaction between PRP and soft tissues, our research team put efforts on muscle tissue repair and rejuvenation. PRP reagents were manufactured following the PRP kit protocol [15]. In vivo models of muscle injury and aging were created by adding dexamethasone (DEX) or galactose (D-gal). PRP can reverse C2C12 atrophy after DEX treated and facilitate myogenic cell hypertrophy. PRP has shown a superior promoting effect on cell proliferation. The senescence β-galactosidase staining showed that PRP can significantly reduce the percentage of senescent C2C12 (Fig. 13.1).

Not only for mono-cell cultures, PRP also demonstrated positive effects on co-cultures. Reinders et al. tested the proliferation potentiality of human dermal microvascular endothelial cells (HDMEC), adipose-derived stem cells (ASC), and the ASC + HDMEC co-culture against irradiation. The colorimetric BrdU assay showed that PRP had a facilitated proliferating effect on radiated cells, indicating that PRP may be an effective wound care management for radiation wounds (Fig. 13.2) [16].

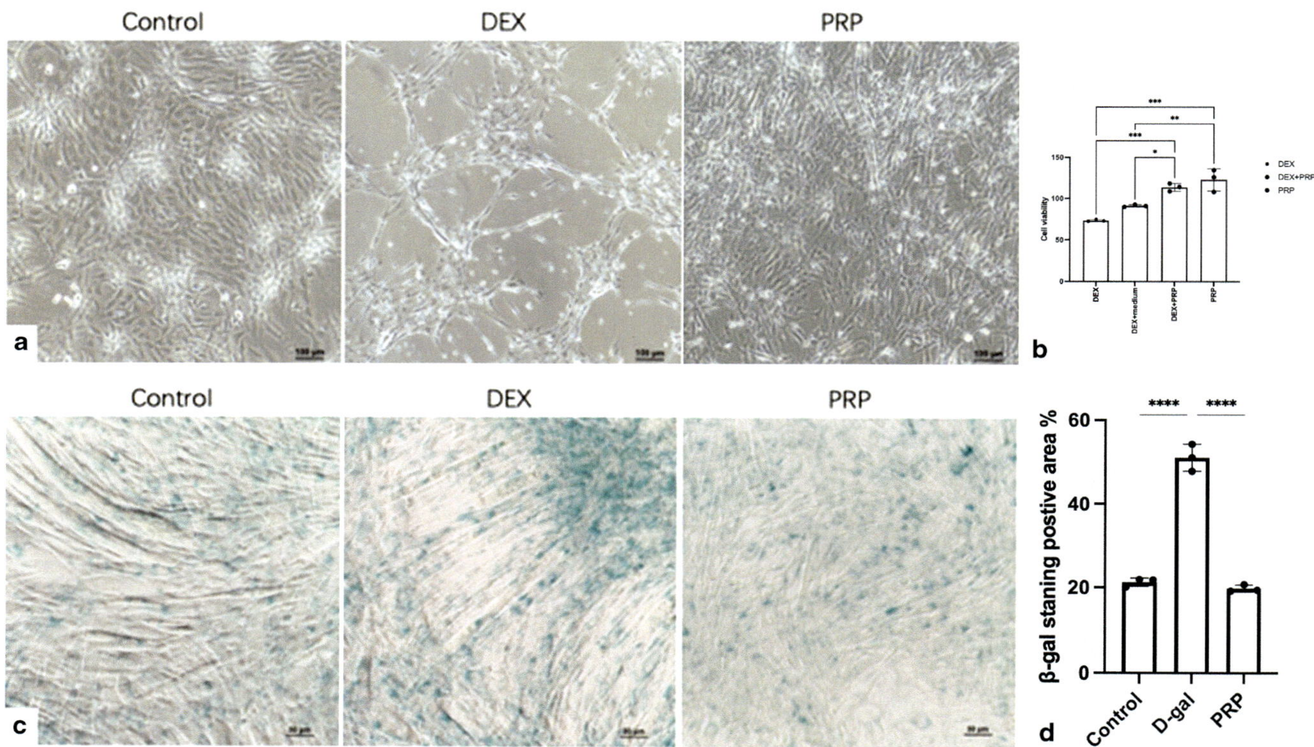

Fig. 13.1 PRP has positive effect on cell proliferation of C2C12. (**a**) Microscopic photographs of C2C12 treated with control, DEX, and PRP after DEX (20×, scale bars 50 μm). (**b**) The MTT assay showed that PRP can effectively protect C2C12, reversing muscle injury. (**c**) Microscopic photographs of senescence β-galactosidase staining for control, D-gal, and PRP after D-gal treatment (10×, scale bars 50 μm). (**d**) PRP reduced the percentage of senescent cell, indicating the possible rejuvenation effect of PRP

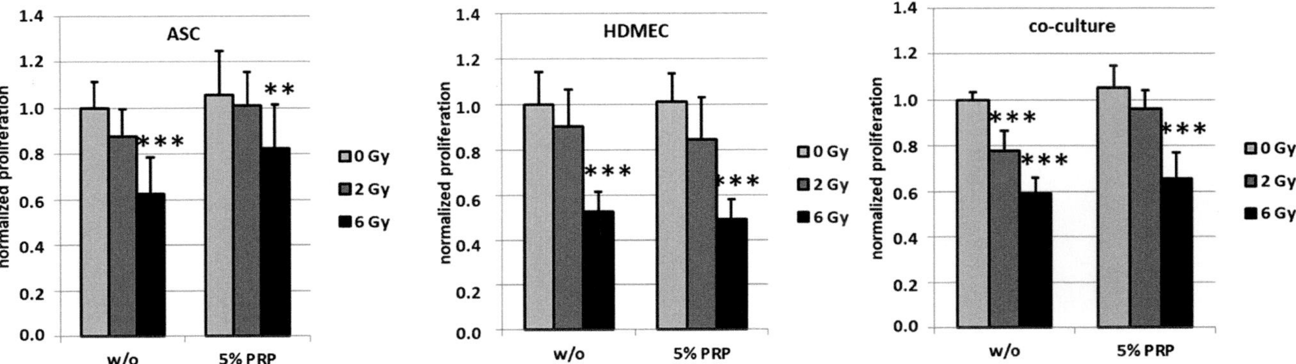

Fig. 13.2 The proliferation rates of mono-cell cultures and co-culture with PRP after irradiation

13.2 Regulate Cell Cycle

The regulation of the cell cycle by signal factors in ECM and intra-cellular molecular pathways has been extensively studied for decades. Research have authenticated that the morphological characteristics and behavior of a single cell are potent regulators of DNA synthesis and cell growth. The launch of mitosis in eukaryotic cells is tightly controlled by several steps, including cyclin B1, CDC2, and phosphorylation of CDC2. After the cell passes the G1/S checkpoint to start DNA synthesis, cyclin E is released, while cyclin A is required for both S-phase and M-phase [2]. Berndt et al. and Misiura et al. reported stimulated human keratinocyte cell cycle progression with PRP treatments. Cell cycle progression could be controlled by PRP through regulating phases G1, S, and G2/M. Similarly, Misiura et al. reported that their studies revealed that the mechanism for PRP stimulating cell proliferation PRP could be due to the upregulated expressions of cell cycle regulatory proteins in target cells [2, 12].

13.3 Promote Cell Migration

Besides cell proliferation, cell migration responses to PRP are also essential in skin tissue regeneration and repair. In order to study migratory patterns of target cells treated with PRP, in vitro scratch assay was usually applied, and then a collective and quicker cell migration was observed [12]. Zheng et al. tested the capacity of PRP to attract the rat SC migration and found that in 20%, 10%, and 5% PRP-treated groups, significantly more cells were induced to migrate than that in the control and 40% PRP groups. Thus, PRP with suitable concentration can support the regeneration of injured nerves by providing bioactive substrates for axonal migration and releasing molecules that regulate axonal outgrowth [11]. However, in the same study conducted by Amaral et al., even 2%, 5%, and 10% PRP were found to improve cell proliferation; no great influence was found on cell migration. Among the molecules found in PRP are fibronectin and vitronectin, which immobilize growth factors within the fibrin and allow the fibrin scaffold to function as a matrix for epithelial migration [17]. Cho et al. reported an in vitro scratch wound assay in which the cell migration ability of HDFs were compared among different cultivation conditions, for example, medium only, with 0.5%, 1%, or 2% PRP. The results demonstrated that prominently increased cell migration distance was recorded with PRP treatment in a concentrated-dependent manner [7]. In our study, HUVECs were employed in the scratch assay for angiogenesis and neovascularization which had been recognized as the fundamental step for wound healing and skin regeneration. PRP treatment demonstrated prominent enhancement on cell migration compared with medium group (Fig. 13.3).

Some studies deemed when PRP integrated with coagulation reagents, such as thrombin or calcium chloride ($CaCl_2$) and fibrinogen within PRP, would form a fibrin network, releasing growth factors and acting as a natural collagen scaffold for seed cell migration and differentiation [18]. Once a PRP gel was formed, it could decelerate the platelet loss and prevent the wound from bacterial infection. In our clinical experiences of applying PRP injection and PRP gel for nonhealing pressure injury in immobilized patients, intra-wound PRP injection and PRP gel could be considered as an effective treatment for accelerating wound healing. PRP and PRP gel were manufactured following the PRP kit protocol [15]. We investigated 15 nonhealing wounds treated with PRP wound therapy (Fig. 13.4), combing intra-wound PRP injection with PRP gel in treating. Wound evaluations showed that wound surface areas had been observed significant reduction, from pretreatment 11.73 ± 12.29 cm^2 to 1.81 ± 3.51 cm^2 afterward. Wound edge tissue samples were acquired before PPR treatment through skin trephine with a diameter of 5 mm. Tissue samples were cut into 4-μm-thick sections for hematoxylin and eosin (H&E) staining, and morphological observation was performed under the inverted phase-contrast microscope. The histological results showed

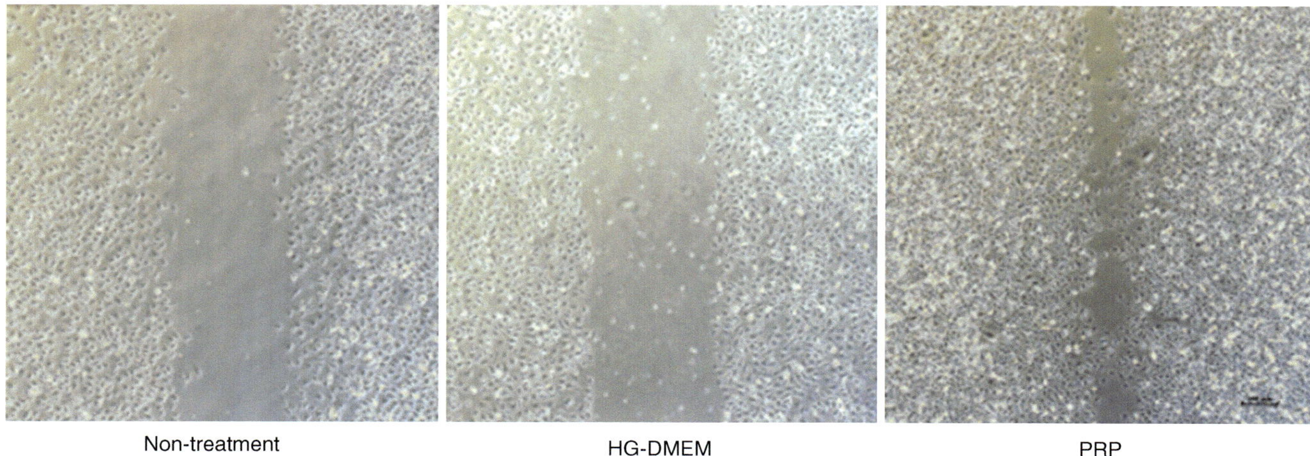

Fig. 13.3 The migration of HUVEC was accelerated by PRP through scratch assay (magnification 20×, scale bars 100 μm)

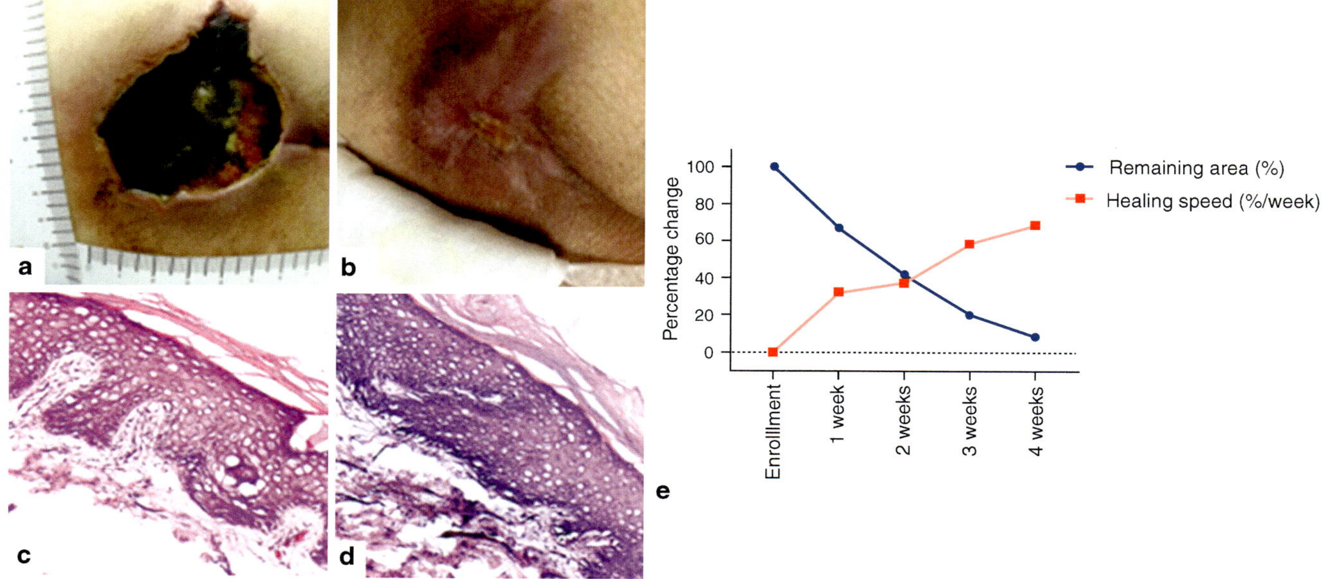

Fig. 13.4. (**a**, **b**) Clinical case photos of one pressure injury healing progress. (**c**, **d**) H&E staining showed accelerated wound skin healing after PRP and PPR gel treatment (20×). (**e**) The percentage changes of wound size. The dot line showed the cumulative percentage of reduced wound surface area compared with baseline. The square line showed the reduced rate of wound size. Healing speed = (wound size-wound size*)/wound size*100

that the structure of the tissue appeared mature and dense after PRP treatment with regularly arranged epidermis.

13.4 Roles in Autophagy and Apoptosis

Autophagy is a catabolic process and involves proteins, organelles, and cytoplasmic components being recycled and degraded in lysosomes and decreasing cellular stress. With the existent of apoptosis in cells, regeneration is necessary to maintain homeostasis and respond to the external environment. Evidence is mounting that autophagy plays a role in the repair of damaged tissues and in the replacement of impaired organs or body parts after injury [19].

In OA chondrocytes, Moussa et al. found that the autophagosome formation was increased in response to increasing PRP concentrates, indicating a concentration-dependent increase in autophagy with PRP. In their study, Moussa et al. detected that over 90% of chondrocytes turned into quiescent cells with 20% PRP. They believed that PRP could increase autophagy and induce chondrocyte quiescence. Due to the strong association between autophagy and apoptosis, the study also reported that compared to the control, PRP at 5%, 10%, and 20% concentrations could significantly decrease 37.63%, 37.97%, and 38.65% apoptotic ratios of OA chondrocytes, respectively [14]. PRP could reverse the senescence of OA chondrocytes by increasing the quiescence in OA chondrocytes. Keshk et al. conducted experiments to evaluate the protective effect of PRP against thioacetamide (TAA)-induced chronic renal damage. The results demonstrated the protective and regenerative effects of PRP by improving mitochondrial biogenesis, metabolism, and autophagy level [20]. PRP can change autophagy and reverse senescence by promoting autophagosome formation. At the same time, PRP can activate in situ progenitor cells to proliferate and differentiate into target cell and restore injured tissue.

In human epidermis tissue, cell death, along with proliferation and differentiation of epidermal cells, is a crucial and tightly controlled mechanism in the human epidermis that maintains tissue homeostasis. Keratinocytes are capable of both apoptosis and differentiation, which are linked to cell death. This process of differentiation of keratinocytes results in cornification with several steps, including degradation of nuclei and organelles. There are some similarities between this process and apoptosis, but the cells are not removed by phagocytosis, which is the case for apoptotic cell death, and this one is hoped to maintain the homeostasis in the skin tissue. Thus, the autophagy is also implicated in cell growth, cancer, aging, and the death of keratinocyte cell.

In brief, the various effects of PRP on cell biological functions, including but not limited to speeding up cell proliferation and regulating cell migration to modulating cell autophagy and apoptosis, have been explored and studied at certain degree. Several cell-cell, cell-ECM, and intercellular signal pathways have been studied. The further mechanisms of interaction between PRP and target cells, especially the intercellular mechanism, still needed more basic research work.

References

1. Xu J, et al. Platelet-rich plasma and regenerative dentistry. Aust Dent J. 2020;65(2):131–42.
2. Misiura M, et al. Platelet-rich plasma promotes the proliferation of human keratinocytes via a progression of the cell cycle. A role of prolidase. Int J Mol Sci. 2021;22(2):936.
3. Xu P, et al. Platelet-rich plasma accelerates skin wound healing by promoting re-epithelialization. Burns Trauma. 2020;8:tkaa028.
4. Guo SC, et al. Exosomes derived from platelet-rich plasma promote the re-epithelization of chronic cutaneous wounds via activation of YAP in a diabetic rat model. Theranostics. 2017;7(1):81–96.
5. Gentile P, Garcovich S. Systematic review-the potential implications of different platelet-rich plasma (PRP) concentrations in regenerative medicine for tissue repair. Int J Mol Sci. 2020;21(16):5702.
6. Do Amaral R, et al. Functionalising collagen-based scaffolds with platelet-rich plasma for enhanced skin wound healing potential. Front Bioeng Biotechnol. 2019;7:371.
7. Cho EB, et al. Effect of platelet-rich plasma on proliferation and migration in human dermal fibroblasts. J Cosmet Dermatol. 2019;18(4):1105–12.
8. Tavassoli-Hojjati S, et al. Effect of platelet-rich plasma concentrations on the proliferation of periodontal cells: an in vitro study. Eur J Dent. 2016;10(4):469–74.
9. Wang K, et al. Optimization of the platelet-rich plasma concentration for mesenchymal stem cell applications. Tissue Eng Part A. 2019;25(5–6):333–51.
10. Amable PR, et al. Mesenchymal stromal cell proliferation, gene expression and protein production in human platelet-rich plasma-supplemented media. PLoS One. 2014;9(8):e104662.
11. Zheng C, et al. Effect of platelet-rich plasma (PRP) concentration on proliferation, neurotrophic function and migration of Schwann cells in vitro. J Tissue Eng Regen Med. 2016;10(5):428–36.
12. Berndt S, et al. Autologous platelet-rich plasma (CuteCell PRP) safely boosts in vitro human fibroblast expansion. Tissue Eng Part A. 2019;25(21–22):1550–63.
13. Atashi F, et al. Autologous platelet-rich plasma: a biological supplement to enhance adipose-derived mesenchymal stem cell expansion. Tissue Eng Part C Methods. 2015;21(3):253–62.
14. Moussa M, et al. Platelet rich plasma (PRP) induces chondroprotection via increasing autophagy, anti-inflammatory markers, and decreasing apoptosis in human osteoarthritic cartilage. Exp Cell Res. 2017;352(1):146–56.
15. Liu X, et al. Exosomes derived from platelet-rich plasma present a novel potential in alleviating knee osteoarthritis by promoting proliferation and inhibiting apoptosis of chondrocyte via Wnt/beta-catenin signaling pathway. J Orthop Surg Res. 2019;14(1):470.
16. Reinders Y, et al. Impact of platelet-rich plasma on viability and proliferation in wound healing processes after external radiation. Int J Mol Sci. 2017;18(8):1819.
17. Kang YH, et al. Platelet-rich fibrin is a bioscaffold and reservoir of growth factors for tissue regeneration. Tissue Eng Part A. 2011;17(3–4):349–59.
18. Gentile P, et al. Impact of the different preparation methods to obtain autologous non-activated platelet-rich plasma (A-PRP) and activated platelet-rich plasma (AA-PRP) in plastic surgery: wound healing and hair regrowth evaluation. Int J Mol Sci. 2020;21(2):431.
19. Song Q, et al. Autophagy and its role in regeneration and remodeling within invertebrate. Cell Biosci. 2020;10:111.
20. Keshk WA, Zahran SM. Mechanistic role of cAMP and hepatocyte growth factor signaling in thioacetamide-induced nephrotoxicity: unraveling the role of platelet rich plasma. Biomed Pharmacother. 2019;109:1078–84.

The Molecular Mechanisms of PRP on Cell Biological Function

14

Weidong Zhu, Yan Peng, and Biao Cheng

Before the cell performs some biological behavior responding to the environment, the signal must be transmitted from extracellular to intracellular by the molecular signaling pathway. Extracellular signals refer to some molecules outside the cell (also called ligand), such as growth factors, cytokines, other small molecule compounds, etc. When the ligand specifically binds to the receptor in the cell membrane or intracellular, the signal will be amplified, dispersed, and regulated by cascade, thus regulating the genes and proteins in the cell. Changes in the body must be caused by changes in cellular biological behavior, and any drug that affects cellular biological behavior must first affect the molecular expression of cellular signaling pathways. Throughout the current development trend of bioscientific research, any research on effector components cannot be separated from the exploration of molecular mechanism, which is fundamental to understand how changes in upstream and downstream molecules of signaling pathways regulate genes. Therefore, the purpose of this chapter is to provide a preliminary understanding of the molecular regulation mechanism of PRP and to provide a more solid theoretical basis for the future clinical application of PRP.

PRP is a kind of autologous blood processing product, and its complex and timely effector components determine that PRP can affect biological behaviors of various cells, such as proliferation, migration, autophagy, apoptosis, and so on, thus producing different physiological effects. Various growth factors and cytokines (currently considered to be the main components of PRP effect) released after the degranulation of α-granule in platelets can act on specific receptors on the cell membrane and cause changes in molecular pathways within the signal. Many cytokines and growth factors transmit signals to intracellular through Janus kinase (JAK)/signal sensor and transcriptional activator (Stat) pathways, while some growth factor receptors (e.g., EGF and PDGF) have inherent tyrosine kinase activity stimulated by ligand binding that directly phosphorylates and activates Stat proteins. It has been reported that blocking the JAK/Stat3 signaling pathway leads to upregulation of P27 and P21, thereby inhibiting CDK-induced cell proliferation [1]. The team of Cheng Biao also found that PRP can significantly improve the proliferation of a variety of stem cells (Zhu Meishu et al. [2] found that platelet lysates promote hair follicle stem cell proliferation; Xu Pengchen et al. [3] found that platelet lysates promote epidermal stem cell proliferation, etc.), thus increasing the evidence level of PRP in the treatment of hair regeneration and wound repair.

Mitogen-activated protein kinase (MAPK) is a highly conserved serine-threonine protein kinase that plays a role in proliferation, differentiation, cell motility, and death in multiple types of cells. Three MAPK family proteins have been identified, including P38, SAPK/JNK1, 2, and 3 and extracellular signal-regulated kinase (ERK). These three MAPK family members all receive signals from extracellular growth factors, so the effect of PRP which is rich in growth factors on cell proliferation largely depends on the MAPK signaling pathway. Guo et al. [4] found that PRP- and PRP-derived exosomes feedback YAP information by activating the PI3K/AKT and ERK1/EKT2 signaling pathways of fibroblasts and endothelial cells to promote cell proliferation.

Platelet-derived growth factor (PDGF) is an effective migration chemokine that is essential for vascular remodeling and induces cell migration through MAPK/P38 and PI3K/Akt pathways. Cell migration is the result of coordination between cells and extracellular matrix. Zhang et al. [5] found that PDGF can induce the synthesis of new Cyr61 and transfer it to the extracellular region to merge with integrin/

W. Zhu
Department of Burn and Plastic Surgery, General Hospital of Southern Theater Command, PLA, Guangzhou, China

Y. Peng
Department of Burn and Plastic Surgery, General Hospital of Southern Theater of PLA, Guangzhou, Guangdong, China

B. Cheng (✉)
Department of Burn & Plastic Surgery, General Hospital of Southern Theater Command, Guangzhou, China

B. Cheng, X. Fu (eds.), *Platelet-Rich Plasma in Tissue Repair and Regeneration*, https://doi.org/10.1007/978-981-99-3193-4_14

Table 14.1 Effect of PRP on cell signaling pathway

Signal pathways	Downstream	PRP type	Cell	Effect	References
RhoA	YAP	PRP-exosome	Fibroblasts	Proliferation and migration	Guo et al. [4]
	ROCK2, LIMK1, and Cofilin	PRP	Adipose-derived stem cells (ADSCs)	Migration	Zhang et al. [6]
PI3K/AKT	YAP	PRP-exosome	Human retinal Muller cells	Proliferation and fibrosis	Zhang et al. [7]
	–	PRP-exosome	Endothelial cells	Vascularization and proliferation	Guo et al. [4]
	–	PL	Hacat	Proliferation	Lee et al. [8]
	NF-κB	PRCR(platelet-rich clot releasate)	Rat bone marrow-derived mesenchymal stem cells	Anti-apoptosis	Peng et al. [9]
	–	PRP(activate supernatant of calcium ion and thrombin)	Rat bone marrow-derived mesenchymal stem cells	Migration	Zhang et al. [10]
NF-κB	p65	i-PRF	Macrophage and dendritic cells	Anti-inflammation	Zhang et al. [11]
CD40L/CD40	–	Platelet-derived microvesicles (PDMV, 20,000 g × 2 h)	T cells and B cells	Inflammation and adaptive immunity	Sprague et al. [12]
MAPK	ERK1/ERK2	PL	ADSCs	Proliferation	Romaldini et al. [13]
	–	PDMV(28,000 g × 1 h)	Hematopoietic cell, CD34+ cells	Survival, proliferation, chemotactic, and fibrinogen adhesion	Baj-Krzyworzeka et al. [14]
	–	PRP-exosome	Endothelial cells	Vascularization and proliferation	Guo et al. [4]
	–	PRP(activate supernatant of calcium ion and thrombin)	Endothelial cells	Proliferation, migration, and vascularization	Kakudo et al. [15]
	ERK1/ERK2, p38 and JNK	PRP(activate supernatant of calcium ion and thrombin)	Human dermal fibroblasts	Proliferation, migration, collagen deposition, and MMP-1/MMP-2 expression	Cho et al. [16]
	–	PRP(activate supernatant of calcium ion and thrombin)	Human dermal papilla cells	Proliferation	Xiao et al. [17]
	ERK1/ERK2, JNK, and not p38	PRP(activate supernatant of calcium ion and thrombin)	ADSCs	Proliferation	Lai et al. [18]
JAK/STAT	p27	PRP(activate supernatant of calcium ion and thrombin)	Rat Achilles tendon cells	Cell cycle and proliferation	Yu et al. [1]
Notch	Notch1, Jagged-1, and Hes1	PL	Endothelial progenitor cells	Proliferation and migration	Zhang et al. [19]

FAK signal transduction and promote cell migration. The signal transduction of PDGF-induced Cyr61 synthesis also involves the activation of intracellular MAPK/ERK and MAPK/JNK signaling pathways. The results showed that PDGF could induce the whole process of a series of molecular signal transductions, that is, from extracellular to intracellular and then to extracellular. PDGF is also one of the main growth factor components in PRP.

The lipid signal released after platelet activation can directly act on the specific receptor in the cytoplasm, causing the activation of the downstream signaling pathway. In addition, platelet activation can also release a variety of small RNA molecules, directly to regulate gene expression. The common molecular signaling pathway changes that PRP can cause to cells involving PI3K/AKT signal pathways, MAPK signal pathways, JAK/STAT signal pathways, RhoA signal pathways, and so on.

Due to the limited content of the chapter, this chapter mainly focuses on the effects of PRP on the signaling pathway of mesenchymal stem cells (MSC), and the regulation of PRP on the cell signaling pathway is shown in the references in Table 14.1.

14.1 Molecular Signals for MSC Proliferation and Migration in PRP

MSC is the most widely used pluripotent stem cell in clinic and has made great contribution to the future development of regenerative medicine and tissue engineering. MSC can be activated when the body needs it, but its activation is very inefficient. In addition, currently commonly used stem cell therapy (often referred to as MSC) has a fatal shortcoming, namely, low survival rate of stem cell transplantation. Therefore, how to improve the survival rate and activation efficiency of MSC transplantation is a hot topic in stem cell therapy research. Cheng Biao's team focused on the research of tissue repair and regeneration and found that PRP could provide significant positive effects on mesenchymal stem cells. Peng Yan et al. [9] (Cheng Biao team) and Zhang Lei et al. [6] (Cheng Biao team) found that PRP can promote the survival of bone marrow mesenchymal stem cells (BM-MSC) by activating the PI3K/AKT/NF-κB signaling pathway and enhancing the migration ability of adipose-derived stem cells (ADSCs) by increasing the expression of Rho family proteins.

The survival of cells depends on the balance between the production and clearance of reactive oxygen species in the body. When any harmful stimulus breaks this balance, the body will enter the state of oxidative stress when the production of reactive oxygen species exceeds the clearance capacity. PRP contains multiple growth factors, so it has a great influence on the PI3K/AKT signaling pathway of cells.

The PI3K/AKT signaling pathway has been extensively studied by researchers in the physiological behaviors of various cells, such as proliferation, differentiation, apoptosis, and migration. As mentioned above, most extracellular signals need to specifically bind to membrane receptors to activate downstream signaling pathways, while PI3K/AKT signaling pathway is one of the most common upstream signaling pathways and also the master switch of several intracellular downstream signaling pathways. Receptor tyrosine kinases (RPTKs) are the largest class of enzyme-linked receptors that bind to both ligands and phosphorylate the tyrosine residues of target proteins, so RPTKs are both receptors and enzymes. RPTKs are high-affinity cell surface receptors for most polypeptide growth factors and cytokines, and PI3K is phosphorylated by RPTKs after receiving the ligand. When RPTK binds to a ligand (such as a growth factor), it fuses with a nearby RPTK that also receives the ligand to form a dimer, which is phosphorylated itself to form an enzyme, and produces an insulin receptor substrate (IRS) docking site, which binds PI3K to activate and phosphorylate it, and then phosphatidylinositol-4,5-diphosphate (PIP2) phosphorylates PIP3 (phosphatidylinositol-3, 4, 5-triphosphate), and PIP3 finally phosphorylates AKT to activate. As a protein kinase B, AKT phosphorylates a large number of downstream sites, resulting in decentralized activation of multiple downstream signaling pathways, such as the mTOR, MAPK, VEGF, and NF-κB pathways.

Peng Yan et al. [9] confirmed in vitro with bone marrow mesenchymal stem cells from mice that PRP reduced the apoptosis rate of MSC in oxidative stress environment and enhanced its survival and proliferation (Fig. 14.1). Further research has found that PRP can enhance the expression of PDGFR-a in MSC and improve the reception of MSC to PDGF signal, thus improving its survivability. After it was proved that PRP can enhance MSC survival, Peng Yan et al. further found that PRP can enhance the tissue repair function of MSC in oxidative stress environment and promote MSC secretion of VEGF and PDGF, thereby enhancing MSC autocrine (self-interest) and paracrine (altruist) ability. Peng continued to confirm that PI3K/AKT/NF-κB signaling pathway plays a key role in PRP affecting MSC through pharmacological blockade in vitro and in vivo studies. Nuclear factor-activated light chain enhancement (NF-κB) of B cells is an important intracellular nuclear transcription factor, involved in inflammatory response, immune response, and regulation of cell apoptosis. Therefore, PRP can activate the nuclear transcription factor NF-κB through the PI3K/AKT signaling pathway, enhancing the survival and function of MSC in harsh environments.

Cell migration ability is one of the decisive factors in whether stem cells can reach the lesion site after transplantation. The process of cell migration involves changes of cytoskeleton, cell basal adhesion, and extracellular matrix. And the cell migration can be divided into four mechanical independent steps: the expansion of flaky pseudopods, the formation of new adhesions, the contraction of the inclusions, and the detachment of the tail.

Rho A/ROCK signaling pathway plays a key role in regulating the above changes during cell migration. The Rho family of small molecules guanosine triphosphate (Rho GTPases) has five subfamilies, namely, Rho, Rac, Cdc42, Rnd, and Rho BTB, most of which are closely related to morphological changes in cell migration. Among them, the Rho subfamily is mainly involved in tension fiber formation and focal adhesion complexes (FACs), the Rac subfamily promotes the formation of lamellar pseudopods and cell membrane folds, and the Cdc42 subfamily promotes filamentous pseudopod formation. As a molecular switch, Rho GTPases family members are also important to signal transduction molecules in the upstream of MAPK signaling pathway. Rho A, a relatively conserved monomer G protein, which is regulated by the inherent activation mechanism, has been extensively studied in cell migration. PRP is rich in growth factors that promote cell migration, such as TGF-β1, bFGF, PDGF, etc.

Zhang Lei et al. [6] (Cheng Biao team) found that PRP can promote the formation of stress fiber of adipose-derived

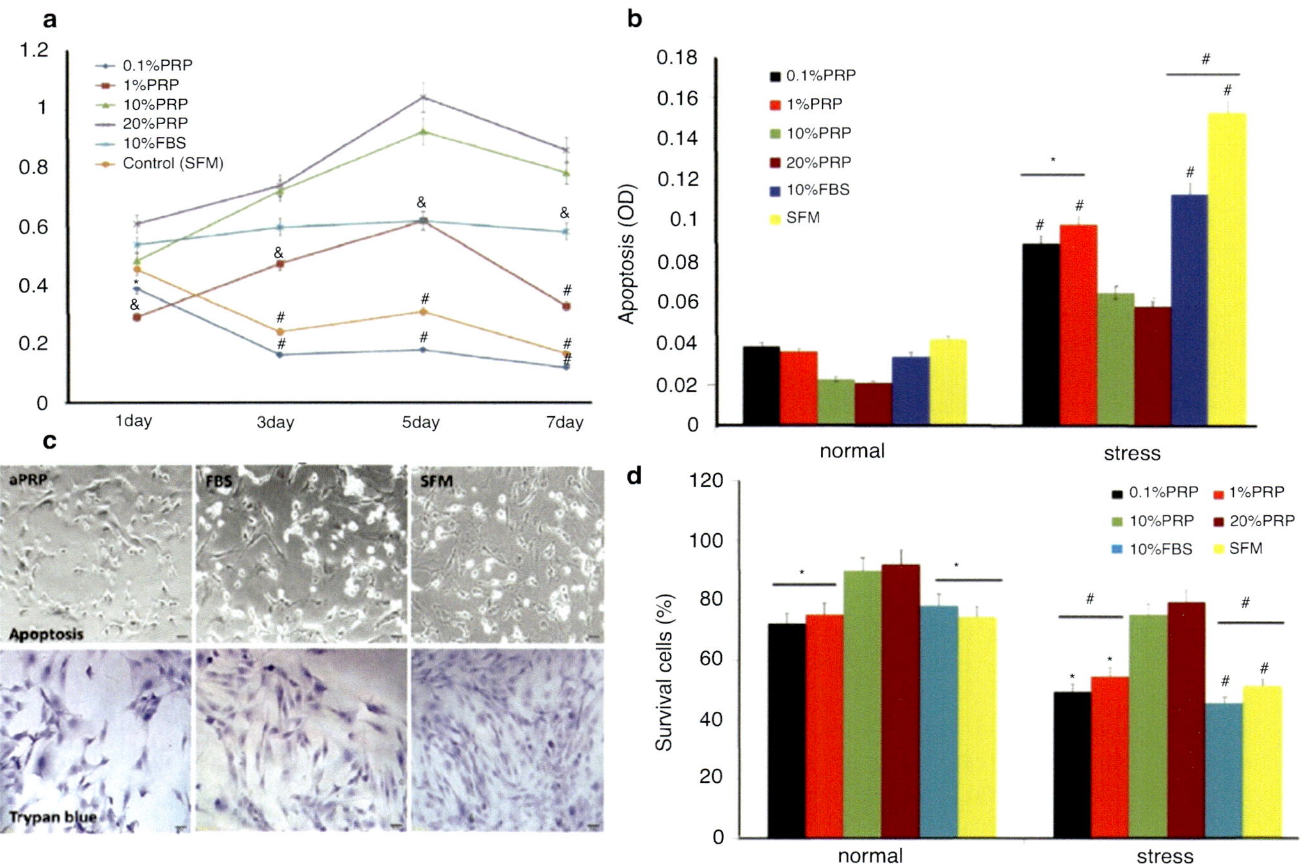

Fig. 14.1 (**a**) MTT assay. (**b**) APOPercentage assay. (**c–d**) Better preserved cell morphology in a PRP group and significantly increased cell viability compared with other groups under stress condition

mesenchymal stem cells (ADSCs) and enhance the migration ability of ADSCs, thus promoting ADSCs to better reach the lesion site and promote wound healing. Further studies have found that PRP enhances the migration of ADSCs by increasing the expression of Rho family proteins including Cdc42, Rac1, and Rho A and promoting the expression of Rho GTP downstream signaling molecules including PAK1, ROCK2, LIMK1, and Cofilin (Fig. 14.2). Rho activation affects phosphorylation of myosin light chains by ROCK (also known as Rho-kinase), including phosphorylation of myosin light chains and inhibiting phosphorylation of myosin light chains. Other research evidence speculates that ROCK and myosin light chain kinase activation are the two coordinates to regulate different directions of cell contraction, because ROCKs manifest as the need for actin light chain phosphorylation in the cell body associated with actin microfilaments, so the cell edge requires actin light chain kinase. LIM kinase 1 (LIMK1), which is a new bispecific kinase family that contains LIM domains with two amino terminals (serine/threonine and tyrosine), has been shown to specifically mediate Rac-induced actin cytoskeletal recombination and focal adhesion complexes. Rac-induced activation of LIMK1 is mediated by PAK1, which phosphorylate limk1 on its Thr508 residue. Other studies have also proposed that Rho- and Cdc42-induced cytoskeletal changes are mediated by Rho-dependent protein kinase ROCK and Cdc42-regulating protein kinase PAK4 phosphorylation LIMK1. Cofilin is an actin-binding protein that is considered a potent regulator in actin dynamics for activity in F-actin depolymerization and is the only known LIMK1 substrate. In addition to Rho A/ROCK, the discovery of the Rho GTP-LIMK1-Cofilin signal axis provides a new idea for PRP to promote cell migration.

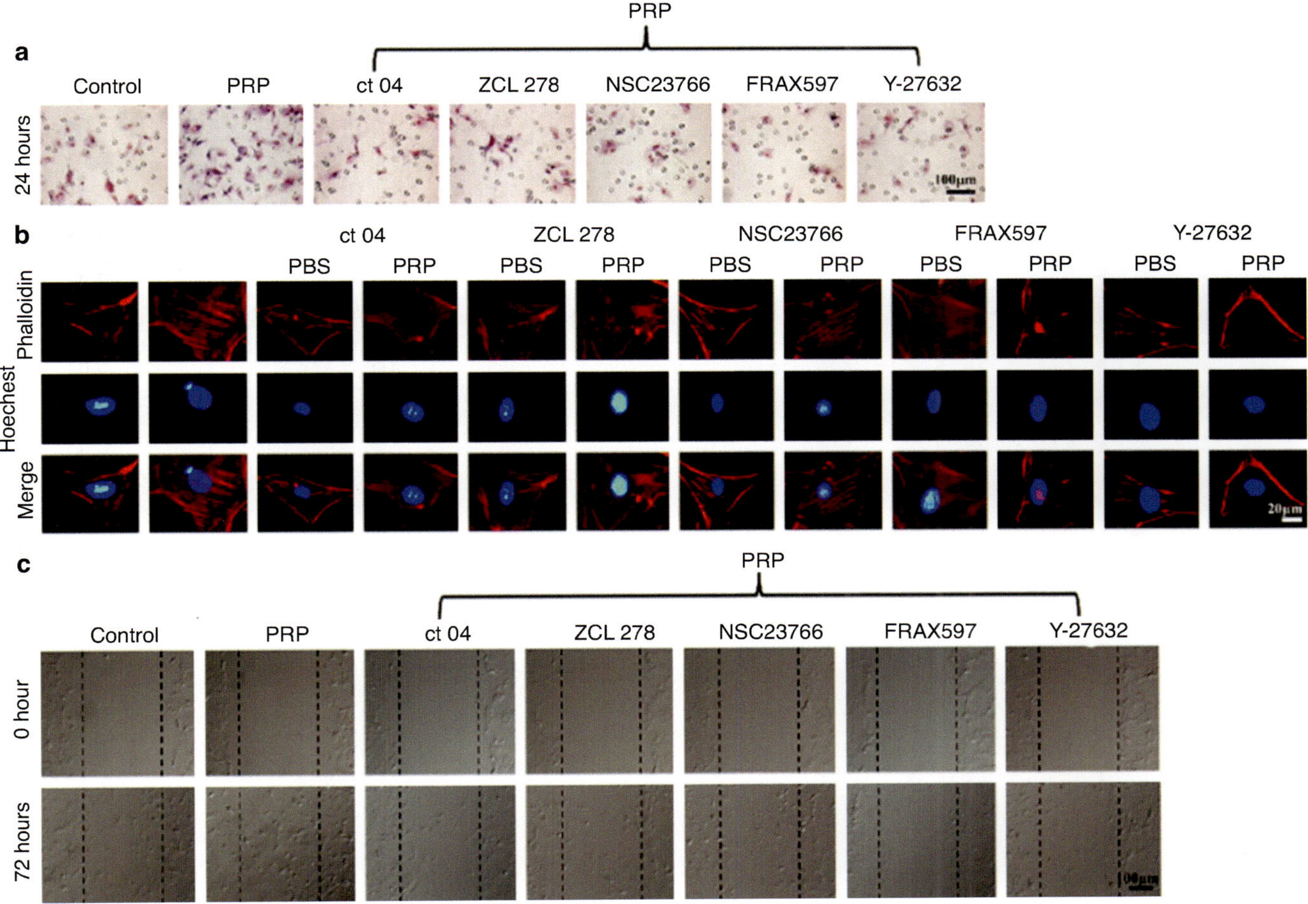

Fig. 14.2 The effects of downstream Rho GTPase signaling molecules on ADSCs, actin stress fiber formation, and migration. (**a**) Transwell assay and quantification of ADSCs. (**b**) Phallotoxin staining (Red) staining actin in ADSCs. (**c**) Scratch wound assay and quantification of ADSCs

14.2 Conclusion

The cellular molecular mechanism is a navigation map in the process of internal changes of an organism. Its exploration helps to explore the deep-seated targeting mechanism of PRP and to select appropriate therapeutic targets for PRP, making PRP a refined, precise, and high-quality treatment method.

References

1. Yu TY, et al. Platelet-rich plasma increases proliferation of tendon cells by modulating Stat3 and p27 to up-regulate expression of cyclins and cyclin-dependent kinases. Cell Prolif. 2015;48(4):413–20.
2. Zhu M, et al. Platelet sonicates activate hair follicle stem cells and mediate enhanced hair follicle regeneration. J Cell Mol Med. 2020;24(2):1786–94.
3. Xu P, et al. Platelet-rich plasma accelerates skin wound healing by promoting re-epithelialization. Burns. Trauma. 2020;8:tkaa028.
4. Guo SC, et al. Exosomes derived from platelet-rich plasma promote the re-epithelialization of chronic cutaneous wounds via activation of YAP in a diabetic rat model. Theranostics. 2017;7(1):81–96.
5. Zhang F, et al. The matricellular protein Cyr61 is a key mediator of platelet-derived growth factor-induced cell migration. J Biol Chem. 2015;290(13):8232–42.
6. Zhang L, et al. Platelet-rich plasma in combination with adipose-derived stem cells promotes skin wound healing through activating rho GTPase-mediated signaling pathway. Am J Transl Res. 2019;11(6):3790.
7. Zhang W, Jiang H, Kong Y. Exosomes derived from platelet-rich plasma activate YAP and promote the fibrogenic activity of Muller cells via the PI3K/Akt pathway. Exp Eye Res. 2020;193:107973.
8. Lee J, et al. Platelet-rich plasma activates AKT signaling to promote wound healing in a mouse model of radiation-induced skin injury. J Transl Med. 2019;17(1):295.
9. Peng Y, et al. Platelet rich plasma clot releasate preconditioning induced PI3K/AKT/NFkappaB signaling enhances survival and regenerative function of rat bone marrow mesenchymal stem cells in hostile microenvironments. Stem Cells Dev. 2013;22(24):3236–51.
10. Zhang J, et al. The effects of platelet-rich and platelet-poor plasma on biological characteristics of BM-MSCs in vitro. Anal Cell Pathol (Amst). 2020;2020:8546231.

11. Zhang J, et al. Anti-inflammation effects of injectable platelet-rich fibrin via macrophages and dendritic cells. J Biomed Mater Res A. 2020;108(1):61–8.
12. Sprague DL, et al. Platelet-mediated modulation of adaptive immunity: unique delivery of CD154 signal by platelet-derived membrane vesicles. Blood. 2008;111(10):5028–36.
13. Romaldini A, et al. Platelet lysate activates human subcutaneous adipose tissue cells by promoting cell proliferation and their paracrine activity toward epidermal keratinocytes. Front Bioeng Biotechnol. 2018;6:203.
14. Baj-Krzyworzeka M, et al. Platelet-derived microparticles stimulate proliferation, survival, adhesion, and chemotaxis of hematopoietic cells. Exp Hematol. 2002;30(5):450–9.
15. Kakudo N, et al. Platelet-rich plasma releasate promotes angiogenesis in vitro and in vivo. Med Mol Morphol. 2014;47(2):83–9.
16. Cho EB, et al. Effect of platelet-rich plasma on proliferation and migration in human dermal fibroblasts. J Cosmet Dermatol. 2019;18(4):1105–12.
17. Xiao S, et al. The mechanism of activated platelet-rich plasma supernatant promotion of hair growth by cultured dermal papilla cells. J Cosmet Dermatol. 2019;18(6):1711–6.
18. Lai F, et al. Platelet-rich plasma enhances the proliferation of human adipose stem cells through multiple signaling pathways. Stem Cell Res Ther. 2018;9(1):107.
19. Zhang C, et al. Platelet-rich plasma with endothelial progenitor cells accelerates diabetic wound healing in rats by upregulating the notch1 signaling pathway. J Diabetes Res. 2019;2019:5920676.

Quality Control and Application Transformation

15

Ju Tian, Biao Cheng, Linying Shi, and Guiqiu Shan

The preparation of PRP (platelet-rich plasma) is divided into methods such as plasma exchange and density gradient centrifugation. Currently, density gradient centrifugation is often used for preparation. When using density gradient centrifugation, some studies believe that single centrifugation can achieve the desired effect, but more studies use two density gradient centrifugation methods. The first centrifugation separates the red blood cells from the plasma and buffy coat layers. The second centrifugation concentrates the platelets and separates them from the platelet-poor plasma.

Whether it is manual preparation or machine preparation, the factors that affect the preparation of PRP include centrifugal force, centrifugation time, number of centrifugation, centrifugation temperature, age, gender, initial concentration of platelets, platelet size, interindividual biological differences, hematocrit variability, and other factors [1–5].

The quality of PPR obtained by different preparation methods and the same preparation method in different individuals and processing different blood volumes is also inconsistent, and it is difficult to evaluate which PRP preparation program is the best. Generally speaking, for the first centrifugation, the number of platelets obtained is more important than the concentration. The second centrifugation to obtain a sufficiently high concentration of platelets is the most important. At present, most studies on the preparation of PRP use the final platelet concentration to determine its effectiveness. Most scholars believe that the minimum concentration of platelets to release growth factors is $1 \times 10^6/\mu L$ [6–7]. The increase of platelet concentration cannot bring about the proportional growth of active substances but may inhibit cell growth [8]. For different tissues, it promotes cell proliferation, migration, and infiltration. The best platelets are needed. The concentration is also different [9–11].

When evaluating the quality of PRP, the age, the gender, the platelet concentration of the donor, the number of centrifugation during preparation, the centrifugal force, the time of centrifugation, and the temperature during the centrifugation should be clearly described. It should also indicate the method and temperature of PRP activation, measure the concentration of platelets in PRP and the concentration of growth factors after activation, and calculate platelet recovery, growth factor release, and other indicators [12], so as to provide objective indicators for comparison with other studies.

There is no PRP preparation method that can meet the requirements of all diseases. The so-called standardization of platelet preparation is not a unified preparation method but an individualized preparation method that is determined according to individual characteristics and specific treatment purposes and other comprehensive considerations. In the treatment process specific to each person being treated, most of the active substances in PRP come from platelets. The factors that determine the efficacy of PRP are essentially the number of platelets in PRP and the function of releasing active substances. The number of platelets is determined by the concentration of platelets in the whole blood of the subject, the amount of blood collected, and the preparation method (whether a high concentration of platelets can be obtained during the preparation process). The function of platelets is determined by the age, gender, disease state, and preparation method of the person being treated (whether it is activated in advance during the preparation process, resulting in a decrease in its function). Therefore, in the treatment process, we should control those controllable factors to the best and then prepare and treat according to these uncontrollable factors.

J. Tian (✉)
Department of Plastic Surgery, People's Hospital of Zhongshan City, Zhongshan, Guangdong, China

B. Cheng
Department of Burn & Plastic Surgery, General Hospital of Southern Theater Command, Guangzhou, China

L. Shi · G. Shan
Department of Transfusion Medicine, General Hospital of Southern Theater of PLA, Guangzhou, China

B. Cheng, X. Fu (eds.), *Platelet-Rich Plasma in Tissue Repair and Regeneration*, https://doi.org/10.1007/978-981-99-3193-4_15

In the treatment process specific to each person being treated, most of the active substances in PRP come from platelets. The factors that determine the efficacy of PRP are essentially the number of platelets in PRP and the function of releasing active substances. The number of platelets is determined by the concentration of platelets in the whole blood of the subject, the amount of blood collected, and the preparation method (whether a high concentration of platelets can be obtained during the preparation process). The function of platelets is determined by the age, gender, disease state, and preparation method of the person being treated (whether it is activated in advance during the preparation process, resulting in a decrease in its function). Therefore, in the treatment process, we should control those controllable factors to the best and then prepare and treat according to these uncontrollable factors.

The author proposed an optimized and standardized secondary centrifugal platelet-rich plasma preparation method with platelet parameters (PLT, PCT, MPV, PDW) as quality control indicators [13]. The whole blood platelet concentration and PCT were used to evaluate and calculate the PLT count in PRP and the amount of PRP prepared. MPV and PDW were used to evaluate the quality of platelets in PRP. In the course of clinical treatment, the amount of PRP used or the number of uses is adjusted according to the patient's age, disease state, and treatment purpose, or the target concentration of platelets in the PRP is determined according to the treatment purpose. This method is both simple and practical, and prepared PRP can promote the healing of complex wounds in the elderly, which is worthy of further research.

15.1 Frozen Storage of Concentrate Platelets

Platelet-rich plasma has been widely used in various aspects of acute and chronic wounds, sports injuries, plastic surgery, and tissue engineering, but the preservation of PRP has not been well solved. The process of PRP treatment is usually long, and patients need to take repeated blood collection or use a platelet apheresis machine for multiple uses, so the preservation of PRP is a current concern for researchers and clinicians. In particular, the platelets contained in PRP contain many active substances but have poor stability and short preservation time and are somewhat limited by the promotion and application of PRP. The current commonly used platelet storage method is to use a special storage bag to save the concentrated platelet amount to 22 °C incubator in the oscillation for 5 days. Expiries of platelets must be discarded due to bacterial contamination and loss of activity, thus causing great waste. Another method of preserving platelets is the long-term preservation of platelet preparations at low or deep low temperatures, extending the platelet preservation time to 1 year. However, the preparation quality of frozen platelets is affected by many factors, the quality is very unstable, and the clinical effect is difficult to guarantee, among which the most important influencing factor is the choice of cryopreservation agent. The quality of platelets during the freezing process directly depends on the slow freezing and fast freezing process, which is mainly slow injury. Frozen was slow and extracellularly crystallized, and the solution was concentrated to form a hypertonic state. Cells were severely dehydrated in a hypertonic environment, causing degeneration of membrane proteins, followed by chemical damage. Freezing too fast, the cells form ice crystals during freezing, causing mechanical damage to the cellular membrane. Deep low-temperature intracellular protective agent can replace and fix the intracellular free water through the cell membrane, change the intracellular freezing conditions, make the crystallization process slow or form no crystallization, and maintain the balance of internal and external osmotic pressure. In addition, it can also increase the viscosity of the platelet suspension, reduce the disguised point of the frozen cells, and reduce the protein degeneration during the freezing process, so as to achieve a protective effect, so that the fast frostbite damage is greatly reduced. Dimethylsulfoxide (DMSO) is the most commonly used platelet cryoprotective agent, which has the characteristics of good protection effect, easy elution, and low toxicity. Clinically, frozen platelets made of added DMSO have been thawed by intravenous infusion to patients needing urgent platelet treatment, which plays a very important role in rescuing the lives of patients. At the same time, no obvious toxic reaction was found, indicating that its safety is guaranteed. This is also an important reason why DMSO is commonly used for frozen platelet preservation. The best effect on platelet protection is 5–6% of the DMSO and has no clinical infusion side effects. But due to its strong permeability, metabolites such as foul odor dimethyl sulfide, teratogenesis, and other reasons, its widespread use is restricted. Therefore, in recent years, some researchers used a mixture of frozen messenger regulator (TS)—second messenger additives composed of multiple components mainly include amilolil (amiloride), adenosine (adenosine), sodium nitrosodium (sodium nitroprusside), pansentine (dipyridamole), thiloropidine (ticlopidine), etc., by inhibiting platelet initiation in vitro and stabilizing intracellular biochemical processes and preventing freezing injury by acting reversibly on specific activation pathways, to improve its in vitro and in vivo function and activity in preservation. The final concentration of DMSO in concentrated platelets with TS preservation was reduced to 2%, with higher in vivo survival than conventional 6% DMSO preserved platelets, and both in vitro recovery and function improved after rewarming. Our previous study found that 2% DMSO

+ TS was frozen as the storage agent for 8 weeks with PLT, MPV, and PH (Fig. 15.1). The content of PDGF, VEGF, and EGF in the freezing platelet gel supernatant(FPGS) was better than the gel supernatant prepared from fresh platelets for 3 days (Fig. 15.2). Animal experiments found that the gel prepared from frozen platelets had the same wound healing effect as that prepared from fresh platelets, and the wound healing rate was better than human recombinant human epidermal growth factor (rhEGF) gels (Fig. 15.3). Therefore, freezing preservation is currently an important method for PRP isolation and preservation. If PRP can be prepared with frozen platelets for treatment, individualiza-

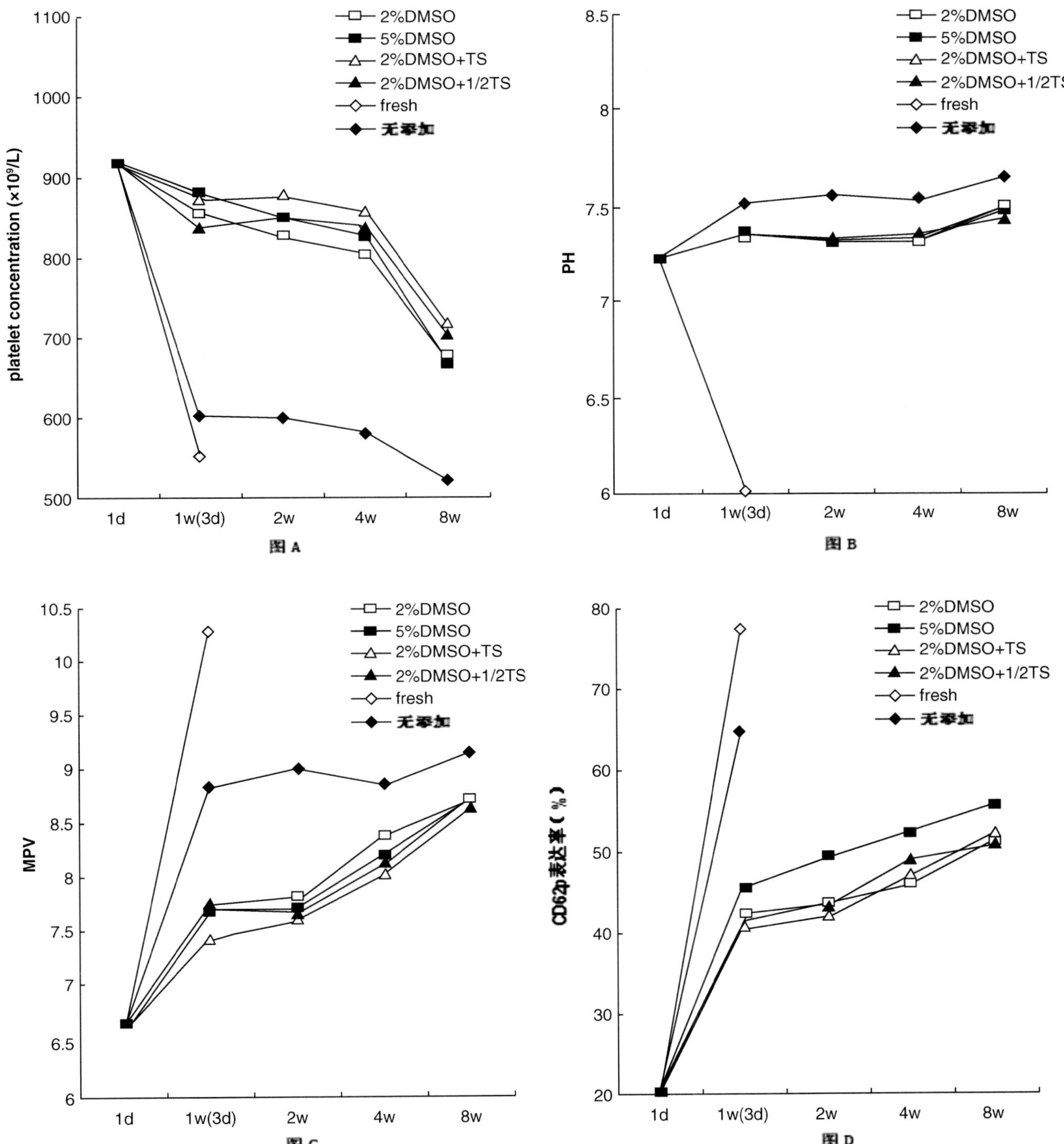

Fig. 15.1 The frozen storage agent has little influence on platelet PLT, MPV, PH and platelet activation, and the preservation effect is better than that of the group without added storage agent and the group with conventional platelet preservation

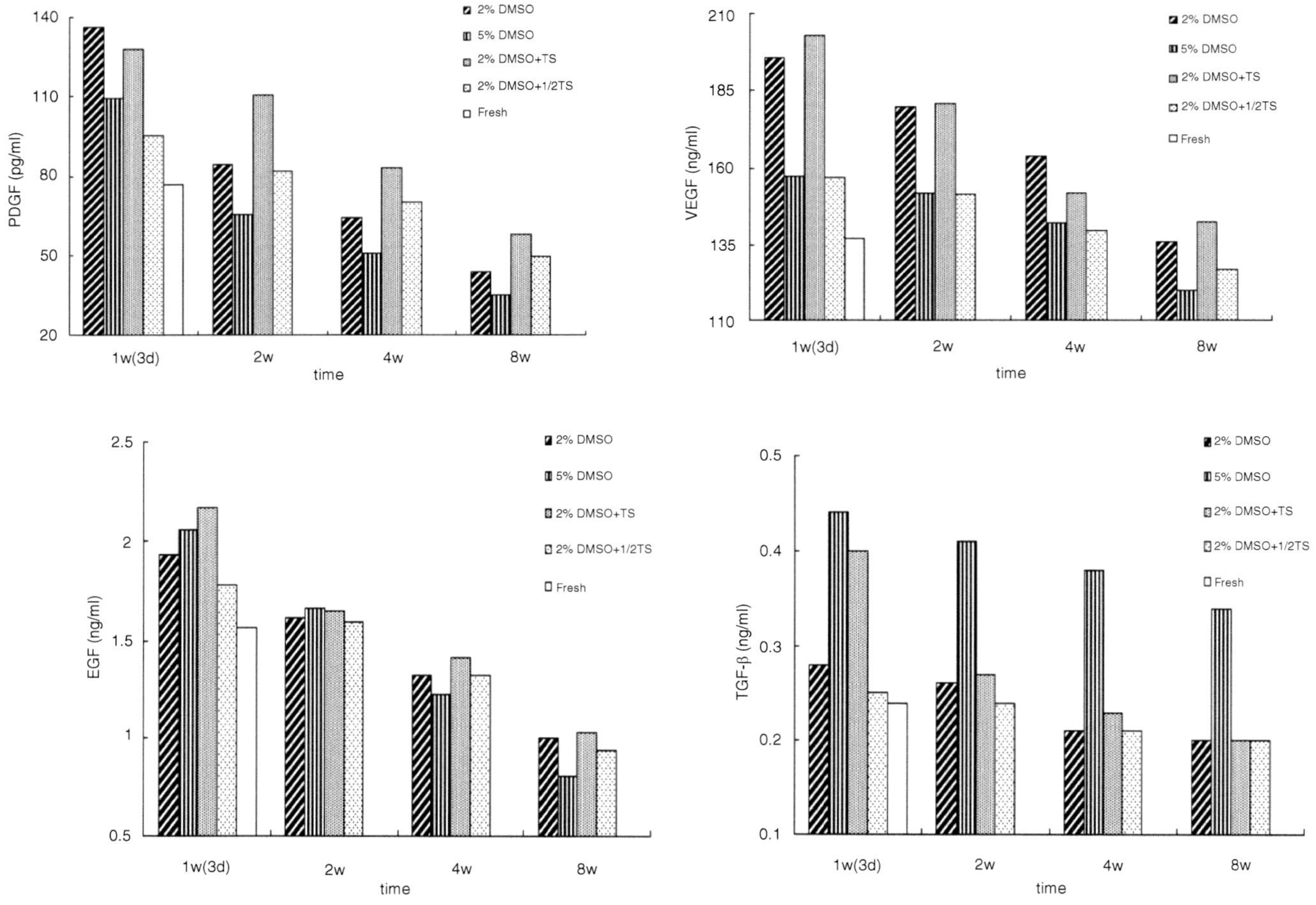

Fig. 15.2 The levels of the growth factors PDGF, VEGF, EGF, and TGF in FPG were significantly higher than fresh PG

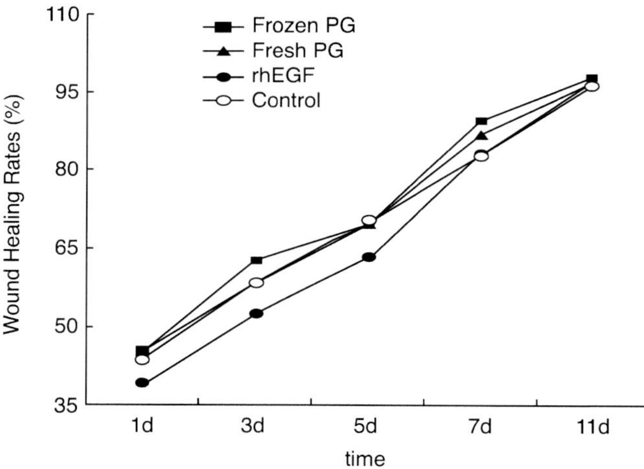

Fig. 15.3 FPG has the same pro-wound healing effect as fresh PG and is superior to a single growth factor

tion of treatment can be achieved: for patients whose autologous PRP can be applied, including patients requiring PRP treatment during major surgery, whole blood can be collected at one time. Platelets were isolated and kept as frozen for use in elective surgery. For chronic refractory ulcer wounds, platelets can be collected once and frozen. For multiple uses, it helps to solve the problem of frequent and repeated blood collection; for patients with unfavorable autologous PRP application, such as old age, weak disease, and physical deficiency, and patients without autologous platelet collection, then PRP treatment can be prepared using allogeneic frozen platelets. This can fully meet the needs of all patients who need PRP treatment. At the same time, doctors can be allowed to take the initiative in time, choose to use autologous or allogeneic PRP according to the specific situation of patients, and realize the personalized treatment plan of PRP treatment, so as to promote and apply it in hospitals at all levels across the country. However, although the cryofreezing method can effectively extend the storage period of platelets, large refrigeration equipment and liquid nitrogen are required to continuously provide the cryogenic environment and cannot achieve PRP product production. Therefore, our research group dried platelet-rich plasma and then dried it at low temperature on the basis of freezing, so as to extend the preservation time to realize the convenience of platelet preservation and use.

At present, freeze-drying technology has been widely used in fields such as the food industry, pharmaceutical industry, and microbe preservation [2–6]. Freeze-drying technology has unique advantages in cell preservation. Freeze-drying process at low temperature and high vacuum degree, cells are dormant, and their own metabolic process is basically stopped, thus ensuring the stability of cell physics and chemical and biological shape. Drying at low temperatures and under higher vacuum, microbial growth and enzyme action are largely inaccessible, eliminating the possibility of microbial contamination. The freeze-dried samples remove the vast majority of the water, greatly reduce the volume, reduce weight, and can also realize time preservation at room temperature. Frozen-drying technology has unique advantages in cell preservation. During the freeze-drying process at low temperature and high vacuum degree, the cells are dormant, and their own metabolic process is basically stopped, thus ensuring the stability of cell physics and chemical and biological shape. Platelet drying preservation technology of platelets is not easy to achieve. Frozen drying preservation research began in the 1950s. However, because platelets are cell structure, it is very difficult to freeze-drying. After freezing and drying, platelet cell structure and activity were basically lost, and the initial exploration ended in failed [7, 8]. To maintain the functional morphology of platelets, the researchers began trying to add protective agents before platelet lyophilization to reduce platelet damage by the freeze-drying process. Many factors in the freeze-drying process will have important effects on the platelet preservation effect, including the selection of protective fluid, freezing and cooling rate, and storage conditions. Therefore, we must evaluate the particularity of platelets, and the success of platelet freeze-drying preservation is based on the recovery rate and functional integrity of platelets after freeze-drying. Research and optimization of the factors affecting the effect and physiological function of platelet lyophilized drying can have great significance for reducing the platelet lyophilized injury and improving the recovery rate and function. The lyophilization process of platelets is a multistep process with multiple effects such as low temperature, freezing, and dehydration. Even if the freeze-drying process is going out relatively smoothly, it is still difficult to ensure that the activity of platelet freeze-drying products is not lost in the long-term storage process. Among the many influencing factors, the final effect of the protective agent system on freeze-drying is most prominent in [9].

Fusion of platelet cell membranes, phase transition, and lateral phase separation during the lyophilization are the main causes of cell damage. Platelet cell membrane protectants can reduce the destruction of the platelet cell membrane by the lyophilization process, and the aldehydes and sugars are all good platelet cell membrane protective agents. The addition of trehalose or some other sugars can inhibit the fusion of the phospholipid bilayer in the dry state and reduce the phase transition temperature of its gel phase-liquid crystal phase and protect the phospholipid from phase change or phase separation during lyophilized rehydration, and trehalose can also protect the dehydrated proteins from aggregation or denaturation. In addition to sugars, other solutes such as salt and polymers are added to the lyophilized preservation of platelets, which can be divided into buffer, platelet activation inhibitor, protein protectant, and permeability cryoprotectant. Platelets are suspended in the buffer solution during the incubation, freezing, and rehydration stages of the salt solute which is required to maintain the osmotic pressure balance of the solution inside and outside the cell, and the PH buffer regulates the PH of the solution. The salt concentration in freeze-drying buffer should be as low as possible to avoid protein degeneration during frozen concentration; PH buffer should select less affected [11] such as potassium phosphate, citrate, Tris, and HEPES. Given that platelets are readily activated during thermal incubation for loading trehalose and rehydration, the addition of platelet activation inhibitors to the loading buffer and rehydration solution is required. Platelet inhibitors of activation generally include EGTA, imidazole, prostaglandin E1, and levoarginine. In addition to trehalins, proteins and other macromolecular polymers are also necessary protective agents for cell freeze-drying and preservation. They increase the solution viscosity, improve the solution glass transition temperature, act as a "spatial blocking agent" to inhibit cell or protein aggregation, and act as a shaping agent to improve the stability of drying samples [12]. In order to reduce the ice crystal damage and solute damage to cells during freezing, some scholars have opted to add permeability cryoprotectants such as DMSO and glycerol to the protective agent solution, which can penetrate into the cells, reduce the intracellular and external salt ion concentration, increase the solution viscosity, and reduce the likelihood of intracellular ice crystal formation.

After a large number of experiments, our research group initially determined that those using sodium chloride and potassium chloride as buffer and those including activator inhibitors and protein protective agents were preferred. Using the optimal platelet aggregation rate, the platelet recovery, platelet activation markers PAC-1 and CD62P, and detecting the changes of platelet structure and growth factor after 8 weeks of normal temperature sealing, we found that the FDP was stable and not significantly different from the previous results (Figs. 15.4 and 15.5).

Our research group conducted a preliminary evaluation of the role of lyophilized PRP in promoting trauma healing and hemostasis through animal models. We established a trauma model of whole layer skin defects in SD rats, treated with FDP, PRP, and rhEGF, to evaluate the effect of FDP in

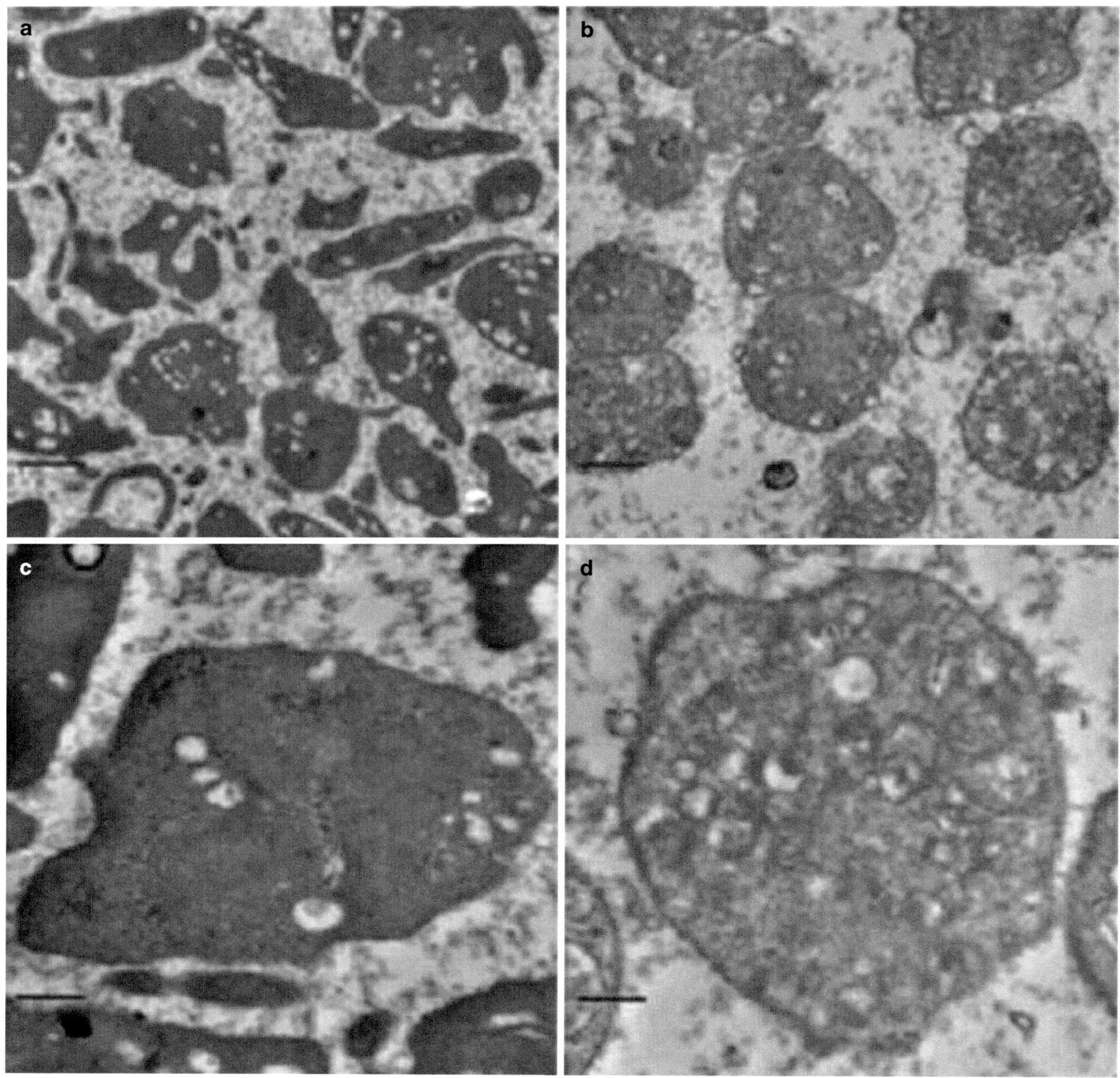

Fig. 15.4 FDP was slightly swollen and stained lightly, but the α-particles, dense granules, lysosomes and open canalicular system did not change significantly compared to the fresh platelets

promoting trauma repair by comparison of trauma healing rates. In the early stage of the experiment (10 days before the wound healing process), the wound healing rate of FDP treatment was similar to that of PRP and rhEGF, both significantly higher than that of blank controls (Fig. 15.6). Pathological section examination suggested that the use of FDP and PRP shortened the period of traumatic inflammation, accelerated wound reepithelialization, and promoted cell proliferation, angiogenesis, and the generation and maturation of collagen fibers (Figs. 15.7 and 15.8). It was inferred that FDP has a similar effect as PRP in promoting the early healing of the acute wound. In the evaluation of hemostasis, a model of New Zealand white rabbit was established to determine the hemostasis effect of FDP and compared with freeze-dried cold precipitation (freeze-dried cryoprecipitate, FDC). The results suggested that FDP was superior to FDC for external wound arteriolar bleeding; and the combination had a more significant hemostatic effect compared with FDP or FDC alone (Fig. 15.9).

In conclusion, the preparation of preserved PRP by freezing or freeze-drying methods can partly retain the activity of therapeutic substances in PRP, giving it a therapeutic effect

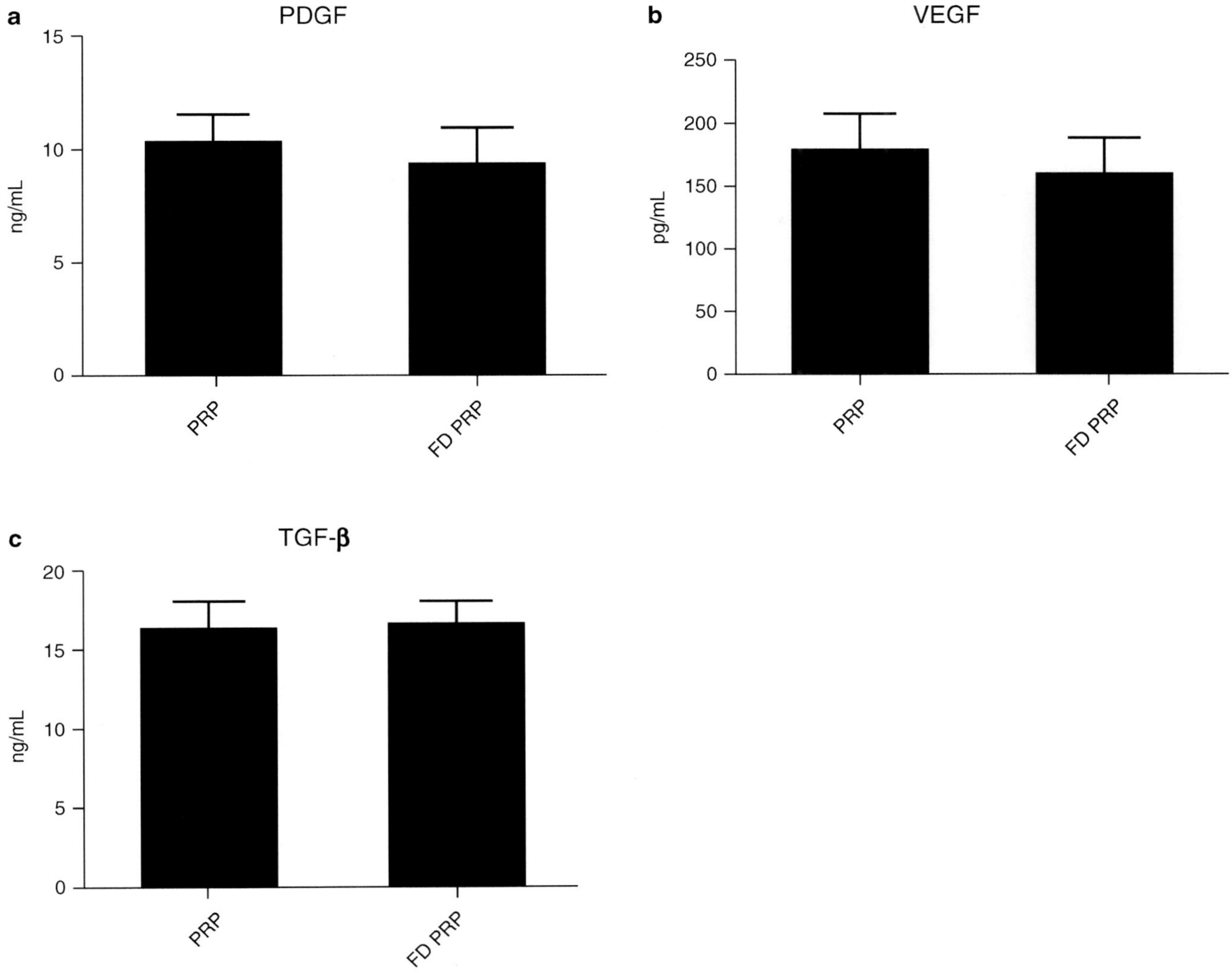

Fig. 15.5 The levels of the growth factors TGF-b, VEGF and PDGF were no significant changes in the levels of these growth factors between before and after freeze-drying

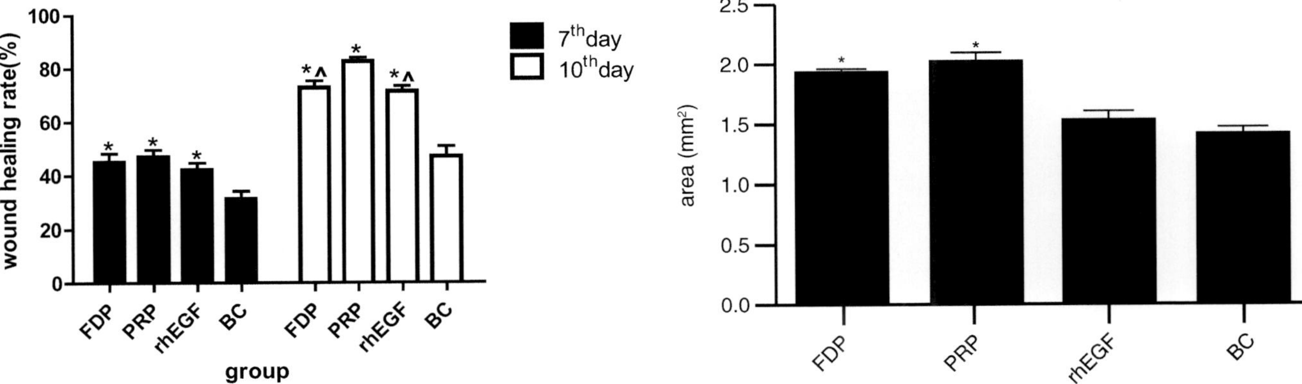

Fig. 15.6 FDP was significantly promote the wound healing rate, and similar to that of PRP and rhEGF in SD rats

Fig. 15.7 FDP significantly promoted collagen fibrillogenesis in the wound tissue and was not significantly different from PRP

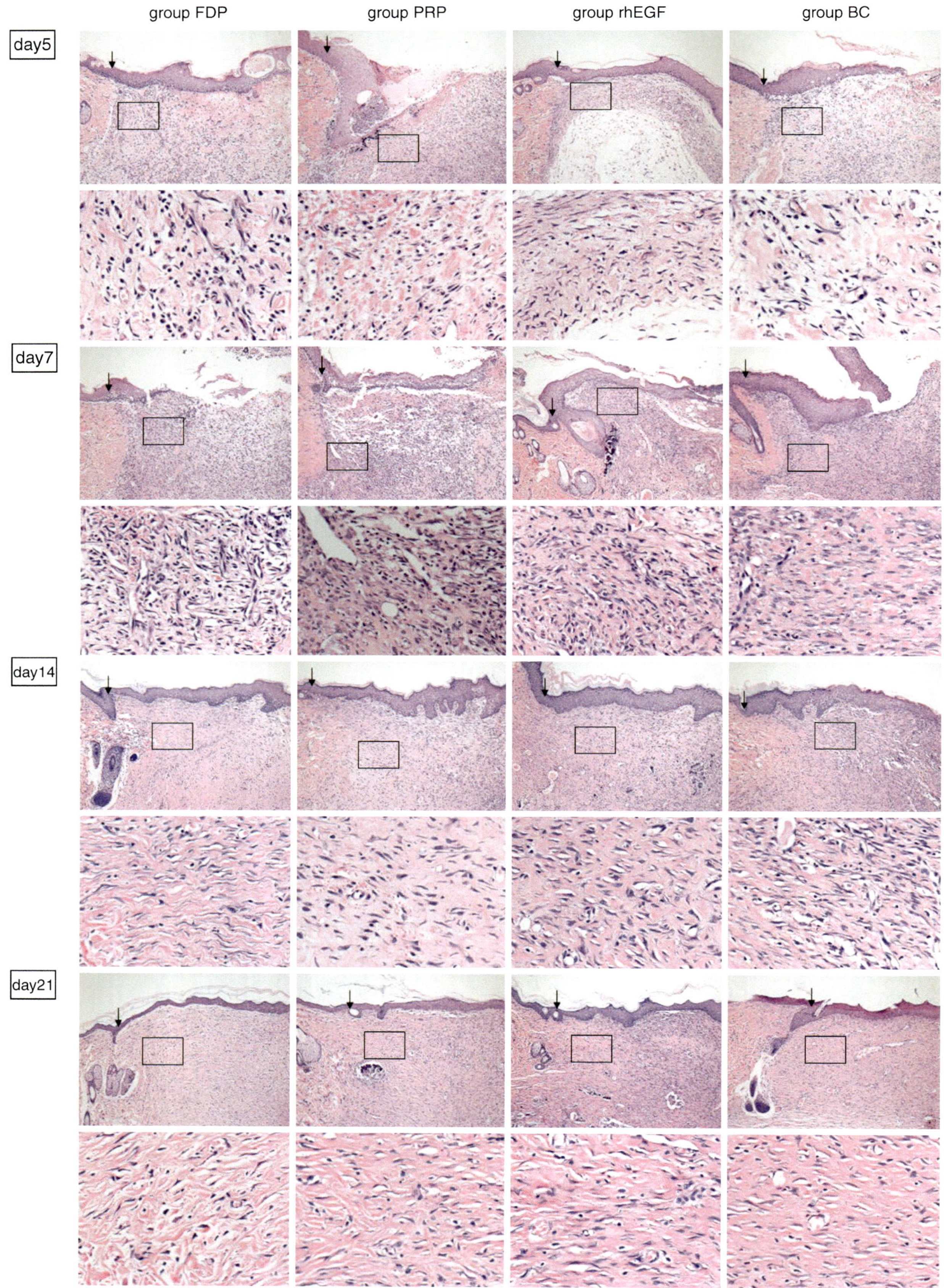

Fig. 15.8 HE staining of wound tissue in SD rats shows FDP shortened the period of traumatic inflammation, accelerated wound reepithelialization, and angiogenesis

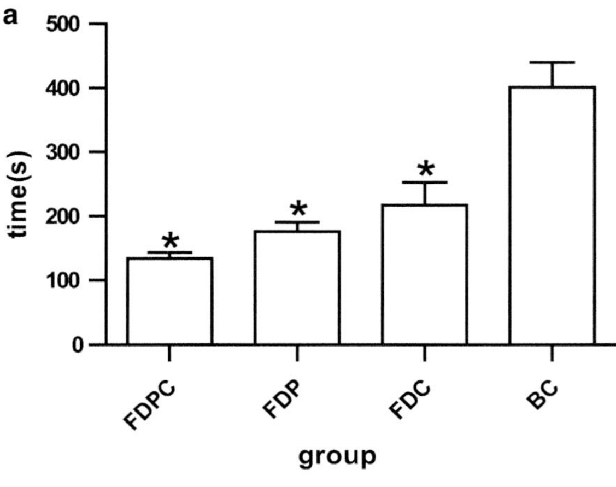

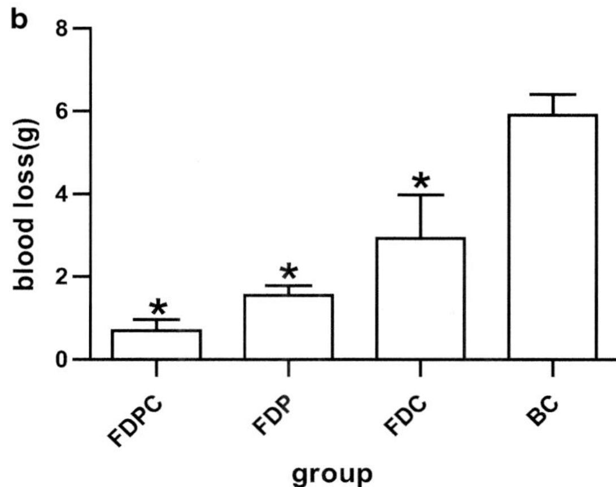

Fig. 15.9 Time of bleeding and blood loss in New Zealand rabbit ear artery (**a**) combination of FDP and FDC shorten the bleeding time (**b**) combination of FDP and FDC reduce blood loss

similar to fresh PRP. Therefore, freezing or freeze-dried preservation preparation methods can expand the scope of clinical application of PRP and increase the convenience and flexibility of PRP use, allowing PRP to serve more patients.

References

1. Sonker A, Dubey A. Determining the effect of preparation and storage: an effort to streamline platelet components as a source of growth factors for clinical application. Transfus Med Hemother. 2015;42:174–80.
2. Bonazza V, Borsani E, Buffoli B, et al. How the different material and shape of the blood collection tube influences the concentrated growth factors production. Microsc Res Tech. 2016;79(12):1173–8.
3. Kushida S, Kakudo N, Morimoto N, et al. Platelet and growth factor concentrations in activated platelet-rich plasma: a comparison of seven commercial separation systems. J Artif Organs. 2014;17(2):186–92.
4. Mazzocca AD, McCarthy MB, Chowaniec DM, et al. Platelet-rich plasma differs according to preparation method and human variability. J Bone Joint Surg Am. 2012;94:308–16.
5. Magalon J, Bausset O, Serratrice N, et al. Characterization and comparison of platelet-rich plasma preparations in a single-donor model. Arthroscopy. 2014;30:629.
6. Suchetha A, Lakshmi P, Divya B, et al. Platelet concentration in platelet concentrates and periodontal regeneration-unscrambling the ambiguity. Contemp Clin Dent. 2015;6(4):510.
7. Piccin A, Di PA, Canzian L, et al. Platelet gel: a new therapeutic tool with great potential. Blood Transfus. 2016;15:333–40.
8. Marx RE. Platelet-rich plasma: evidence to support its use. J Oral Maxillofac Surg. 2004;62(8):1047–8.
9. Jalowiec JM, D'Este M, Bara JJ, et al. An in vitro investigation of PRP-gel as a cell and growth factor delivery vehicle for tissue engineering. Tissue Eng Part C Methods. 2015;22:229–30.
10. Anna R, Ilaria G, Sandra D, et al. Platelet gel-released supernatant modulates the angiogenic capability of human endothelial cells. Blood Transfus. 2008;6(1):12–7.
11. Fajardo V, González I, Dooley J, et al. Identification of an optimal concentration of platelet gel for promoting angiogenesis in human endothelial cells. Transfusion. 2010;49(4):771–8.
12. Fresno L, Fondevila D, Bambo O, et al. Effects of platelet-rich plasma on intestinal wound healing in pigs. Vet J. 2010;185(3):322–7.
13. Tian J, Hang H, Cheng L, et al. Application of standardized platelet-rich plasma in elderly patients with complex wounds. Wound Repair Regen. 2019;27(3):268–76.

Platelet-Rich Plasma and Tissue Regeneration and Rehabilitation

16

Zhuo Xu, Yali Wang, and Biao Cheng

16.1 Definition, Preparation Process, and Component Analysis of PRP

PRP (platelet-rich plasma) is a platelet concentrate extracted from autologous blood by centrifugation. Therefore, PRP not only contains high levels of platelets but also contains complete clotting factors, which the latter usually maintain normal physiological levels. PRP is rich in a series of growth factors, chemokines, cytokines, and other plasma proteins [1].

Nowadays, there is no general consensus regarding the preparation of the optimal PRP for blood component concentrations, and there are lots of various commercial PRP systems on the market. The quality, efficiency, and function of platelets are highly dependent on the protocols that are used to prepare PRP. Numerous attempts have been made to standardize PRP preparation protocols. However, there is considerable variation in methods between studies in terms of rotational speed, centrifugal time, the volume of blood, temperature, and anticoagulant agonists, making it difficult to directly compare the advantages and disadvantages of these different protocols [2]. Usually, before centrifugation, whole blood is collected and mixed with anticoagulant factors to separate red blood cells (RBCs) from platelet-poor plasma and the "buffy layer," which contains concentrated platelets and white blood cells. Platelets are separated in a variety of ways and can then be injected directly into the patient, or be "activated" by the addition of calcium chloride or thrombin, which then causes the platelets to degranulate and release growth factors.

Usually, PRP can be obtained by either a single step of centrifugation or two-step centrifugation procedure. The Anitua plasma-rich growth factor procedure is the most commonly used one-step centrifugation procedure for preparation of PRP, which obtains a PRP suspension with very few white blood cells and lower platelet concentrations, comparing with other PRP preparations [3]. In the most commonly used two-step centrifugation procedure, three layers are formed after centrifugation: the bottom red blood cell (RBC) layer, the middle PRP layer containing leukocytes, and the platelet-poor plasma top layer. Then, the RBCs are removed and centrifuged again to form platelet pellets. Furthermore, there are many commercial PRP kits that help prepare ready-to-use platelet-rich suspensions in a reproducible manner.

In PRP, in addition to higher platelet concentrations and other parameters such as the presence or absence, activation of leukocytes needs to be considered. This will define different types of PRP used in the different pathologies, such as leukocyte-rich PRP, pure PRP, leukocyte-poor PRP, leukocyte- and platelet-rich fibrin, and pure platelet-rich fibrin.

Totally, a standardized procedure is lacking in application in regeneration medicine. Such variables can finally influence the clinical efficacies of individual PRP preparations. Thus, studies on PRP preparations should highlight the concentration of PRP components and the optimal concentration of platelets, white blood cells, and growth factors for regenerative medicine.

16.2 History and Development of PRP in the Field of Regeneration

PRP begins with the discovery of plate growth factors and is developed by fibrin glue. The fibrin glue was extracted from autologous or allogeneic plasma by centrifugal method and contains high concentrations of fibrinogen, which can be

Z. Xu (✉)
Department of Rehabilitation Medicine, China-Japan Union Hospital, Jilin University, Changchun, China
e-mail: xuzhuo@jlu.edu.cn

Y. Wang
Department of Blood Transfusion, China-Japan Union Hospital, Jilin University, Changchun, China

B. Cheng
Department of Burn & Plastic Surgery, General Hospital of Southern Theater Command, Guangzhou, China

B. Cheng, X. Fu (eds.), *Platelet-Rich Plasma in Tissue Repair and Regeneration*, https://doi.org/10.1007/978-981-99-3193-4_16

used to seal wounds and stop bleeding, strengthen wound contraction, and promote wound healing.

Most of the early fibrin glue was extracted from allogeneic blood in the blood bank. The first application of fibrin glue in maxillofacial surgery in 1982 achieved good clinical results. However, with the rejection of allogeneic fibrin glue, the complexity of the production process, and the high cost of autologous fibrin glue and other factors, people have gradually begun to look for and study autologous, simplified, and more effective alternatives.

Before the 1970s, platelets were thought to have only blood clotting functions. ROSS discovered that the supernatant after platelet activation can accelerate cell mitosis and promote cell proliferation in 1974. In 1978, Witte named this factor, which promotes cell proliferation, as PDGF. In the following 20 years, growth factors in platelets were successively discovered, such as TGF-β in 1983, IGF-1 in 1989, and bFGF in 1993. Around 1990, some scholars used platelet concentrate to treat chronic wounds successfully, which established a good start for the widespread application of PRP.

With the gradual deepening of research on platelets, the consensus is that platelets contain a variety of growth factors, which can be used to promote tissue repair and tissue regeneration. These growth factors mainly include transforming growth factor (TGF-β), platelet-derived growth factor (PDGF), vascular endothelial growth factor (VEGF), insulin growth factor (IGF-1), epidermal growth factor (EGF), etc.

Compared with fibrin glue, PRP is simple to operate, derives from autologic body, and has nonimmune rejection response and the possibility of disease transmission. It contains a large number of high concentrations of growth factors which theoretically supports that PRP can more effectively promote bone and soft tissue repair and regeneration.

The earliest research reports show that Witman and Marx applied PRP to repair bone tissue in 1997 and 1998, respectively. PRP was then mainly used in the musculoskeletal field of sports injury. With its application in professional athletes, PRP has been widely used in this field. Other medical fields that also use PRP are cardiac surgery, pediatric surgery, gynecology, urology, orthopedics, and ophthalmology.

16.3 The Status and Clinical Applications of PRP in the Field of Regeneration

Recently, PRP has been broadly explored and studied in regenerative medicine. It contains many important growth factors that affect wound healing, so it can greatly promote tissue repair. Bleeding can be effectively reduced by using PRP during surgery, meanwhile enhancing soft tissue healing and bone regeneration. In addition, the use of PRP can reduce the cost of regenerative therapy. Therefore, PRP is becoming more and more popular in the medical field, especially in the field of regenerative medicine.

16.3.1 Applications of PRP in Wound Healing

Generally, wound healing is one of the complex and normal processes in human beings, involving various signal transduction pathways activated by different cellular and chemical factors. Usually, the process of wound healing is divided into four distinct phases, hemostasis, inflammation, proliferation or re-epithelialization, and remodeling or maturation, which are regulated by many factors. The biological factors that play a vital role in the healing process of platelets released in PRP include fibrin as coagulants and other factors involved in different stages including TGF-β1, interleukin-1 (IL-1), platelet-derived epidermal growth factor (PDEGF), IGF-2, etc. Many of these biological factors can induce cell proliferation and division by attracting undifferentiated cells to form a new matrix, thereby promoting wound healing. In addition, by inhibiting cytokine secretion to reduce inflammation, PRP can improve the healing, regeneration, re-epithelialization, and angiogenesis of damaged and injured tissues. Another function of PRP is their defense mechanism against certain bacteria at the wound site, thereby reducing microbial infections.

PRP repairs wound healing and has shown significant repair effects in clinical treatment. In a randomized controlled trial, the healing time for the treatment of diabetic foot ulcers with PRP gel was significantly shorter compared with those in the control group. In addition, studies on application of autologous PRP support its beneficial and safe role in chronic wound healing and provide accumulating evidence that it can actually reverse the trends of nonhealing. After trauma and when combined with hyaluronic acid, PRP promotes the healing of ulcers and the rapid re-epithelialization of lower extremity wounds through bone exposure, which can be used as an effective cell growth scaffold to cover the exposed tendons of acute and chronic open wounds of the foot and ankles. Suthar et al. found that PRP treatment can decrease wound size, pain, and inflammation in 23 patients with nonhealing ulcers. Furthermore, in a study of 150 patients with diabetes-induced foot ulcers by Babaei, PRP treatment after 4 weeks has been shown to reduce wound size and improve healthy budding tissue formation. Prabhu's study demonstrated that the treatment with PRP resulted in the healing of 81.73% of patients, while 12.5% of cases presented healing after skin grafting [4, 5]. Recently, Wang et al. found PRP loaded with antibiotics as an affiliated treatment for infected bone defects by combining wound healing property and antibacterial activity [6]. Totally, PRP might be a safe and effective treatment method that can improve the healing rate of wounds.

16.3.2 Application of PRP in Bone Fracture Healing

Bone is a key and primary component of the body's motor system and is also unique and dynamic scaffold organ. Segmental bone defects are usually caused by open fractures, tumor resection, and osteomyelitis debridement [7]. Furthermore, damage related to the blood circulation around the site of fracture can lead to the failure of repairing and critical-size-long bone defects. These defects usually lead to nonunion or delayed healing of the bone in the clinic, which represents the transformation of acute injury to chronic bone disease. Therefore, repairing bone defects is a clinical challenge that needs to be overcome [8]. The bone healing process mainly consists of three stages: the early inflammatory stage [9], the repair stage, and the late remodeling stage. The condition of the blood vessel at the fracture site is critical to determining the success of the healing during bone healing process [10]. Accumulating data has demonstrated that PRP's remarkable healing power is attributed to the growth factors and cytokines that it contains, which play a key role in inflammation and promote the differentiation of bone marrow mesenchymal stem cells in the microenvironment of the reconstruction defect site. Therefore, PRP is particularly useful for preventing nonunion and delayed connection.

In clinical studies, platelet-rich products can significantly promote fusion in spinal surgery and have been successfully used to treat clavicle nonunion [11, 12]. PRP reduces the time required for bone regeneration of intraosseous defects and was used to treat osteonecrosis of the mandible caused by radiotherapy [13–15]. Furthermore, Liebergall et al. found that the fracture healing time was shorter by using the PRP combined with MSC and considered this treatment to be a safe and effective method [16]. Moreover, multiple studies have showed that the application of PRP in combination with biomaterial scaffolds is an advantageous approach to immobilize large and highly concentrated amounts of bioactive growth factors, thereby providing an optimized and favorable microenvironment for tissue regeneration [17]. Studies also showed that PRP-based tissue engineering has demonstrated significant advantages and promise for the treatment of bone and articular cartilage defects [18, 19]. Collected, the application of PRP in bone fracture healing has obtained good results.

16.3.3 The Application of PRP in Aesthetic and Regenerative Medicine.

In recent years, the use of PRP in aesthetic and beauty interventions has been steadily increasing. A large number of studies have shown that PRP treatment has shown its broad prospects in safe and effective aesthetic and cosmetic interventions, including skin rejuvenation, hand rejuvenation, and hair repair [20].

In terms of skin and facial rejuvenation, various factors, including multiple growth factors and cytokines, are crucial in the process of cell regeneration and rejuvenation in the skin, so an effective antiaging strategy will be to increase the content of these factors in the skin. Processes such as wound healing and cell replacement in the facial epidermis diminish with age, leading to sagging and wrinkling of the skin. The most important contributor to skin aging is the reduction of fibroblast and collagen production [21]. In addition, during the skin aging process, the interaction between fibroblasts and dermal mast cells, epidermal keratinocytes, and adipocytes is also vital [22]. These intercellular spaces are filled with extracellular matrix (ECM) proteins, glycoproteins, cytokines, and growth factors, which maintain their integrity and youthful appearance via enhancing skin cell interactions [23]. The process of skin cell replacement requires a variety of growth factors and cytokines to continuously stimulate the synthesis of collagen. The degradation of ECM and subsequent skin aging will gradually occur with aging. The degradation of ECM and subsequent skin aging will gradually occur in the process of aging. As an important source of growth factors, cytokines, and other bioactive substances related to tissue regeneration and remodeling, PRP is an effective strategy to restore skin vitality. PRP can significantly increase the expression of matrix metalloproteinase (MMP) protein, finally causing ECM remodeling and improving skin cell proliferation and differentiation [24]. In addition, PRP also can increase the secretion and release of hyaluronic acid, which promotes skin firming and improves its elasticity through hydration [25]. Recently, a single-center, prospective, uncontrolled study evaluated the efficacy of injectable platelet-rich fibrin on facial skin rejuvenation through using an objective skin analysis system and verified the outcome indicators reported by patients. The study included 11 healthy female individuals who were given injectable platelet-rich fibrin intradermal injections in 3 facial areas every month for 3 months. During the three-month follow-up, the spots and pores on the skin surface improved significantly. Other variables, such as skin texture, wrinkles, UV spots, and porphyrin, showed numerical improvements. Therefore, this study showed that intradermal injection of platelet-rich fibrin is a safe intervention, which is related to the objective beauty of the facial skin and improved patient satisfaction [26].

Furthermore, accumulating data has confirmed that PRP therapy is an effective choice for treating hair loss in both men and women through stimulating the hair follicles, increasing the number of hairs, hair growth, and hair thickening. For example, Shapiro and colleagues performed a randomized, placebo-controlled, split-scalp clinical study to evaluate the treatment effects of PRP on hair restoration and regrowth [27]. They found that the hair density in the PRP-treated area was significantly increased compared with baseline at all visits. However, there was no significant difference in hair density change between the PRP-treated and placebo-treated groups. Recently, Zhou and colleagues also found that autologous activated PRP can promote hair growth, and PRP injection is a safe and effective method for the treatment of androgenetic alopecia [28].

In regard to hand rejuvenation, PRP injections can significantly stimulate angiogenesis, and the synthesis of collagen provides a firm, smooth, and youthful appearance. However, knowledge on the clinical studies in this area are very limited.

16.3.4 The Application of PRP in the Tendons, Ligament, and Muscle

The application of PRP in clinical trials to treat the injuries of the ligament, muscle, and tendon has shown significant clinical effects. Tendon stem cells play a critical function in tendon regeneration. When activated, platelets release a variety of growth factors that promote the proliferation, growth, and differentiation of tendon stem cells and produce tenocytes and abundant collagen. In a study evaluating the application of PRP to enhance the repair of complete Achilles tendon tears, Sanchez et al. found that six PRP-treated athletes who underwent open suture repair took significantly less time to take light running and return to training activities compared to a control group that underwent conventional surgery [29]. PRP has also been shown to reduce pain in patients with chronic tendinopathy, with effects lasting at least 2 years from the start of treatment [30]. The benefit of PRP as a second-line, nonsurgical treatment for elbow tendinopathy resistant to physical therapy was further demonstrated in a prospective randomized trial [31]. A clinical trial involving PRP injections for Achilles tendinopathy showed, under ultrasound guidance, that tendon thickness could be increased with PRP relative to the tendon thickness observed in the placebo group [32]. In another clinical trial, the arthroscopic hip arthroplasty group treated with PRP injections had significantly changed tissue characteristics of the rotator cuff, with decreased cellularity and vascularity, along with increased apoptosis [33]. A study of 34 athletes treated for ulnar lateral ligament anterior bundle injury showed that 88% of these athletes returned to sport after an average of 12 weeks without any complaints [34]. Anterior cruciate ligament (ACL) reconstruction treated with PRP therapy is another high-profile application of PRP. Figueroa et al. reported that PRP may have a role in enhancing ACL reconstruction [35]. Furthermore, Vogrin et al. found that ACL grafts treated with platelet gels had significantly higher levels of vascularization at the osseous ligament interface 4–6 weeks postoperatively compared to control grafts [36, 37]. However, some of the data showed that PRP is not beneficial alongside ACL reconstruction. For example, Everhart et al. found that PRP provides no benefit for meniscal repairs with ACL reconstruction.

Regarding the application of PRP in the treatment of acute muscle injuries, a trial study conducted on patients undergoing arthroscopic rotator cuff repair showed that intraoperative use of PRP significantly enhanced function and reduced pain, with no adverse reactions. Moreover, athletes with small muscle tears achieved a full recovery in half of the expected time after receiving PRP. Recently, Mohamad et al. evaluated the clinical effects of PRP in the treatment of acute grade-2 hamstring tear in high-performance athletes, which will help to identify the most effective and best protocol of PRP application for muscle injuries [38].

16.3.5 The Application of PRP in Articular Cartilage Lesions and Osteoarthritis

Articular cartilage disease and osteoarthritis are the most common diseases in orthopedic department. Changes in synovial and synovial fluid composition lead to inadequate healing associated with inflammation and vascular pathology, apoptosis, meniscal changes, bone reconstruction, and subchondral sclerosis, resulting in periodic progressive joint degeneration and ultimately osteoarthritis (OA). OA is unique in terms of joint biology, steady-state, metalloproteinase, and inflammatory cytokine levels and has an impact on patient symptoms [39]. The clinical application of PRP in cartilage injury mainly involves patients with knee or hip OA. In 14 randomized clinical trials, Shen et al. performed a meta-analysis and showed that multiple injections of PRP improved Western Ontario and McMaster Universities Osteoarthritis Index (WOMAC) scores at 3-, 6-, and 12-month follow-ups. Finally, their results have shown that PRP is more effective in patients with OA based on pain relief and patient-reported outcomes than other alternative injections [40]. Furthermore, Riboh et al. performed a meta-analysis and compared LP-PRP and LR-PRP in the treatment of knee OA; they found that compared with hyaluronic acid or placebo, LP-PRP injection can significantly improve WOMAC scores [41].

In terms of PRP application to treat hip OA, several studies have demonstrated that PRP initially has better pain reduction compared to hyaluronic acid (HA), and the initial advantage appears to diminish over time as PRP and HA have very similar efficacy up to 12 months of treatment. For example, Dallari et al. evaluated the effects of PRP and HA injections for hip OA and also compared the effects of a combination of PRP and HA injections with those of injections alone. They found that the PRP group had the lowest VAS scores at 2-, 6-, and 14-month follow-ups and also had significantly better WOMAC scores at 2 and 6 months but not at 12 months. Moreover, Di Sante et al. found that compared with HA treatment group for OA, the PRP treatment group for OA had the lower VAS scores at 4 weeks but not at 16 weeks, suggesting an initial but not sustained reduction in pain [42]. Collectedly, PRP may be effective for early and temporary pain relief in hip OA, and overall is very similar to the efficacy of HA injections [43].

16.3.6 The Application of PRP in Regenerative Dentistry

PRP has been extensively used in many dental regeneration procedures with promising results, including periodontal regeneration procedures, oral and maxillofacial surgery, sinus floor augmentation, and bone remodeling.

The goal of periodontal regenerative surgery is to promote new bone formation by grafting material to repair bone defects and restore the anatomical shape of the alveolar bone in order to achieve desired bone regeneration or newly attached healing. PRP is thought to improve the predictability and success of periodontal regenerative surgery. The delivery of autologous platelets to the periodontal wound during the healing process after exogenous application of PRP increases the concentration of local growth factors, which in turn exerts a regulatory effect on the steady state of periodontal tissues, alters the response of the periodontal soft and hard tissues, and improves the healing effect [2]. Due to the limited space provision potential of PRP, PRP must be used in combination with bone grafts or substitutes. Multiple data has shown that the use of PRP in periodontal regenerative surgery has produced controversial results ranging from significant to invalid. For example, Bhardwaj and colleagues demonstrated that the application of PRP to bone grafting appears to be beneficial for treatment of human periodontal intraosseous bone defects [44]. Moreover, another data showed that the addition of PRP to bone graft material did not significantly increase positive results, independent of barrier or graft type. PRP polypeptide proteins do not increase the clinical regenerative effects of enamel matrix proteins [45].

Regarding the application of PRP in the oral and maxillofacial surgery, it opens up new ways and methods for tissue repair and regeneration in oral surgery. The main purpose of using PRP in oral surgery is to regenerate new tissue during the healing process. Platelets in PRP have been shown to release large amounts of growth factors that attract and recruit repair cells and facilitate several biological processes required for soft tissue repair and alveolar bone regeneration. A study on the healing of extraction sockets by Alissa and colleagues showed that compared with the control group, patients treated with PRP had significantly reduced postoperative pain and clinically significant soft tissue healing. Moreover, Prataap's study found that autologous PRP could improve soft tissue healing, relieve pain, and reduce the incidence of alveolar osteitis in the extraction socket [46]. Additionally, Ruktowski"s study demonstrated that the radiographic density over baseline level after tooth extraction has a significant increase [47].

In terms of PRP application to sinus floor augmentation and bone remodeling, this is still controversial about the beneficial application of PRP as an auxiliary material for bone replacement material for sinus floor eminence surgery. For instance, Torres' study found that PRP can increase the regeneration potential of organic bovine bone via increasing the amount of new bone formation [48]. Stumbras' study also found that the combination of PRP with bone graft materials can effectively increase the bone formation and blood vessels of the maxillary sinus floor elevation [49]. Nikolidakis' study, however, showed that the addition of PRP to β-tricalcium phosphate grafts did not provide an additional contribution to new bone formation [50].

16.3.7 Problems and Challenges of PRP in Clinical Applications of Regeneration Medicine

Though much progress has been made on PRP in clinical applications of regeneration medicine, the study and application of PRP also face enormous challenges, and there are still some questions regarding PRP that need further exploration in future research.

First, the optimal processing time of PRP and method of separating platelets and leukocytes, as well as the optimal concentration of PRP for maximum beneficial effects, are still unknown. Multiple papers attempt to characterize and classify the multiple technologies available on the market based on preparation (including centrifugation speed, optimal relative centrifugal force and centrifugation time, use of anticoagulants), contents (e.g., platelets, leukocytes, and growth factors), and application. Nowadays, these aspects described above are strongly discussed in the growing literature, and no consensus has yet been reached [51].

Second, the challenge of optimizing PRP is to identify the main bioactive components responsible for beneficial clinical outcomes. In fact, we should consider neither the platelets themselves nor the growth factors of platelets but rather the synergistic effects of both. For example, in vivo degranulation of platelets is considered essential for the progressive release of growth factors and bioactive proteins, which are important roles in tendon healing. Therefore, in the context of sports regenerative medicine, the ability of preparation to preserve the greatest number of resting and activatable platelets may be of specific advantage for sports regenerative recovery and healing [51].

Third, the presence or absence of platelet activators and the type of activator used are important factors to document. How platelets are applied to the tissue will undoubtedly influence the tissue response. For example, an exogenous platelet activator may be required to generate clots in some procedures, whereas endogenous platelet activation without the use of external coagulation factors may be desirable in other indications. In addition to documenting the composition of the final PRP product, it is also important to document the delivery technique and whether other factors are assigned to the tissue sites [52].

Fourth, since the use of certain types of PRP may be important in the administration of different conditions, all commercial kits should be validated for cells and PRP types, but this is not always the case. Furthermore, studies have shown that the pH of the sample may be decreased due to the addition of citrate to the blood collected, and it was discussed whether the pH of the resulting PRP affects platelet function and therefore whether the produced PRP should be "buffered" [53].

Fifth, a potential limitation to prepare PRP by using the method of centrifugation is the risk of bacterial contamination during transfer between tubes. Therefore, the transfer should be performed in a laminar flow hood to reduce the opportunity of bacterial contamination.

Sixth, the role of WBC in PRP therapy remains unclear in the literature. There are insufficient data in the clinical trial to determine whether WBCs are beneficial for PRP treatment in regeneration medicine. In terms of their WBC content, additional studies are necessary to optimize PRP. Some studies found that PRP with higher WBC concentrations can impede tissue regeneration and healing. Moreover, the presence of WBCs in PRP is closely associated with increased scar tissue and collagen degradation ex vivo. High concentrations of WBCs may negatively affect the matrix production in tendons. However, some studies suggest that the presence of WBCs in PRP may also be beneficial, as WBCs can increase growth factor production. PRP containing a sufficient number of WBCs is recommended for another therapeutic purpose, as WBCs trigger growth factor secretion from tissues treated with PRP [54].

Seventh, nowadays, multiple commercially available kit claimed to yield consistent liquid end products and higher platelet count than manual laboratory preparation. However, the difference in the concentration of platelets and other blood components between commercial PRP kits affects the clinical treatment effect. Furthermore, these commercial kits are expensive. Therefore, commercial PRP kits for clinical use need to be standardized.

Eighth, a variety of reports have revealed various controversial results regarding the therapeutic effects of PRP in regenerative medicine. Indeed, many factors influence the outcome of regenerative treatment, including study design, clinical parameters, and the period of observation. Moreover, when combined with different graft materials, the additional role of PRP has been controversial in a portion of controlled clinical studies. Therefore, when using PRP as a clinical regenerative treatment option, consideration should be given to appropriate study designs, carefully identifying surgical procedures, and increased observation time.

Ninth, abundant high-quality level evidence to PRP efficacy in regeneration medicine is currently lacking, for example, the application of PRP to treat ACL reconstruction and OA of the hip and knee. In particular, the molecular mechanisms by which PRP plays a role in tissue regeneration are not fully understood. Thus, there are multiple unknown properties and mechanisms waiting to be discovered [55].

Taken together, although many challenges and questions remain unanswered with respect to treatment of PRP in regeneration medicine, we believe, accompanied by the development of research strategies, future multicenter studies of the effects of PRP over multiple follow-ups and the interactions of growth factor must contribute to understanding of PRP in regeneration medicine.

References

1. Alves R, Grimalt R. A review of platelet-rich plasma: history, biology, mechanism of action, and classification. Skin Appendage Disord. 2018;4:18–24.
2. Xu J, Gou L, Zhang P, Li H, Qiu S. Platelet-rich plasma and regenerative dentistry. Aust Dent J. 2020;65:131–42.
3. Franchini M, Cruciani M, Mengoli C, Marano G, Pupella S, Veropalumbo E, Masiello F, Pati I, Vaglio S, Liumbruno GM. Efficacy of platelet-rich plasma as conservative treatment in orthopaedics: a systematic review and meta-analysis. Blood Transfus. 2018;16:502–13.
4. Babaei V, Afradi H, Gohardani HZ, Nasseri F, Azarafza M, Teimourian S. Management of chronic diabetic foot ulcers using platelet-rich plasma. J Wound Care. 2017;26:784–7.
5. Prabhu R, Vijayakumar C, Bosco Chandra AA, Balagurunathan K, Kalaiarasi R, Venkatesan K, Santosh Raja E, T S. Efficacy of Homologous. Platelet-rich plasma dressing in chronic non-healing ulcers: an observational study. Cureus. 2018;10:e2145.
6. Wang S, Li Y, Li S, Yang J, Tang R, Li X, Li L, Fei J. Platelet-rich plasma loaded with antibiotics as an affiliated treatment for infected bone defect by combining wound healing property and antibacterial activity. Platelets. 2020;32:1–13.
7. Di Martino A, Di Matteo B, Papio T, Tentoni F, Selleri F, Cenacchi A, Kon E, Filardo G. Platelet-rich plasma versus hyaluronic acid injections for the treatment of knee osteoarthritis: results at 5 years of a double-blind, randomized controlled trial. Am J Sports Med. 2019;47:347–54.
8. Fang J, Jiang W, Zhu Y, Hu Y, Zhao Y, Song X, Zhao J, Wang Y, Zhang W, Peng J. Platelet-rich plasma therapy in the treatment of diseases associated with orthopedic injuries. Tissue Eng Part B Rev. 2020;26:571.
9. Kasten P, Beverungen M, Lorenz H, Wieland J, Fehr M, Geiger F. Comparison of platelet-rich plasma and VEGF-transfected mesenchymal stem cells on vascularization and bone formation in a critical-size bone defect. Cells Tissues Organs. 2012;196:523–33.
10. Schlundt C, Bucher CH, Tsitsilonis S, Schell H, Duda GN, Schmidt-Bleek K. Clinical and research approaches to treat non-union fracture. Curr Osteoporos Rep. 2018;16:155–68.
11. Hartmann EK, Heintel T, Morrison RH, Weckbach A. Influence of platelet-rich plasma on the anterior fusion in spinal injuries: a qualitative and quantitative analysis using computer tomography. Arch Orthop Trauma Surg. 2010;130:909–14.
12. Seijas R, Santana-Suarez RY, Garcia-Balletbo M, Cusco X, Ares O, Cugat R. Delayed union of the clavicle treated with plasma rich in growth factors. Acta Orthop Belg. 2010;76:689–93.

13. Nagaveni NB, Praveen RB, Umashankar KV, Pranav B, Sreedevi R, Radhika NB. Efficacy of platelet-rich-plasma (PRP) in bone regeneration after cyst enucleation in pediatric patients—a clinical study. J Clin Pediatr Dent. 2010;35:81–7.
14. Scala M, Gipponi M, Mereu P, Strada P, Corvo R, Muraglia A, Massa M, Bertoglio S, Santi P, Cafiero F. Regeneration of mandibular osteoradionecrosis defect with platelet rich plasma gel. In Vivo. 2010;24:889–93.
15. Alsousou J, Ali A, Willett K, Harrison P. The role of platelet-rich plasma in tissue regeneration. Platelets. 2013;24:173–82.
16. Liebergall M, Schroeder J, Mosheiff R, Gazit Z, Yoram Z, Rasooly L, Daskal A, Khoury A, Weil Y, Beyth S. Stem cell-based therapy for prevention of delayed fracture union: a randomized and prospective preliminary study. Mol Ther. 2013;21:1631–8.
17. Rohman G, Langueh C, Ramtani S, Lataillade JJ, Lutomski D, Senni K, Changotade S. The use of platelet-rich plasma to promote cell recruitment into low-molecular-weight Fucoidan-functionalized poly (Ester-urea-urethane) scaffolds for soft-tissue engineering. Polymers (Basel). 2019;11:11.
18. Zhang ZY, Huang AW, Fan JJ, Wei K, Jin D, Chen B, Li D, Bi L, Wang J, Pei G. The potential use of allogeneic platelet-rich plasma for large bone defect treatment: immunogenicity and defect healing efficacy. Cell Transplant. 2013;22:175–87.
19. Kazem-Arki M, Kabiri M, Rad I, Roodbari NH, Hosseinpoor H, Mirzaei S, Parivar K, Hanaee-Ahvaz H. Enhancement of osteogenic differentiation of adipose-derived stem cells by PRP modified nanofibrous scaffold. Cytotechnology. 2018;70:1487–98.
20. Samadi P, Sheykhhasan M, Khoshinani HM. The use of platelet-rich plasma in aesthetic and regenerative medicine: a comprehensive review. Aesthet Plast Surg. 2019;43:803–14.
21. Kim DH, Je YJ, Kim CD, Lee YH, Seo YJ, Lee JH, Lee Y. Can platelet-rich plasma be used for skin rejuvenation? Evaluation of effects of platelet-rich plasma on human dermal fibroblast. Ann Dermatol. 2011;23:424–31.
22. Mine S, Fortunel NO, Pageon H, Asselineau D. Aging alters functionally human dermal papillary fibroblasts but not reticular fibroblasts: a new view of skin morphogenesis and aging. PLoS One. 2008;3:e4066.
23. Hsu YC, Li L, Fuchs E. Emerging interactions between skin stem cells and their niches. Nat Med. 2014;20:847–56.
24. Browning SR, Weiser AM, Woolf N, Golish SR, SanGiovanni TP, Scuderi GJ, Carballo C, Hanna LS. Platelet-rich plasma increases matrix metalloproteinases in cultures of human synovial fibroblasts. J Bone Joint Surg Am. 2012;94:e1721–7.
25. Papakonstantinou E, Roth M, Karakiulakis G. Hyaluronic acid: a key molecule in skin aging. Dermatoendocrinol. 2012;4:253–8.
26. Hassan H, Quinlan DJ, Ghanem A. Injectable platelet-rich fibrin for facial rejuvenation: a prospective, single-center study. J Cosmet Dermatol. 2020;19:3213.
27. Shapiro J, Ho A, Sukhdeo K, Yin L, Lo SK. Evaluation of platelet-rich plasma as a treatment for androgenetic alopecia: a randomized controlled trial. J Am Acad Dermatol. 2020;83:1298–303.
28. Zhou Y, Liu Q, Bai Y, Yang K, Ye Y, Wu K, Huang J, Zhang Y, Zhang X, Thianthanyakij T, Wang J, Zhu Y, Lin J, Wu W. Autologous activated platelet-rich plasma in hair growth: a pilot study in male androgenetic alopecia with in vitro bioactivity investigation. J Cosmet Dermatol. 2020;20:1221.
29. Gaweda K, Tarczynska M, Krzyzanowski W. Treatment of Achilles tendinopathy with platelet-rich plasma. Int J Sports Med. 2010;31:577–83.
30. Volpi P, Quaglia A, Schoenhuber H, Melegati G, Corsi MM, Banfi G, de Girolamo L. Growth factors in the management of sport-induced tendinopathies: results after 24 months from treatment. A pilot study. J Sports Med Phys Fitness. 2010;50:494–500.
31. de Vos RJ, Weir A, van Schie HT, Bierma-Zeinstra SM, Verhaar JA, Weinans H, Tol JL. Platelet-rich plasma injection for chronic achilles tendinopathy: a randomized controlled trial. JAMA. 2010;303:144–9.
32. Dallari D, Stagni C, Rani N, Sabbioni G, Pelotti P, Torricelli P, Tschon M, Giavaresi G. Ultrasound-guided injection of platelet-rich plasma and hyaluronic acid, separately and in combination, for hip osteoarthritis: a randomized controlled study. Am J Sports Med. 2016;44:664–71.
33. Carr AJ, Murphy R, Dakin SG, Rombach I, Wheway K, Watkins B, Franklin SL. Platelet-rich plasma injection with arthroscopic Acromioplasty for chronic rotator cuff tendinopathy: a randomized controlled trial. Am J Sports Med. 2015;43:2891–7.
34. Podesta L, Crow SA, Volkmer D, Bert T, Yocum LA. Treatment of partial ulnar collateral ligament tears in the elbow with platelet-rich plasma. Am J Sports Med. 2013;41:1689–94.
35. Figueroa D, Figueroa F, Calvo R, Vaisman A, Ahumada X, Arellano S. Platelet-rich plasma use in anterior cruciate ligament surgery: systematic review of the literature. Arthroscopy. 2015;31:981–8.
36. Vogrin M, Rupreht M, Dinevski D, Haspl M, Kuhta M, Jevsek M, Knezevic M, Rozman P. Effects of a platelet gel on early graft revascularization after anterior cruciate ligament reconstruction: a prospective, randomized, double-blind, clinical trial. Eur Surg Res. 2010;45:77–85.
37. Davey MS, Hurley ET, Withers D, Moran R, Moran CJ. Anterior cruciate ligament reconstruction with platelet-rich plasma: a systematic review of randomized control trials. Arthroscopy. 2020;36:1204–10.
38. Hamid MSA, Hussein KH, Helmi Salim AM, Puji A, Mat Yatim R, Yong CC, Sheng TWY. Study protocol for a double-blind, randomised placebo-controlled trial evaluating clinical effects of platelet-rich plasma injection for acute grade-2 hamstring tear among high performance athletes. BMJ Open. 2020;10:e039105.
39. Le ADK, Enweze L, DeBaun MR, Dragoo JL. Current clinical recommendations for use of platelet-rich plasma. Curr Rev Musculoskelet Med. 2018;11:624–34.
40. Shen L, Yuan T, Chen S, Xie X, Zhang C. The temporal effect of platelet-rich plasma on pain and physical function in the treatment of knee osteoarthritis: systematic review and meta-analysis of randomized controlled trials. J Orthop Surg Res. 2017;12:16.
41. Riboh JC, Saltzman BM, Yanke AB, Fortier L, Cole BJ. Effect of leukocyte concentration on the efficacy of platelet-rich plasma in the treatment of knee osteoarthritis. Am J Sports Med. 2016;44:792–800.
42. Di Sante L, Villani C, Santilli V, Valeo M, Bologna E, Imparato L, Paoloni M, Iagnocco A. Intra-articular hyaluronic acid vs platelet-rich plasma in the treatment of hip osteoarthritis. Med Ultrason. 2016;18:463–8.
43. Le ADK, Enweze L, DeBaun MR, Dragoo JL. Platelet-rich plasma. Clin Sports Med. 2019;38:17–44.
44. Kaushick BT, Jayakumar ND, Padmalatha O, Varghese S. Treatment of human periodontal infrabony defects with hydroxyapatite + beta tricalcium phosphate bone graft alone and in combination with platelet rich plasma: a randomized clinical trial. Indian J Dent Res. 2011;22:505–10.
45. Dori F. Effect of combined therapeutic methods on healing of periodontal vertical bone defects in regenerative surgery. Orv Hetil. 2009;150:517–22.
46. Prataap N, Sunil PM, Sudeep CB, Ninan VS, Tom A, Arjun MR. Platelet-rich plasma and incidence of alveolar osteitis in high-risk patients undergoing extractions of mandibular molars: a case-control study. J Pharm Bioallied Sci. 2017;9:S173–9.
47. Rutkowski JL, Johnson DA, Radio NM, Fennell JW. Platelet rich plasma to facilitate wound healing following tooth extraction. J Oral Implantol. 2010;36:11–23.
48. Torres J, Tamimi F, Martinez PP, Alkhraisat MH, Linares R, Hernandez G, Torres-Macho J, Lopez-Cabarcos E. Effect of

platelet-rich plasma on sinus lifting: a randomized-controlled clinical trial. J Clin Periodontol. 2009;36:677–87.
49. Stumbras A, Krukis MM, Januzis G, Juodzbalys G. Regenerative bone potential after sinus floor elevation using various bone graft materials: a systematic review. Quintessence Int. 2019;50:548–58.
50. Nikolidakis D, Meijer GJ, Jansen JA. Sinus floor elevation using platelet-rich plasma and beta-tricalcium phosphate: case report and histological evaluation, vol. 27. Dent Today; 2008. p. 66, 68, 70; quiz 71.
51. Bausset O, Giraudo L, Veran J, Magalon J, Coudreuse JM, Magalon G, Dubois C, Serratrice N, Dignat-George F, Sabatier F. Formulation and storage of platelet-rich plasma homemade product. Biores Open Access. 2012;1:115–23.
52. DeLong JM, Russell RP, Mazzocca AD. Platelet-rich plasma: the PAW classification system. Arthroscopy. 2012;28:998–1009.
53. Fitzpatrick J, Bulsara MK, McCrory PR, Richardson MD, Zheng MH. Analysis of platelet-rich plasma extraction: variations in platelet and blood components between 4 common commercial kits. Orthop J Sports Med. 2017;5:2325967116675272.
54. Shin HS, Woo HM, Kang BJ. Optimisation of a double-centrifugation method for preparation of canine platelet-rich plasma. BMC Vet Res. 2017;13:198.
55. Zhang C, Cheng B, Yuan T. Clinical application of platelet-rich plasma technology. First ed. Shanghai Jiao Tong University Press; December 2018.

17 Outlook

Xiaobing Fu, Biao Cheng, Ting Yuan, and Hongchen He

With the development of regenerative medicine, PRP (platelet-rich plasma) is gradually showing its advantages in tissue engineering, the medical technology that promotes self-repair and regeneration of the body or constructs new tissue and organs to repair and regenerates or replaces damaged tissues and organs which involves three main factors: cells, active factors, and scaffolds. Moreover, PRP is attracting more and more attention for its unique role and some new mechanisms, such as tissue regeneration and immune regulation which hold great potential application. The multiple roles of PRP in antiaging, genetic engineering, tissue engineering, and other aspects (PRP is active factor, secretory cell, and also scaffold material) deserve further exploration and recognition. Vast basic and clinical researches on PRP have been done in the past 10 years, which confirms that PRP is of great potential use.

17.1 Key Areas of Plastic and Aesthetic Surgery Where Concentrated Platelets Are Widely Used

Due to the differences in nomenclature and classification, on the one hand, the use and reporting of platelet concentrates have increased sharply, while on the other hand, controlled systematic studies are still lacking. In terms of safety, it is difficult to obtain standardized products due to the differences in the use of activators and properties. Therefore, most applications of platelet concentrates are still limited to autologous mode to avoid the risk of infectious disease transmission. Patients with impaired platelet function or contraindications to self-donation will not benefit from PRP treatment. In recent years, with the expansion of the application scope of PRP, successful attempts have been made in clinical application in dermatology, ophthalmology, ENT (eyes, nose, and throat) department, obstetrics and gynecology, and sexual medicine. At the same time, great breakthroughs have been made in its release products and targeted therapy in the laboratory. In this chapter, tentative application of PRP in plastic and aesthetic surgery in recent years will be summarized.

The use of concentrated platelets is not limited to simple wound repair; its advantages in restoring the skin barrier make it possible to maintain the complete structure of the skin. The use of bioactive agents to enhance the initiation of wound repair accelerates the healing process and improve the quality of healing which is one of the great challenges facing regenerative medicine, and it becomes a focus and difficult in the fields of innovative research. It has been recognized that platelet concentrates can accelerate wound repair and even improve healing outcomes for chronic wounds.

The use of PRP in combination with mesenchymal stem cells (MSCs) can improve the effectiveness of cell therapy on tissue repair. Studies have confirmed that the mechanisms of the combined use of adipose mesenchymal stem cells and human PRP on stimulating skin repair are mainly related to the pro-angiogenesis properties. Moreover, PRP improves the elasticity of newborn skin by accelerating the wound healing process, and PRP in combination with MSCs plays a positive role in rebuilding the skin's barrier.

In a broad sense, the skin barrier includes physical barrier, nerve barrier, immune barrier, pigment barrier, etc., while in a narrow skin sense, the skin barrier refers to the physical or

X. Fu (✉)
Academician of the Chinese Academy of Engineering (CAE, Division of Medicine and Health), International Academicians of National Academy of Engineering (NAE) of USA and Franch Academy of Medicine, PLA General Hospital and PLA Medical College, Beijing, China

B. Cheng
Department of Burn & Plastic Surgery, General Hospital of Southern Theater Command, Guangzhou, China

T. Yuan
Department of Orthopaedics, Shanghai JiaoTong University Affiliated Sixth People's Hospital, Shanghai, China

H. He
Department of Rehabilitation Medicine, West China Hospital, Sichuan University, Chengdu, China

B. Cheng, X. Fu (eds.), *Platelet-Rich Plasma in Tissue Repair and Regeneration*, https://doi.org/10.1007/978-981-99-3193-4_17

mechanical barrier of the epidermis (stratum corneum), also known as the permeable barrier (epidermal permeation barrier function). Studies have found that PRP can reverse the damage of the skin's permeable barrier caused by irradiation (K10 expression reflects the level of stratum corneal envelope protein expression, which is the marker of the skin's permeable barrier). Expression of cornified envelope protein and TEWL (transepidermal water loss) values both increased in irradiated skin treated with PRP. In mouse models of radiation-induced skin damage, PRP can accelerate the repair of the skin barrier. Yuan Sha et al. used the model of suckling mouse to observe the intervention of platelet-rich plasma (platelet concentrate) in the growth of skin barrier keratin sheath and skin structure and found that PRP has a significant role in promoting the development of the early epidermis and dermis and making the skin barrier function mature and complete in suckling mice.

Skin attachments are one of the characteristics of the skin integrity. With the rapid development of the society and the great pressure of life brought by it, the number of alopecia patients is increasing year by year, and hair regeneration has become one of the fastest-growing fields of plastic surgery. Using concentrated platelets to treat baldness has achieved amazing results and has attracted people's attention. But the exact mechanism remains to be explored. The fact that there exist a large number of positive clinical results has given people boundless hope, but how to choose the right population, the type and level of baldness, the course of treatments, and the intervention method (combined use of injection and microneedling) need to be further refined and standardized.

Different mechanisms of PRP in the treatment of atrophic scar and hypertrophic scar show the characteristics of its multiple effects, which has the advantages of comprehensively improving the quality of repair and ameliorating fibrosis. There have been a large number of clinical reports concerning the treatment of PRP for atrophic scar, adhesion scar, acne scar, and striae gravidarum. The early intervention of concentrated platelets on healing is mainly reflected in the regulation of type I collagen, the improvement of the microenvironment of scars, the acceleration of scar tissue remodeling, and the reduction of scar formation. It even plays a role in improving pain and itching symptoms of hypertrophic scar and even keloids. The mechanism may be related to the PRP-triggered signal negative feedback mechanism of TGF-β1, which reduces the gene transcription CTGF (connective tissue growth factor).

Peyronie's disease (PD) is a condition concerning the chronic cavernitis of the penis, in which a fibrous thickening mass caused by the inflammatory changes in the spongiosa of the penis causes the spongiosa to shrink and lose its elasticity and interspace, resulting in the curvature of the penis during erection. The first clinical observation of "PRP in the treatment of PD" was made in 2014 and turned out to be safe. Subsequently, some scattered studies confirmed the unique efficacy of PRP in this particular type of fibrotic disease. But more large sample studies are needed to determine the therapeutic effect and promotion value of PRP for Peyronie's disease.

At the same time, concentrated platelets can be used in combination with various photoelectronic devices (such as plasma radiofrequency, fractional laser, etc.), as well as (stem) cells, hyaluronic acid, fat transplantation, microneedling, surgery, and other methods to treat various types of scars. In general, platelet concentrate can be used as a direct or adjunctive therapy for scars. Also, more studies with a longer duration of follow-up are needed to find the most appropriate method for treating different types of scars.

The repair regulation of platelet concentrates on multiple tissues (fat, lymph, nerves, etc.) shows the prospect for tissue regeneration: autologous fat transplantation has been widely used in recent years, but the high absorption rate after transplantation has become a difficult point hindering its wide application, thus improving the retention rate after autologous fat transplantation becomes a research hotspot in plastic surgery in recent years. A variety of studies have shown that platelet concentrate can provide nutrients such as plasma for transplanted adipose tissue, secrete growth factors, promote the proliferation and differentiation of adipose stem cells into lipolysis, and promote the angiogenesis of transplanted adipose tissue, thereby improving the survival rate of fat cells after autologous fat transplantation. However, at present, the key problem of concentrated platelets applied to fat transplantation is that the ratio between concentrated platelets and fat cells varies greatly in different studies, and too high or too low ratio may have adverse or even negative effects. Therefore, it is necessary to further determine the concentration, proportion, and activation method of concentrated platelets in fat and concentrated platelet transplantation.

The blood and lymphatic systems are the two main circulatory systems of the human body. Lymphatic capillaries help maintain homeostasis of tissue fluid by absorbing the exudate and transporting it back to the venous circulation through larger lymphatic vessels. In addition, lymphatic vessels play an important role in mammalian immune monitoring, being the main conduit for antigens and antigen-presenting cells to enter the lymph nodes from the periphery, thereby initiating the immune response. The lymphatic system is essential for the absorption of dietary fats. Lymphatic vessel damage is associated with the pathogenesis of many diseases, including lymphedema, fibrosis, inflammation, and metastasis of malignant tumors. In recent years, there has been a growing focus on lymphangiogenesis. For example, hair follicle stem cells secrete key molecules that control lymph capillaries in order to control the composition of fluids and cells in the surrounding environment and ultimately affect the regeneration of entire tissues. Studies have confirmed that PRP can improve lymph node growth and regeneration in autologous transplantation. The combined use of PRP and fat-derived mesenchymal stem cells (ADMSCs) has a positive effect on improving the symptoms of lymphedema, promoting wound repair and formation of vascular structures.

The role of concentrated platelets in antiaging and rejuvenation treatment: The aging of the body includes many aspects, in which plastic and aesthetic surgeries are most concerned about the skin. The skins of the face, neck, or hands are all related to rejuvenation. Due to various reasons, skin aging can lead to weakened skin elasticity, sagging skin, pigmentation, wrinkles, enlarged pores, telangiectasia, loss of facial tissues (thinning of red lips, collapse in the middle of the face, etc.), and other problems. Concentrated platelets can secrete a variety of growth factors and cytokines, which quickly activate the proliferation of fibrin. Fibrin itself is an important scaffold in the skin, which is necessary for maintaining cell proliferation, increasing skin elasticity, reducing edema, increasing the length of dermal-epidermal junction, increasing the number of fibroblasts, promoting the synthesis of hyaluronic acid, and reshaping the extracellular matrix, and has been widely used in the field of skin rejuvenation. Studies have shown that in the treatment of facial rejuvenation, activated PRP is more effective than nonactivated PRP. In the future, the application of skin rejuvenation will mainly focus on more refined areas such as the treatment needs (wrinkles, pigmentation, skin elasticity, etc.), the way of administration (activated or not? direct injection? load material), optimal concentration (number of cells per unit volume), cost performance, and removal of nucleated cells. In addition to the aging of the skin, its antiaging effect in the reproductive system has attracted more and more attention, and improving sexual potential has become a hot topic of research and application in recent years.

Erectile dysfunction in men refers to the failure to achieve or maintain an erection during sexual intercourse. With the increase of age, men over the age of 40 begin to experience a gradual decline in erectile ability. Although there are some medications that can help and maintain an erection, their effects are mostly temporary and may have serious side effects including the risk of heart attack and stroke. As a quick, safe, and effective natural remedy, platelet concentrate can increase blood flow to the sexual organs, improve sexual sensitivity, and restore sexual health in men. Four preclinical trials and six clinical trials of platelet concentrates for the treatment of male sexual dysfunction have been analyzed. Although the existing studies have small sample sizes, short follow-up periods, or lack control groups and quality and quantitative analysis of platelet concentrates, the available data still shows that platelet concentrates have great potential for the treatment of male sexual dysfunction, with no adverse reactions detected at present.

The treatment of female reproductive dysfunction has also attracted the attention of both doctors and patients, and PRP is of great help to awaken female sexual potential and improve the symptoms of female postpartum sexual dysfunction. Of course, there is still much work to be done in this area of reproductive plastic surgery, and we feel that it is necessary to give the reader a comprehensive, scientific, and rational understanding.

Others: Plastic and aesthetic surgery, injection, and even laser treatment may lead to complications such as skin necrosis. The treatment of such complications is difficult, but the use of platelet concentrates serves as a new therapeutic option for those complications. Even some intractable skin diseases, such as scleroderma and melasma, have been reported to be successfully treated with platelet concentrates in small samples or individual cases.

17.2 Outlook and Thinking

Platelet concentrates can provide xeno-free media for stem cell therapy, which are more in line with medical ethics: Cell expansion in vitro is often applied for advanced therapeutic drugs for clinical use, so it must comply with good preparation practices. The use of standardized animals and xeno-free compounds during preparation is critical for the clinical safety of biological products. Fetal bovine serum is the most common source of growth factors and is often used as a medium additive in research to promote cell expansion. However, fetal bovine serum contains heterogeneous carbohydrates and proteins, which may lead to adverse clinical effects. Substitutes of fetal bovine serum for cell products have long been strongly recommended in Europe and the United States. Human platelet concentrate is a suitable, abundant, low-cost alternative source of growth factors. In previous studies, human growth factors extracted through repeated freeze-thaw cycles have been successfully used to amplify cells in vitro. Mixing multiple single donor agents together minimizes product variability.

17.2.1 According to the Therapeutic Needs, Different Compositions and Forms of Platelet Concentrates Can Be Used to Construct Different Tissue Engineering Biological Scaffolds

The application of platelet-rich plasma in tissue engineering is a research hotspot in recent years, and it is also an important direction for the future research. At present, there have been studies on platelet-rich plasma combined with other drugs or biological materials constructing degradable tissue engineering to complete the repair and regeneration of soft tissues. The various forms of platelet concentrates (gels or liquids, such as platelet lysate, platelet secretion fluid, and exosomes) make their application in tissue engineering extremely flexible and can be loaded with different degradable biomaterials (hydrogels, decellularized matrices, etc.) according to the needs of tissue regeneration. However, the active time of concentrated platelets is short, and storage and sustained release are another focus of the research field. In addition, for the purpose of standardized application, it is recommended that researchers and clinicians fully describe the type of platelet concentrates they use in the articles: the preparation method (centrifugal force, centrifugal time), the concentration and dose, activation methods (activate or not? Activator? ultrasonic or photoelectric stimulus?), and the very noteworthy time windows.

17.2.2 Rational View of Platelet Concentrate in the Clinical Application of Plastic Surgery

The clinical applications of platelet concentrate have enjoyed a huge surge in recent years, expanding to the treatment of incurable diseases such as infertility, sclerosis, and even tumors. However, scholars believe that the use of platelet concentrate for the treatment of cancer should be cautious. Due to the effect of platelet concentrates on immune regulation, especially the regulation of innate immunity and adaptive immunity, as well as the regulation of oxygen, and oxidation-reduction rebalancing, platelet concentrates may become therapeutic targets for many diseases. However, they should be carried out cautiously prudently on the basis of medical ethics and evidence of EBM.

Although the application of platelet concentrates has achieved exciting results in plastic surgery, there should be a clear understanding of this explosive growth. In some cases, the use of autologous concentrated platelets is also not absolutely safe. Although it is safe to use platelet concentrates derived from autologous tissue itself; its safety will be reduced during the process of extraction and preparation. Compared to other common side effects, pain, swelling, and bruising are temporary and recoverable. There have been reports of skin reactions to calcium preparations and even anaphylactic shock. There was one case report of a healthy woman who suffered from serious complications of permanent blindness in one eye after receiving PRP injection, as well as pigmentation caused by platelet concentrate. Although it is still uncertain whether these are caused by platelet concentrate itself, activators, or other factors, how to avoid and reduce the occurrence of such things in the process of plastic and aesthetic treatment still requires continuous attention. It is necessary to strengthen standardized training and operation concerning PRP. Only in this way can we make the application of platelet concentrate be scientific, reasonable, and long-lasting.

GPSR Compliance

The European Union's (EU) General Product Safety Regulation (GPSR) is a set of rules that requires consumer products to be safe and our obligations to ensure this.

If you have any concerns about our products, you can contact us on ProductSafety@springernature.com

In case Publisher is established outside the EU, the EU authorized representative is:

Springer Nature Customer Service Center GmbH
Europaplatz 3
69115 Heidelberg, Germany

Batch number: 10372219

Printed by Printforce, the Netherlands